| Country | Map Abbreviation |
|---|---|
| Afghanistan | Afg. |
| Austria | Aut. |
| Azerbaijan | Aze. |
| Bangladesh | Bgd. |
| Belarus | Blr. |
| Benin | Ben. |
| Bhutan | Btn. |
| Botswana | Bwa. |
| Bulgaria | Bgr. |
| Burkina Faso | Bfa. |
| Burundi | Bdi. |
| Cambodia | Khm. |
| Cameroon | Cmr. |
| Central African Republic | C.A.R. |
| Congo | Cog. |
| Costa Rica | Cri. |
| Cote d'Ivoire | Civ. |
| Democratic Republic of the Congo | Drg. |
| Denmark | Dnk. |
| Djibouti | Dji. |
| Dominican Republic | Dom. |
| East Timor | Etm. |
| Equatorial Guinea | Gnq. |
| Eritrea | Eri. |
| Estonia | Est. |
| Finland | Fin. |
| France | Fra. |
| French Guiana | Guf. |
| Gabon | Gab. |
| Georgia | Geo. |
| Germany | Deu. |
| Ghana | Gha. |
| Greece | Grc. |
| Guatemala | Gtm. |
| Guinea | Gin. |
| Guinea Bissau | Gnb. |
| Guyana | Guy. |
| Haiti | Hti. |
| Honduras | Hnd. |
| Ireland | Irl. |
| Israel | Isr. |
| Italy | Ita. |
| Jordan | Jor. |
| Kenya | Ken. |
| Kuwait | Kwt. |
| Kyrgyzstan | Kgz. |
| Laos | Lao. |
| Latvia | Lva. |
| Lebanon | Lbn. |
| Liberia | Lbr. |
| Lithuania | Ltu. |
| Madagascar | Mdg. |
| Malawi | Mwi. |
| Malaysia | Mys. |
| Mauritania | Mrt. |
| Morocco | Mar. |
| Mozambique | Moz. |
| Myanmar | Mmr. |
| Namibia | Nam. |
| Nepal | Npl. |
| Netherlands | Nld. |
| Nicaragua | Nic. |
| North Korea | N. Kor. |
| Norway | Nor. |
| Oman | Omn. |
| Pakistan | Pak. |
| Panama | Pan. |
| Poland | Pol. |
| Portugal | Prt. |
| Qatar | Qat. |
| Republic of Moldova | Mda. |
| Romania | Rom. |
| Rwanda | Rwa. |
| Senegal | Sen. |
| Sierra Leone | Sle. |
| Somalia | Som. |
| South Korea | S. Kor. |
| Spain | Esp. |
| Suriname | Sur. |
| Swaziland | Swz. |
| Sweden | Swe. |
| Syria | Syr. |
| Tajikistan | Tjk. |
| Thailand | Tha. |
| Tunisia | |
| Turkmenistan | n. |
| Uganda | |
| Ukraine | |
| United Arab Emirates | |
| United Kingdom | |
| United Republic of Tar | |
| Uzbekistan | |
| Vietnam | |
| Western Sahara | |
| Yemen | |
| Yugoslavia | |
| Zambia | |
| Zimbabwe | Zwe. |

# THE NUTRITION TRANSITION:

## Diet and Disease in the Developing World

# Food Science and Technology
## International Series

Series Editor

Steve L. Taylor
*University of Nebraska*

Advisory Board

Bruce Chassy
*University of Illinois, USA*

Patrick Fox
*University College Cork, Republic of Ireland*

Dennis Gordon
*North Dakota State University, USA*

Robert Hutkins
*University of Nebraska, USA*

Ronald Jackson
*Quebec, Canada*

Daryl B. Lund
*University of Wisconsin, USA*

Connie Weaver
*Purdue University, USA*

Louise Wicker
*University of Georgia, USA*

Howard Zhang
*Ohio State University, USA*

*A complete list of the books in this series appears at the end of this volume.*

# The Nutrition Transition:

## Diet and Disease in the Developing World

Editors

**Benjamin Caballero and Barry M. Popkin**

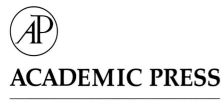

## ACADEMIC PRESS

An imprint of Elsevier Science

Amsterdam • Boston • London • New York • Oxford • Paris
San Diego • San Francisco • Singapore • Sydney • Tokyo

Academic Press
*An Imprint of Elsevier Science*
84 Theobald's Road, London WC1X 8RR, UK
http://www.academicpress.com

Academic Press
*An Imprint of Elsevier Science*
525 B Street, Suite 1900, San Diego, California 92101-4495, USA
http://www.academicpress.com

ISBN 0-12-153654-8

Library of Congress Control Number: 2002103917

A catalogue record for this book is available from the British Library

Typeset by Charon Tec Pvt. Ltd, Chennai, India
Printed and bound in China by RDC Group Limited

02 03 04 05 06 07 RD 9 8 7 6 5 4 3 2 1

# Contents

Contributors List . . . . . . . . . . . . . . . . . . . . . . . . . . . . . . . . . . . vii
Foreword . . . . . . . . . . . . . . . . . . . . . . . . . . . . . . . . . . ix
About the Editors . . . . . . . . . . . . . . . . . . . . . . . . . . . . . . xiii

1     Introduction . . . . . . . . . . . . . . . . . . . . . . . . . . . . . . . . 1
       *Benjamin Caballero and Barry M. Popkin*

**Part I The Global Context** . . . . . . . . . . . . . . . . . . . . . . . **7**

2     Economic and technological development and their
       relationships to body size and productivity . . . . . . . . . . . . . . . . . 9
       *Robert W. Fogel and Lorens A. Helmchen*

3     Food production . . . . . . . . . . . . . . . . . . . . . . . . . . . . 25
       *Vaclav Smil*

4     Can the challenges of poverty, sustainable consumption
       and good health governance be addressed in
       an era of globalization? . . . . . . . . . . . . . . . . . . . . . . . . 51
       *Tim Lang*

5     Demographic trends . . . . . . . . . . . . . . . . . . . . . . . . . . 71
       *Hania Zlotnik*

**Part II Biological Factors Affecting the Nutrition Transition** . . . . . . . . . **109**

6     The dynamics of the dietary transition in the
       developing world . . . . . . . . . . . . . . . . . . . . . . . . . . . . 111
       *Barry M. Popkin*

7     Early nutrition conditions and later risk of disease . . . . . . . . . . . . 129
       *Linda S. Adair*

8   Obesity in the developing world . . . . . . . . . . . . . . . . . . . . . . . . .   147
    *Reynaldo Martorell*

9   Diabetes . . . . . . . . . . . . . . . . . . . . . . . . . . . . . . . . . . . . . . . . . . .   165
    *Kerin O'Dea and Leonard S. Piers*

10  Cardiovascular diseases . . . . . . . . . . . . . . . . . . . . . . . . . . . . . .   191
    *K. Srinath Reddy*

11  The nutrition transition in China: a new stage of
    the Chinese diet . . . . . . . . . . . . . . . . . . . . . . . . . . . . . . . . . . . .   205
    *Shufa Du, Bing Lu, Fengying Zhai, and Barry M. Popkin*

12  Trends in under- and overnutrition in Brazil . . . . . . . . . . . . . . . .   223
    *Carlos A. Monteiro, Wolney L. Conde, and Barry M. Popkin*

13  Policy implications . . . . . . . . . . . . . . . . . . . . . . . . . . . . . . . . . .   241
    *Benjamin Caballero and Barry M. Popkin*

**Index** . . . . . . . . . . . . . . . . . . . . . . . . . . . . . . . . . . . . . . . . . . . . . .   251

# Contributors List

Linda S. Adair
Associate Professor of Nutrition
University of North Carolina at Chapel Hill
University Square, CB # 8120
123 West Franklin Street
Chapel Hill, NC 27516-3997, USA

Benjamin Caballero
Director, Center for Human Nutrition
Johns Hopkins University
Suite No 2205
615 N Wolfe St
Baltimore, MD 21205, USA

Wolney L. Conde
Carolina Population Center
CB # 8120 University Square
University of North Carolina at Chapel Hill
Chapel Hill, NC 27516-3997, USA

Shufa Du
Nutrition Evaluation Laboratory
School of Public Health
University of São Paulo
Av. Dr. Arnaldo 715
São Paulo 01246-904, Brazil

Robert W. Fogel
Graduate School of Business
The University of Chicago
1101 E. 58th Street
Chicago, IL 60637, USA

Lorens A. Helmchen
Department of Economics
The University of Chicago
1126 E. 59th Street
Chicago, IL 60637, USA

Tim Lang
Director of Centre for Food Policy
Thames Valley University
Wolfson Institute of Health Sciences
Centre for Food Policy, 32–38 Uxbridge Road
Westel House, Ealing W5 2BS, UK

Bing Lu
Carolina Population Center
CB # 8120 University Square
University of North Carolina at Chapel Hill
Chapel Hill, NC 27516-3997, USA

Reynaldo Martorell
Robert W. Woodruff Professor of International
Nutrition, Rollins School of Public Health
Emory University, International Health
1518 Clifton Road, NE
Atlanta, GA 30322, USA

Carlos Monteiro
Director, Center for Epidemiological Studies in
Health and Nutrition (NUPENS/USP)
School of Public Health
University of São Paulo
Av. Dr. Arnaldo, 715
São Paulo 01246-904 SP, Brazil

Kerin O'Dea
Director, Menzies School of Health Research
PO Box 41096
Casuarina, NT 0811, Australia

Leonard S. Piers
Division of Population Health and Chronic Diseases
Menzies School of Health Research
PO Box 41096
Casuarina, N.T. 0811, Australia

Barry M. Popkin
Professor of Nutrition
Carolina Population Center
CB # 8120 University Square
University of North Carolina at Chapel Hill
Chapel Hill, NC 27516-3997, USA

K. Srinath Reddy
Professor of Cardiology
Cardiothoracic Centre
All India Institute of Medical Sciences
Ansari Nagar
New Delhi 110 029, India

Nevin S. Scrimshaw
Institute Professor Emeritus
Massachusetts Institute of Technology
Senior Advisor of Food and Nutrition Program
United Nations University, Box 330
Campton, NH 03223, USA

Vaclav Smil
The University of Manitoba
N306 Duff Roblin Bldg
Winnipeg R3T 2N2, Canada

Fengying Zhai
Professor of Nutrition
Deputy Director
Institute of Nutrition and Food Safety
Chinese Center for Disease Control and Prevention
29 Nanwei Road
Beijing 100050, China

Hania Zlotnik
Estimates and Projections Sections
Population Division
United Nations
Room DC2-1918
New York, NY 10017, USA

# Foreword

There have always been transition periods in human history, although they have come at different times for different countries and regions and have in the past been widely spread out over time. The transitions described in this book have few precedents in both the rapidity of the change and the large proportion of the world's population involved. The shift from hunting and gathering to agriculture was spread over thousands of years and the industrial revolution over about 200 years, but transitions are now occurring within developing countries over a few decades. They are determining the future health and welfare of human kind and the nature of the environment in which we all must live. This book contains informative descriptions of past changes and trends, but its importance lies in its characterization of dynamic current processes and their probable impact on future history.

It is difficult to conceive that from the 15th to 18th centuries in all of Europe frequent local famines led to starvation, riots, and migrations in search of food (Scrimshaw, 1987). Mortality rates were far higher than in developing countries today, life expectancy was about 25 years, and the populations were severely stunted. Improvement took centuries. In every industrialized country height increased steadily in the 19th and most of the 20th centuries, for example, from about 166 cm to nearly 180 cm in Sweden (Steckel, 2001). The 1993 Nobel Prize winner in Economics, Robert Fogel, points out that the mean height of the Dutch in 1860 of 164 cm is one percentile of their current mean height and that this percentile is the mean height in India today (Fogel, 2000). Clearly the anthropometric transition for India still lies ahead.

The high death rates that were associated with infectious disease dropped precipitously in the late 19th and early 20th centuries well before there were specific therapies and in some cases before the causative agent was known. McKeown (1976) in *The Modern Rise of Population* concluded that this was due, almost entirely, to improving nutrition and not to any other major factors that could be identified. The further decreases in mortality from diseases such as measles, diphtheria, whooping cough, tuberculosis, and pneumonia with the advent of antibiotics and immunizations were relatively very small.

In the 1960s, cases of severe protein-calorie malnutrition, kwashiorkor, could still be demonstrated in children in almost any hospital in the developing world. Only 20 years later, kwashiorkor had essentially disappeared. Earlier this occurred for scurvy, pellagra, and beri-beri. In the 1930s pellagra was still a major problem in the United States. Beri-beri persisted in Southeast Asia into the 1950s. The ocular signs of vitamin A deficiency leading to blindness were still a serious concern in the 1970s but are now rare even in poor countries. Except for scurvy which largely disappeared earlier, these transitions occurred in the 20th century. Unfortunately these nutritional disorders have returned in some refugee populations.

Thirty years ago obesity was rare in developing countries and it is now increasing rapidly in both industrialized and developing countries with seriously adverse impacts on health. The InterAmerican Atherosclerosis Study published in 1968 examined aortas and coronary vessels from serial autopsies for three years in eight general hospitals in Latin America and the Caribbean (McGill, 1968). In the populations studied at that time, atherosclerosis progressed so slowly that cardiovascular disease was almost unknown. Four decades later, coronary heart disease is a growing problem in these same countries.

A characteristic of these successive transitions is that they are coming more frequently, are progressing more rapidly, and are increasingly global in scope. This book documents and interprets the current transition that is occurring in both nutrition and related socioeconomic conditions in developing nations. They are associated with a demographic transition in an increasing number of these countries. The nutrition transition is taking place so rapidly that undernutrition and micronutrient deficiencies coexist with overnutrition. As a consequence, many developing countries still face the need to prevent undernutrition and malnutrition at a time when they are facing an increasing burden of chronic degenerative disease.

The dynamics of the current dietary change and the increasing obesity and diabetes in the developing world are well described in early chapters. A relatively new theme, the relationship between early malnutrition and the later occurrence of chronic degenerative disease, is also covered. Low birth weight due largely to poor nutrition during pregnancy and malnutrition during infancy have been shown to increase the risk of diabetes, hypertension, and coronary heart diseases in later life. Populations with a relatively high frequency of fetal and infant malnutrition whose rising affluence led them to more dietary fat and less exercise appear to be at a particularly high risk of chronic disease as they age. This is a further burden on developing countries in transition.

Other important topics covered are the roles of governance, globalization, demographic behavior, and disease trends. China and Brazil are presented as case studies of what may be happening or will happen to diet, activity levels and health in other parts of the developing world. The chapter on food wisely avoids predictions of global food shortages but does express concern that the developing world may not be able to derive the full benefit from current and future scientific and technical advances in food production.

This book comes at a time when multiple transitions are coming with great rapidity and globalization has become a dominant theme. It is a valuable documentation of the food and nutrition components of the most accelerated set of major transitions in human history. Readers will find it a fascinating and insightful glimpse into the benefits and threats to health of the unprecedented nutrition, demographic, and economic changes that are so strongly and rapidly affecting the health and welfare of the populations of developing countries.

Nevin S. Scrimshaw
Professor Emeritus, Massachusetts Institute of Technology
Senior Advisor, UNU Food and Nutrition Program
Winner of the World Food Prize, 1991

# References

Fogel, R. (2000). "The Fourth Great Awakening and the Future of Egalitarianism". University of Chicago Press, Chicago.

McGill, H. (ed.) (1968). "The Geographic Pathology of Atherosclerosis". Williams & Wilkins, Baltimore.

McKeown, T. (1976). "The Modern Rise of Population". Academic Press, New York.

Scrimshaw, N.S. (1987). The phenomenon of famine. *Ann. Rev. Nutr.* **7**, 1–21.

Steckel, R.H. (2001). Health and nutrition in the preindustrial era: insights from a millennium of average heights in Northern Europe. Working Paper 8452. National Bureau of Economic Research, Boston.

# About the Editors

**Benjamin Caballero, MD, PhD** is Professor of International Health and of Pediatrics, and Director of the Center for Human Nutrition at the Schools of Public Health and of Medicine, Johns Hopkins University. He is a member of the Food and Nutrition Board of the Institute of Medicine, National Academy of Sciences, and of the Nutrition and Metabolism Study Section, National Institutes of Health. Dr Caballero's research on childhood nutrition encompasses protein-energy malnutrition, nutrition and infection interactions, and obesity, particularly in minorities and developing country populations.

**Barry M Popkin, PhD** is Professor of Nutrition at UNC-CH where he heads the Division of Nutrition Epidemiology in the School of Public Health. His special research focus is the dynamic changes in diet, physical activity and inactivity and body composition and the factors responsible for these changes. Much of his work on the nutrition transition focuses on the rapid changes in obesity and their causes. He is actively involved in research in the US and a number of other countries around the world; included are detailed longitudinal studies that he directs in China and Russia, active involvement with longitudinal studies in the Philippines and South Africa, and related work in Brazil and several other countries. Dr Popkin has an active US research program in understanding dietary behavior with a focus on eating patterns, trends, and socio-demographic determinants. Dr Popkin serves on several scientific advisory organizations including Chair, the Nutrition Transition Committee for the International Union for the Nutritional Sciences; he has published more than 150 journal articles, book chapters, and books, and has a PhD in economics.

# Introduction

*Benjamin Caballero and Barry M. Popkin*

Evolution is transition. Fueled by ideas, war, scientific breakthroughs, and chance, the relationship of humans with their environment is in constant change, in an endless quest for equilibrium. Food, as a central component of survival, has always been at the center of that evolution. But if we are in constant transition, what does the term "nutrition transition" really define?

Arguably, the concept of transition in the study of human populations was first introduced by Omran in 1971, in an article entitled "The Epidemiologic Transition" (Omran, 1971). In that paper, the author attempted to offer a systematic process by which to identify and characterize change, and in doing so, to be able to predict future trends. Another concept of transition often seen in the literature is the demographic transition – the shift from a pattern of high fertility and high mortality to one of low fertility and low mortality, typical of modern industrialized countries. Interpretations of the demographic and epidemiologic transition share a focus with the nutrition transition on the ways in which populations move from one pattern to the next. This concept of transition may also be applied to the study of changes in the food–diet environment and its impact on health. The concept of nutrition transition, however, goes beyond diet, recognizing that most of the health effects of diets in human populations are also strongly affected by lifestyle, particularly physical activity. We therefore use the term nutrition transition to encompass these shifts not only in diet but also in physical activity and their effects on body composition. In other words, we must explicitly recognize the role of the other nonnutritional factors closely related to the health outcomes of interest. These three relationships are presented in Fig. 1.1.

Why does the current nutrition transition merit special attention, and define a specific area of research in nutrition science? First, our ability to identify different patterns of intake in populations, and to correlate these with health indicators has advanced substantially over the past decades. Thus, the necessary data have reached a critical mass from which study can progress and inferences can be made. Second, the rate of change is such that its effects can frequently be identified in the population within a generation or two, facilitating their identification and quantification. Third, many of the changes in the area of nutrition and health are closely connected to economic and political changes, thus linking the nutrition transition with key determinants of the historical evolution of countries and regions.

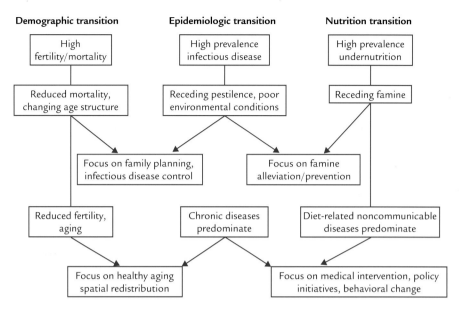

**Figure 1.1**  Stages of health, nutritional, and demographic change (from Popkin, 2002).

This book focuses on the developing world. Our interest centers on the rapid shifts from a stage often termed the period of receding famine to one dominated by nutrition-related noncommunicable diseases (NR-NCD). The periods encompassing this transition are outlined in Fig. 1.2. Our focus is increasingly on patterns 3 to 5, in particular on the rapid shift in much of the world's low and moderate income countries from the stage of receding famine to NR-NCD. The importance of the shift from pattern 3 to 4 is such that for many this is synonymous with the Nutrition Transition.

The most dramatic impact of the changes in food supply, dietary intake and lifestyle can be observed in the developing world. There are several reasons for this. First, the projected growth in world population for the next 30 years will occur almost exclusively in the developing world. Even more importantly, most of that population growth will occur in urban areas, where, as will be shown, the impact of the nutrition transition is most evident. Second, the health consequences of the nutrition transition, a continuing increase in the prevalence of NR-NCD, is having and will continue to have a dramatic impact in countries that, for the most part, have not yet solved the burden of nutritional deficiencies.

Traditionally, the diets of poor countries have been considered insufficient in quantity, and inadequate in quality. One reason for this has been the predominance of higher fiber, lower fat plant sources, which are known to be limited in certain essential nutrients, to have poor bioavailability for essential nutrients, and a low energy density. Paradoxically, the hunter–gatherer and the subsequent diet of countries in phase of receding famine, which are both low in fat and rich in fiber, are today considered the desired pattern for disease prevention in higher income industrialized countries. However, the diet of developing countries also has natural contaminants (goitrogenic substances, natural toxins, pesticides, microbial agents) that are undesirable.

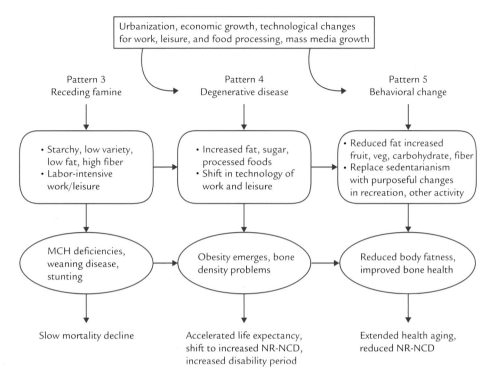

**Figure 1.2**   Stages of the nutrition transition (from Popkin, 2002).

What fuels the rapid shift in the stage of the nutrition transition? Critical elements include urbanization, internationalization (globalization) of food production and marketing, expansion of mass media and communications, and changes in the work market with predominance of low-energy output labor.

Almost 90% of the projected world population growth over the next 20 years will take place in the developing world. Even more striking is the fact that almost all this growth will occur in urban areas. Thus, today's developing world, still largely defined by the rural poor, will change dramatically in the next two decades, with the progressive dominance of an urban population. Urban dwelling is associated with an array of behaviors and lifestyles that are associated with higher levels of obesity and other NR-NCD.

*Globalization* is a term that generates strong reactions, in spite (or perhaps because) of its vague definition. Included in what we term globalization is a shift in dominance on the economic, technological, cultural, and consumption level of goods that are mass produced by modern techniques and a system that is market driven. Although the term usually applies to recent trends in international trade, globalization has been an essential element for the continuing expansion of market economies since the industrial revolution. For example, by 1840, after the consolidation of the industrial revolution in England, 530 million yards of British cottons were exported to the "underdeveloped" regions of the world, compared to only 200 million for all of Europe (Hobsbawm, 1996). Thus, economic expansion of industrialized countries has historically depended on expansion of markets into the developing world. Market expansion is achieved by selling goods to increasing numbers of people, and also by creating new needs. Culture plays a key role in fulfilling this task; linking products to lifestyles, celebrities, and movies is one of the most effective means of increasing sales of nonessential products. The importance of culture for trade is such that the opinion-shaping industry (ad agencies, entertainment, media) is one of the leading exports of the US and other developed countries. Television is one of the major purveyors of this cultural context, and it is not surprising that TV ownership and watching are increasing at high pace throughout the developing world (cf. the China case study). Television has a double impact on NR-NCD: as a vehicle for dissemination of unhealthy eating habits, and by promoting physical inactivity.

Globalization of food production affects the nutrition transition in a number of ways. Use of modern technologies for mass production reduces the price of selected food items and worldwide distribution and marketing facilitate the introduction of processed foods to a wide range of countries. In turn, driven by the population growth mentioned above, a large proportion of global food production will be driven by the demands of developing countries. A recent study concluded that over the next 20 years, 85% of the increase in the demand for cereals and meat will come from developing countries (Pinstrup-Andersen *et al.*, 1999).

Because the food share of the household budget is substantially higher in developing than in developed countries (55% vs. 16% in 1997), changes in food prices and income tend to have a much stronger impact on people's dietary intake in developing than in developed countries. This effect is reinforced by the stronger price elasticity associated with lower than with higher incomes. Thus, technological advances and aggressive marketing strategies that reduce prices of certain food items in developing markets result in increased consumption. A clear example of this is the increase in consumption of vegetable oils in the developing world (Drewnowski and Popkin, 1997).

## Poverty and the nutrition transition

Data from the past decade and projections for the next 20 years (Murray and Lopez, 1996) indicate a continuing rise in the contribution of noncommunicable diseases to mortality rates in developing countries, where a large proportion of the global poor lives. But within the developing world population, there are clear differences between the upper and lower socioeconomic groups. Among the poorest 20%, communicable diseases still account for about 60% of deaths, whereas they account for only 8% among the richest 20% (Gwatkin *et al.*, 1999). A confounding factor may be the difference in population patterns between richer and poorer countries, with the latter having as much as twice the number of under-15 population, which has higher rates of communicable disease than older groups. Although it is likely that the younger population of the developing world still faces infectious diseases as a major threat to health and quality of life, the burden of noncommunicable diseases continues to mount for the older poor.

As economic status and education improve, populations in developing countries around the world respond quite consistently by demanding more animal protein in their diet. In many cases, this demand is justified, since their typical diet is usually low in zinc, iron, selenium, retinol, and other essential nutrients found primarily in animal sources. However, increases in the animal protein content of diets almost invariably increases the content in saturated fats, which is undesirable.

The role of genes in the human adaptation to rapid environmental changes has been postulated for many decades, but only with advances in molecular genetics can we identify with some clarity the interactions between genes and environmental components such as diet. Populations living under subsistence conditions are forced to maximize their potential for survival, and it is likely that specific sets of genes are activated to facilitate this process. Thus, rapid changes in the environment, even when positive (e.g., more food available) will tend to perturb that precarious equilibrium between the genome and the environment. If the genetic makeup of some individuals does not allow for a rapid shift to the new environmental conditions, adverse health effects may result. This hypothetical but probable phenomenon can be seen within the same generation, i.e., children who were malnourished early in life becoming more prone to obesity as adults. The particular genetic makeup of populations in developing countries, of which we know so little, adds a unique and important element to the impact of the nutrition transition on health. Individuals "mis-adapted" to the new dietary conditions may have a higher risk of adverse health effects.

## Summary

The rapid shifts in the stages of the nutrition transition seen in the developing world today clearly relate to major changes in food production, urbanization, and globalization of trade. This book provides an overview of these factors, as well as the resulting health outcomes of obesity, diabetes, and cardiovascular diseases. The role of nutrition during pregnancy and infancy in affecting each person's risk of later disease is also addressed. Finally, the impact of the nutrition transition in China and Brazil is presented in more detail, to highlight the individual characteristics of this process and the policy responses in these countries. As discussed in the final chapter, a major focus on prevention in a multinational dimension will be necessary to reduce NR-NCD in the developing world.

## References

Drewnowski, A., and Popkin, B.M. (1997). The nutrition transition: new trends in the global diet. *Nutr. Rev.* **55**, 31–43.

Gwatkin, D.R., Guillot, M., and Heuveline, P. (1999). The burden of disease among the urban poor. *Lancet* **354**, 586–589.

Hobsbawm, E. (1996). The industrial revolution. *In* "The Age of Revolution". Vintage Books, New York.

Murray, C.J.L., and Lopez, A.D. (1996). "The Global Burden of Disease". Harvard University Press, Cambridge, MA.

Omran, A.R. (1971). The epidemiologic transition. A theory of the epidemiology of population change. *The Milbank Memorial Fund Q.* **49**, 509–538.

Pinstrup-Andersen, P., Pandya-Lorch, R., and Rosegrant, M.W. (1999). World food prospects: critical issues for the early twenty-first century. Food Policy Report, IFPRI, Washington, DC.

Popkin, B. (2002). An overview on the nutrition transition and its health implications: The Bellagio meeting. *Public Health Nutr.* **5**, 93–103.

Popkin, B.M., Horton, S., Kim, S., Mahal, A., and Shuigao, J. (2001). Trends in diet, nutritional status and diet-related noncommunicable diseases in China and India: The economic costs of the nutrition transition. *Nutr. Rev.* **59**, 379–390.

# The Global Context

2. Economic and technological development and their relationships
   to body size and productivity . . . . . . . . . . . . . . . . . . . . . . . . . . . . . . . 9
3. Food production . . . . . . . . . . . . . . . . . . . . . . . . . . . . . . . . . . . . . . . . 25
4. Can the challenges of poverty, sustainable consumption and good health
   governance be addressed in an era of globalization? . . . . . . . . . . . . . . . . . 51
5. Demographic trends . . . . . . . . . . . . . . . . . . . . . . . . . . . . . . . . . . . . . . 71

PART

I

# Economic and technological development and their relationships to body size and productivity

*Robert W. Fogel and Lorens A. Helmchen*

## Introduction

From 1948 to 1998, real per capita income nearly tripled in the United States, growing at an average annual rate of 2.17% (US Department of Commerce, 2000; US Census Bureau, 2000)

Between 1780 and 1979, British per capita income grew at an annual rate of about 1.15% (Maddison, 1982; Crafts, 1985)

The enormous increase in productivity that these figures reflect is also found when output per capita is measured in physical units. A case in point is the number of cars in the United States, which rose from eight thousand in 1900 to more than 200 million in 2000, providing on average each American adult with a car at the end of the millennium (Caplow *et al.*, 2000).

The growth in material wealth has been matched by changes in body size over the past 300 years, especially during the twentieth century. Perhaps the most remarkable secular trend has been the reduction in mortality. Between 1900 and 1998, life expectancy at birth in the United States increased by 65% for women, from 48.3 years to 79.5 years, and by 60% for men, from 46.3 years to 73.8 years (National Center for Health Statistics, 2001). Table 2.1 provides an overview of the long-term trend in life expectancy at birth for seven nations. The data show that in England life expectancy has more than doubled since the early eighteenth century. France has recorded even larger gains in longevity. French children born today can expect to live nearly three times longer than their ancestors 250 years ago.

**Table 2.1** Life expectancy at birth (years) in seven nations, 1725–1990 (both sexes combined)

| Country | 1725 | 1750 | 1800 | 1850 | 1900 | 1950 | 1990 |
|---|---|---|---|---|---|---|---|
| England or UK | 32 | 37 | 36 | 40 | 48 | 69 | 76 |
| France | | 26 | 33 | 42 | 46 | 67 | 77 |
| US | 50 | 51 | 56 | 43 | 47 | 68 | 76 |
| Egypt | | | | | | 42 | 60 |
| India | | | | | 27 | 39 | 59 |
| China | | | | | | 41 | 70 |
| Japan | | | | | | 61 | 79 |

Source: Fogel (in press).

**Table 2.2** Estimated average final heights (cm) of men who reached maturity between 1750 and 1875 in six European populations, by quarter centuries

| Date of maturity by century and quarter | Great Britain | Norway | Sweden | France | Denmark | Hungary |
|---|---|---|---|---|---|---|
| 18-III | 165.9 | 163.9 | 168.1 | | | 168.7 |
| 18-IV | 167.9 | | 166.7 | 163.0 | 165.7 | 165.8 |
| 19-I | 168.0 | | 166.7 | 164.3 | 165.4 | 163.9 |
| 19-II | 171.6 | | 168.0 | 165.2 | 166.8 | 164.2 |
| 19-III | 169.3 | 168.6 | 169.5 | 165.6 | 165.3 | |
| 20-III | 175.0 | 178.3 | 177.6 | 172.0 | 176.0 | 170.9 |

Source: Author's calculations.

Although not as significant numerically, final heights of European men who reached maturity have also been increasing over the past two centuries, as shown in Table 2.2. In some countries, average heights increased by as much as 10 cm per century.

Body weight has also increased. Figure 2.1 shows that for some age groups, the body mass index (BMI), a measure of weight adjusted for height (equal to $kg/m^2$), increased by about 10–15% within the past 100 years.

This chapter aims to elucidate the long-run relationship between labor productivity and body size. In particular, it will be shown that improvements in the nutritional status of a number of societies in Western Europe since the early eighteenth century may have initiated a virtuous circle of *technophysio* evolution. The theory of *technophysio* evolution posits the existence of a synergism between technological and physiological improvements that has produced a form of human evolution that is biological but not genetic, rapid, culturally transmitted, and not necessarily stable over time. In the context of the present study, we suggest that an increase in agricultural efficiency and labor productivity improved human physiology, in turn leading to further gains in labor productivity.

The next two sections identify how the early modern advances in agriculture and the increased availability of calories per capita raised labor productivity over the course of successive generations. This is followed by an analysis of the determinants and consequences of accelerating productivity gains in American agriculture after World War II to illustrate the changing relationship among nutrition, body size, and labor productivity.

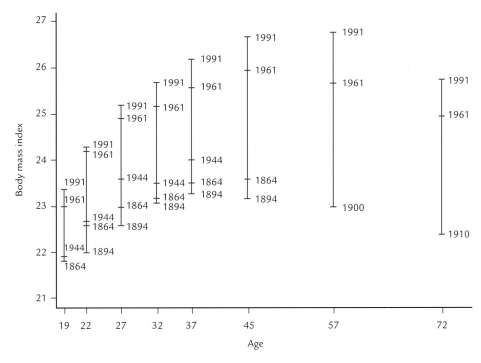

**Figure 2.1**   Mean body mass index by age group and year, 1863–1991 (from Costa and Steckel, 1997). The age groups, which are centered at the marks, are ages 18–19, 20–24, 25–29, 30–34, 35–39, 40–49, 50–64, and 65–79. For some years BMI is not available for a specific age group. Costa and Steckel (1997). Reproduced with kind permission from The University of Chicago Press. © 1997 by the National Bureau of Economic Research.

These recent changes serve as a backdrop to define and track the nutrition transition. The chapter concludes with a summary of the findings, which outlines possible scenarios for further nutrition-induced changes in body size and labor productivity.

# The effect of improved nutrition on productivity and output

To understand the relationship between the secular trends in body size and productivity, it is useful to begin by examining changes in nutritional status that took place over the same period.

## Energy cost accounting

Nutritional status is most commonly measured by the amount of calories available per person balanced against caloric requirements, also referred to as *net nutrition*[1].

---

[1] By contrast, the total amount of calories ingested is referred to as *gross nutrition*.

The principal component of the total energy requirement is represented by the basal metabolic rate (BMR). The BMR, which varies with age, sex, and body size is the amount of energy required to maintain body temperature and to sustain the functioning of the heart, liver, brain, and other organs. For adult males aged 20–39 years living in moderate climates, BMR normally ranges between 1350 and 2000 kcal/day depending on height and weight. For comparison across time and different populations, it is convenient to standardize for the age and sex distribution of a population by converting the per capita consumption of calories into consumption per equivalent adult male aged 20–39, also referred to as a consuming unit.

Since the BMR does not allow for the energy required to eat and digest food, or for essential hygiene, an individual cannot survive on the calories needed for basal metabolism. The energy required for these additional essential activities over a period of 24 hours is estimated at 0.27 of BMR or 0.4 of BMR during waking hours. In other words, a survival diet is 1.27 BMR, or between 1720 and 2540 kcal/day for a consuming unit. A maintenance diet contains no allowance for the energy required to earn a living, prepare food, or any other activities beyond those connected with eating and essential hygiene.

Whatever calories are available beyond those claimed for basal metabolism and maintenance can be used at the discretion of the individual, either for work or for leisure activities.

## Chronic malnutrition in late-eighteenth century Europe

According to recent estimates, the average caloric consumption in France on the eve of the French Revolution was about 2290 kcal per consuming unit, that for England was about 2700 kcal per consuming unit. These averages, however, do not reveal the variation in caloric consumption within the French and English populations. Table 2.3 shows the probable French and English distributions of the daily consumption of kcal per consuming unit toward the end of the eighteenth century.

The principal finding that emerges from this table is the exceedingly low level of food production, especially in France, at the start of the Industrial Revolution. The French distribution of calories implies that 2.48% of the population had caloric consumption below basal metabolism, whereas the proportion of the English population below basal metabolism was 0.66%. For the remainder of the population, the level of work capacity permitted by the food supply was very low, even after allowing for the reduced requirements for maintenance because of small stature and reduced body mass. In France the bottom 10% of the labor force lacked the energy for regular work and the next 10% had enough energy for less than 3 hours of light work daily (0.52 hours of heavy work). Although the English situation was somewhat better, the bottom 3% of its labor force lacked the energy for any work, while the balance of the bottom 20% had enough energy for only about 6 hours of light work (1.09 hours of heavy work) each day.

Thus, at the end of the eighteenth century, the lack of access to sufficient calories effectively restricted the amount of activity (whether for income or leisure) that most laborers could perform, and it effectively precluded others from working at all.

**Table 2.3** A comparison of the probable French and English distributions of the daily caloric consumption (kcal) per consuming unit toward the end of the eighteenth century

| Decile | France c. 1785 $\bar{X} = 2290$ $(s/\bar{X}) = 0.3$ | | England c. 1790 $\bar{X} = 2700$ $(s/\bar{X}) = 0.3$ | |
| --- | --- | --- | --- | --- |
| | Daily kcal consumption | Cumulative % | Daily kcal consumption | Cumulative % |
| 1. Highest | 3672 | 100 | 4329 | 100 |
| 2. Ninth | 2981 | 84 | 3514 | 84 |
| 3. Eighth | 2676 | 71 | 3155 | 71 |
| 4. Seventh | 2457 | 59 | 2897 | 59 |
| 5. Sixth | 2276 | 48 | 2684 | 48 |
| 6. Fifth | 2114 | 38 | 2492 | 38 |
| 7. Fourth | 1958 | 29 | 2309 | 29 |
| 8. Third | 1798 | 21 | 2120 | 21 |
| 9. Second | 1614 | 13 | 1903 | 13 |
| 10. First | 1310 | 6 | 1545 | 6 |

Sources and procedures: Author's calculations.

**Table 2.4** Secular trends in the daily caloric supply in France and Great Britain 1700–1989 (kcal per capita)

| Year | France | Great Britain |
| --- | --- | --- |
| 1700 | | 2095 |
| 1705 | 1657 | |
| 1750 | | 2168 |
| 1785 | 1848 | |
| 1800 | | 2237 |
| 1803–12 | 1846 | |
| 1845–54 | 2480 | |
| 1850 | | 2362 |
| 1909–13 | | 2857 |
| 1935–39 | 2975 | |
| 1954–55 | 2783 | 3231 |
| 1961 | | 3170 |
| 1965 | 3355 | 3304 |
| 1989 | 3465 | 3149 |

Source: Fogel *et al.* (in press).

## How better nutrition raised output per capita

Table 2.4 shows secular trends in the daily caloric supply in France and Great Britain from 1700 to 1989. Per capita availability of calories more than doubled in this period in France, and increased by about 50% in Great Britain, where caloric supply was 30% larger than that in France at the beginning of the period.

### Framework

How did the substantial increase in calories per capita affect labor productivity? Labor productivity can be defined as the output of marketable goods and services that a typical worker can produce over the span of one day. Daily output per worker, in turn, can be decomposed into the output per calorie expended at work and the daily amount of calories expended on the job by a typical worker. By multiplying the daily output per worker by the number of workers per inhabitant (which is called the labor force participation rate) output per worker is transformed into output per capita, which is used as a measure of the standard of living:

Output of goods and services produced per capita per day
   = daily output of goods and services per calorie expended in their production
      × daily amount of calories expended in production per worker
      × labor force participation rate

In this decomposition, the technological breakthroughs in farming raised yields for a given effort level, represented here as increases in the output per calorie expended in production. At given levels of annual calories expended in production per worker and labor force participation rate, this must have raised the volume of agricultural output per capita. Higher levels of labor productivity in agriculture also allowed parts of the labor force to be employed in nonagricultural sectors of the economy without reducing farm output per person, thus diversifying the range of goods and services produced domestically.

To understand the full effect of gains in agricultural efficiency, however, it is necessary to take into account how the additional calories were used. Those adults who had been working before the development and diffusion of more productive farming methods could now increase the annual amount of calories expended while working, either by performing more energy-intensive tasks or by working additional hours, or both. This increase in calories expended in production by a typical worker further increased the amount of calories produced (and ultimately consumed) per capita.

In addition to boosting the calories available to workers, the expansion of the food supply also made more calories available for members of the poorest segment of the adult population who had had only enough energy above maintenance for a few hours of strolling each day – about the amount needed by a beggar – but less on average than that needed for just one hour of the heavy manual labor required in agriculture. To the extent that these persons now had the energy to work, they raised the labor force participation rate, which led to a further increase in per capita output. Table 2.5 summarizes the daily amount of energy available for work in France, and England and Wales from 1700 to 1980. The most impressive gains are reflected by the data for France, where calories available for work increased nearly fivefold within less than 200 years.

In total, by increasing agricultural yields per calorie expended, the Second Agricultural Revolution expanded the availability of calories per capita, drawing more people into the labor force and raising on-the-job calorie expenditures of those working. This boost in the population's productive capacity in turn fueled further growth not only in food output per capita. It also helped to raise the output in all other, nonagricultural sectors of the economy that benefited from an increase in workers and hours worked.

**Table 2.5** A comparison of energy available for work daily per consuming unit in France, and England and Wales, 1700–1980 (in kcal)

| Year | France | England and Wales |
| --- | --- | --- |
| 1700 | | 720 |
| 1705 | 439 | |
| 1750 | | 812 |
| 1785 | 600 | |
| 1800 | | 858 |
| 1803–12 | | |
| 1840 | | |
| 1845–54 | | |
| 1850 | | 1014 |
| 1870 | 1671 | |
| 1880 | | |
| 1944 | | |
| 1975 | 2136 | |
| 1980 | | 1793 |

Source: Fogel *et al.* (in press).

### Empirical estimate

Time series of anthropometric and macroeconomic statistics can be combined to estimate the contribution of better nutrition to the growth of output per person. The most reliable and complete data in this regard have been collected for England. As noted in the introduction, between 1780 and 1979 British per capita income grew at an annual rate of about 1.15% (Maddison, 1982).

Data are now available to measure the changes in calories available for work and the labor force participation rate. For Britain, it has been estimated that the increases in the supply of calories lifted as much as one fifth of all consuming units above the threshold required for work. As a result, the labor force participation rate increased by 25% over 200 years, contributing 0.11% to the annual British growth rate between 1780 and 1980 ($1.25^{0.005} - 1 = 0.0011$).

The increased supply of calories also raised the average consumption of calories by those in the labor force from 2944 kcal per consuming unit in c.1790 to 3701 kcal per consuming unit in 1980. Of these amounts, 1009 kcal were available for work in c. 1790 and 1569 in 1980, so that calories available for discretionary activities increased by about 56% during the two centuries. If it is assumed that the proportion of the available energy devoted to work has been unchanged between the end points of the period, then the increase in the amount of energy available for work contributed about 0.23% per annum to the annual growth rate of per capita income ($1.56^{0.0053} - 1 = 0.0023$). Thus, in combination, bringing the ultrapoor into the labor force and raising the energy available for work by those in the labor force, explains about 30% of British growth in per capita income over the past two centuries [$(0.0023 + 0.0011) \div 0.0115 \cong 0.30$].

As incomes in OECD countries have risen, the share of discretionary time devoted to working for income has declined. Consequently, it is unlikely that further increases in the amount of calories available per person in those countries will raise labor force participation rates or hours worked[2]. However, the immediate effect of better nutrition on labor productivity still holds enormous potential in poor countries where malnutrition is widespread.

# The self-reinforcing cycle of greater body size and higher productivity

In addition to the direct effect of better nutrition on the growth of output per person, the conquest of chronic malnutrition has had a long-term effect on human physiology, which has taken several generations to unfold.

The role of long-term changes of nutritional status in altering body size is inferred from applying energy cost accounting to an analysis of food balance sheets. In particular, to have the energy necessary to produce the national product of either France or England c. 1700, the typical adult male must have been quite short and very light in weight. The smaller body size reduced the basal metabolic rate and thereby freed up calories that could be used for work. As per capita food supplies expanded, so did not only hours worked but also body size. The increase in body size, in turn, improved health and the capacity of individuals to raise labor productivity further, thus reinforcing the initial increase in labor productivity.

## The effect of improved nutrition on body size, morbidity and mortality

### The gain in weight

As was pointed out earlier, the energy that an individual takes in through food consumption will be spent to maintain body temperature and vital organ functions, as well as for eating, sleeping, and essential hygiene. The remainder is available for discretionary use, such as work and leisure. It was also shown that the additional calories that became available in the wake of the Second Agricultural Revolution were used to engage in more energy-intensive tasks and increase labor force participation. Energy not used is stored, leading to weight gain. As such, the body mass index may be interpreted as a measure of net nutrition, which is defined as the excess of calories ingested over calories claimed for maintenance and discretionary use. Figure 2.1 documents the secular increase in body mass index for white men between 1864 and 1991.

---

[2] In the United States, the labor force participation rate (LFPR) increased from 58.8% to 67.1% between 1948 and 1998. This trend masks important differences between men and women: while the LFPR for men fell from 86.6% to 74.9%, the labor force participation of women rose from 32.7% to 59.8%. These differences are even more pronounced for the group of 55–64-year olds and imply that men tend to retire at earlier ages than before, whereas women continue to expand their participation in the labor market. The increase of the female LFPR has been facilitated by the introduction and adoption of labor-saving technology in the household. As household work became less time consuming, women could reduce the hours spent working at home and seek paid employment in the labor market.

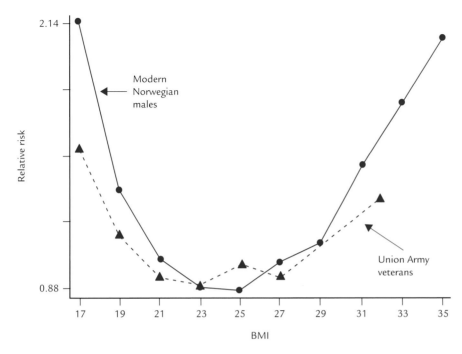

**Figure 2.2**   Relative mortality risk by BMI among men 50 years of age, Union Army veterans around 1900 and modern Norwegians (from Costa and Steckel, 1997). In the Norwegian data BMI for 79 084 men was measured at ages 45–49 and the period of risk was 7 years. BMI of Union Army veterans was measured at ages 45–64 and the observation period was 25 years. Costa and Steckel (1997). Reproduced with kind permission from The University of Chicago Press. © 1997 by the National Bureau of Economic Research.

It has been shown that eliminating chronic hunger will strengthen the body's defenses against infectious diseases, thus lowering the risk of contracting diseases and premature death. The relationship between weight, as measured by the Body Mass Index, and mortality was established empirically by Hans Waaler (1984) for Norwegian men aged 45–49 and confirmed for a sample of Union Army veterans measured at ages 45–64 and followed for 25 years. Figure 2.2 shows a U-shaped relationship between BMI and the relative risk of death for both samples. Among both modern Norwegians and Union Army veterans the curve is quite flat within the range 22–28, with the relative risk of mortality hovering close to 1.0, which represents the average risk of death in the population. However, at BMIs of less than 22 and over 28, the risk of death rises sharply as BMI moves away from its mean value.

## The gain in height

A larger and better survival diet allowed adult members of the generation that first witnessed the rise in agricultural efficiency to increase weight, and, consequently, to improve health and extend life. Better nutrition of pregnant women also improved the nutritional status of fetuses and infants. Access to sufficient amounts of calories and other vital nutrients *in utero* and developmental ages has been shown to affect the offspring's final height. Thus, whereas the immediate effect of the improvements in food

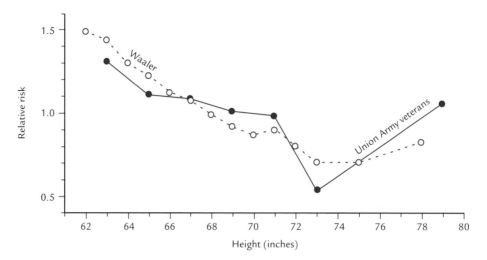

**Figure 2.3**  Relative mortality risk among Union Army veterans and among Norwegian males. Author's calculations.

supply was to raise the amount of energy spent at work and to boost body *weight*, the long-run impact over the course of several generations has been an increase in *stature*. This conclusion is supported by the time series on mean final heights for various European populations, shown in Table 2.2.

Waaler (1984) also identified the role of body height as a factor influencing morbidity and mortality. Figure 2.3 plots the relationship between relative mortality risk and height found among Norwegian men aged 40–59 measured in the 1960s and among Union Army veterans measured at ages 23–49 and at risk between ages 55 and 75. Short men, whether modern Norwegians or nineteenth-century Americans, were much more likely to die early than tall men. Height has also been found to be an important predictor of the relative likelihood that men aged 23–49 would be rejected from the Union Army between 1861 and 1865 because of chronic diseases. Despite significant differences in ethnicity, environmental circumstances, the array and severity of diseases, and time, the functional relationship between height and relative risk are strikingly similar in the two cases.

To gauge the relative importance of height and weight for an individual's risk of mortality, an isomortality surface that relates the risk of death to both height and weight simultaneously is needed. Such a surface, presented in Fig. 2.4, was fitted to Waaler's data. Transecting the isomortality map are iso-BMI lines that give the locus of BMI between 16 and 34. The heavy line transecting the minimum point of each isomortality curve represents the weight that minimizes mortality risk at each height.

Since an individual's height cannot be varied by changes in nutrition after maturity, adults can move to a more desirable BMI only by changing their weight. Therefore, the *x*-axis is interpreted as a measure of the effect of the current nutritional status of mature males on adult mortality rates. Moreover, since most stunting takes place before age three, the *y*-axis is interpreted as a measure of the effect of nutritional

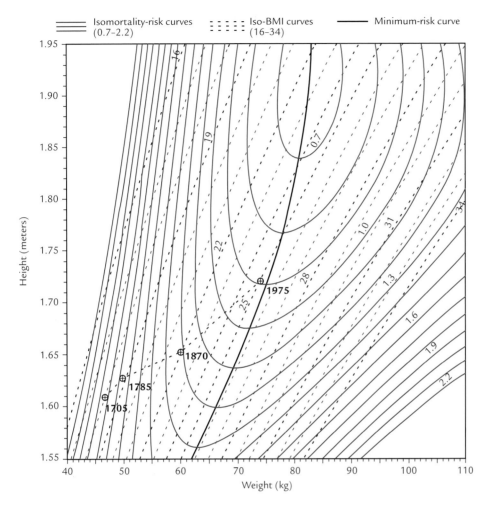

**Figure 2.4** Isomortality curves of relative risk for height and weight among Norwegian males aged 50–64 years, with a plot of the estimated French height and weight at four dates. Author's calculations.

deprivation during developmental ages (including *in utero*) on the risk of mortality at middle and late ages.

Superimposed on Fig. 2.4 are rough estimates of heights and weights in France at four dates. In 1705 the French probably achieved equilibrium with their food supply at an average height of about 161 cm and BMI of about 18. Over the next 270 years the food supply expanded fast enough to permit both the height and the weight of adult males to increase. Figure 2.4 shows that the increase in available food per person translated mostly into weight gain during the eighteenth and nineteenth centuries. During the twentieth century the gains in calories per capita served mainly to increase height. Between 1870 and 1975 height increased at more than twice the rate that it did during the previous 165 years.

Figure 2.4 implies that although factors associated with height and weight jointly explain about 90% of the estimated decline in French mortality rates over the period between 1785 and c. 1870, they only explain about 50% of the decline in mortality rates during the past century.

### The effect of lower morbidity and mortality on labor productivity

The unprecedented gains in life expectancy over the past 300 years, the reductions in disease prevalence, and the increasing age at onset of disability have all contributed to raise the number of years free of disease and disability that a person born today can expect to live. In addition, the development of cures for many conditions and the provision of effective symptom management for those conditions that cannot be cured have eliminated or reduced significantly the age-specific rates of functional impairment that used to be associated with many diseases.

The immediate effect of longer lives is that now more people will be able to use their accumulated experience longer, and that they are more likely to share more of their life span with their children and grandchildren.

As a result of improvements in human physiology and major advances in medicine, the number of disability and symptom-free years of life that remain at any given age is now much larger than it has ever been. This creates strong incentives for individuals to undertake measures aimed at preserving physical functioning and cognitive ability, also referred to as investments in human capital. Individuals respond by undertaking more of these investments, which include purchases of preventive and rehabilitative medical services as well as the acquisition of new skills and knowledge. For instance, in 1910, only 13% of adults in the United States were high school graduates and only 3% were college graduates. By 1998, the comparable percentages were 83 and 24, respectively (Caplow *et al.*, 2000). It is no coincidence that, at the beginning of the twenty-first century, healthcare and educational services constitute two of the fastest growing sectors of the US economy, as they do in most other OECD nations. Not only do these activities maintain or improve the quality of life but they also enhance labor productivity.

## Productivity-induced demographic and economic change in the USA

The relationships between technological development, nutrition, body size, and economic change have become most apparent over the course of the past century. They are perhaps best illustrated by examining the consequences of the dramatic improvements in labor productivity experienced by the agricultural sector in the United States since the end of World War II.

From 1948 to 1994, agricultural output more than doubled, expanding at an average annual rate of 1.9% (Ahearn *et al.*, 1998). During the same period, total hours worked in agriculture, adjusted for quality, fell by more than two-thirds, or 2.7% annually.

These figures imply that between 1948 and 1994 US agricultural output per hour rose at an average rate of 4.6% per annum, a more than ninefold increase over the span of fifty years[3].

This surge in agricultural labor productivity is attributable to steadily improving yields and an increase in the acreage cultivated per hour. For instance, the introduction of pesticides, herbicides, and fertilizer, combined with higher-yielding crop varieties raised the amount of potatoes per harvested acre by a factor of almost 2.5 between 1948 and 1994 (US Department of Agriculture, 2000). Similarly, the number of acres cultivated per hour has been raised dramatically by the mechanization of agriculture, at an average annual rate of about 3%.

As agricultural labor became more productive, the number of annual hours per worker as well as the number of workers were cut without curtailing agricultural output. Although annual hours per agricultural worker declined by 1% per year, the number of agricultural workers fell even more rapidly, by 1.7% per year (Ahearn *et al.*, 1998).

Those workers who were released from the agricultural sector found employment in other sectors of the economy, where they helped to raise output of other goods that consumers wanted, or they stopped working altogether. The fraction of the labor force employed in agriculture fell from 13% in 1948 to 3.2% in 1998 (US Bureau of the Census, 1976; Braddock, 1999; Bureau of Labor Statistics, 2001)[4].

Despite the sharply declining number of hours worked, the growth of US agricultural output has been outpacing the growth of the population during the past 50 years. Whereas from 1948 to 1994 agricultural output grew by 1.9% annually, the population of the United States grew on average by 1.2% per annum (US Department of Commerce, 2000). As a result, agricultural output per capita increased at an annual rate of approximately 0.7%. Compounded over the second half of the twentieth century, therefore, agricultural output per capita, which can be used to assess a country's capacity to supply its inhabitants with calories, increased by about 40%.

# Conclusion and outlook

The sections above have documented how advances in agricultural efficiency after 1700 allowed the societies of Europe and North America to expand and improve their diets by an unprecedented degree. The rise in agricultural efficiency set off a self-reinforcing cycle of improvements in nutrition and gains in labor productivity, leading to a substantial increase in per capita output, which has come to be known as "modern economic growth". It was shown how the initial increase in agricultural

---

[3] A century earlier, output per man-hour had increased 2.16 times in 60 years, or 1.3% annually: whereas in 1840 the production of 100 bushels of wheat required 233 man-hours, in 1900 the same output could be produced with less than half that amount, 108 man-hours. It follows that the growth rate of agricultural productivity accelerated, perhaps doubled, after World War II (cf. Clark, 1993).

[4] This drop in agriculture's employment share was already underway in the nineteenth century; from 1870 to 1920, the fraction of the labor force employed in agriculture fell from 53% to 27%.

efficiency was magnified by providing the population with enough additional calories to boost the number of acres cultivated per hour, annual hours worked, and the labor force participation rate. Based on the notion that variations in the size of individuals have been a principal mechanism in equilibrating the population with the food supply, improved net nutrition has been identified as the primary long-term determinant of the sharp increase in the number of disability-free years of life. The gains in longevity, in turn, have created an incentive for individuals to maintain and upgrade skills and personal health. This line of argument underpins the prediction that the conquest of malnutrition may continue to raise the productivity and innovative capacity of the labor force in the West.

The time series of various components of agricultural output per capita in the United States since World War II has been analyzed and combined with the data presented, the following conclusions emerge for the advanced economies of Western Europe and North America.

- Output per acre cultivated has been increasing throughout the period under study.
- Acres cultivated per hour have been increasing throughout this period, first because human energy available for work increased, then because animal and inanimate power complemented and eventually substituted for human energy.
- Annual hours worked per agricultural worker increased at first, as more calories became available for discretionary use, but have been declining recently and are expected to continue to decline.
- The rise in agricultural labor productivity has permitted the number of agricultural workers per inhabitant to decline without lowering the amount of calories available per person.
- The declining share of agricultural workers in the labor force permitted other sectors of the economy to grow, thus greatly diversifying and expanding the range of nonagricultural goods and services.

The recent reversal of some key trends in energy intensity of work and labor force participation rates suggests that the economic and epidemiologic consequences from the unprecedented improvement of human nutrition in the rich countries are still being played out.

Up to World War II the energy intensity and quantity of work in Europe was limited by the availability of food per capita. Since then, however, caloric intake has not only matched individual caloric requirements but tends to exceed calorie expenditure in an increasing portion of the population. One indicator of this tendency is the growing prevalence of obese adults in the United States, which between 1960 and 1994 increased from 13.3% to 23.3% (National Center for Health Statistics, 2001)[5].

This trend is compounded by the fact that the progressive substitution of human energy by inanimate power and the concomitant expansion of sedentary work have led to a gradual reduction of calories expended per hour worked. The continued increase in agricultural output per person coupled with lower energy requirements on the job

---

[5] A person is considered to be obese if that individual's Body Mass Index is equal to or greater than 30 (National Center for Health Statistics, 2001).

may portend two, not mutually exclusive, scenarios for the next stage of the nutrition transition in the world's richest countries.

1. As more and more people work in occupations that do not place high demands on calorie supply, they may decide to increase energy spent during leisure hours. In addition, further gains in stature and weight will raise the calories needed for maintenance.

2. Alternatively, workers may decide to reduce their overall calorie intake to bring it into line with the decreased amounts of calories at work. Although expenditure on food may not decline in absolute terms, consumers may opt to substitute increasingly away from quantity toward quality of calories and become choosier regarding those calories that they decide to purchase and ingest. To the extent that pressure for advances in productivity and greater per capita supply of calories wanes in rich countries, it is conceivable that forms of agriculture that are less productive in calories will gain popularity to accommodate other criteria in the selection of agricultural products and processes. For example, organic agriculture, which renounces the use of certain herbicides, pesticides and fertilizers, accepts lower yields per acre in order to reduce environmental hazards. Similarly, a shift in consumer preferences may prompt the cultivation of crops that sell at a premium but require more care or are less nutritious, thus lowering the amount of calories per hour worked.

The situation is very different in poor countries where more than 800 million people are chronically undernourished (FAO, 1999). Progress in agricultural productivity remains the focus of most programs aimed at raising the per capita supply of calories and other vital nutrients. Yet even in countries where average food consumption is deemed adequate, an unequal distribution of income may effectively preclude the poorest parts of the population from obtaining sufficient calories, as was shown for late eighteenth-century England and France. Recent data from developing countries confirm the association of greater income inequality with increased food insecurity and smaller body size (Steckel, 1995; Shapouri and Rosen, 1999).

Whatever the approach to alleviating chronic hunger in developing countries, improving the food supply could unlock the short-term and long-term effects of better nutrition on labor productivity that have had such a lasting impact on the growth trajectories of Europe and North America.

# References

Ahearn, M., Yee, J., Ball, E., and Nehring, R. (1998). "Agriculture Information Bulletin 740". US Department of Agriculture, Washington, DC.

Braddock, D. (1999). *Monthly Labor Rev.* **122**, 51–77.

Bureau of Labor Statistics (2001). "Labor Force Statistics from the Current Population Survey". Available: http://146.142.4.24/cgi-bin/surveymost?lf

Caplow, T., Hicks, L., and Wattenberg, B.J. (2000). "The First Measured Century: An Illustrated Guide to Trends in America, 1900–2000". American Enterprise Institute for Public Policy Research, Washington, DC.

Clark, G. (1993). *In* "The British Industrial Revolution – An Economic Perspective" (J. Mokyr, ed.), pp. 227–266. Westview Press, Boulder.

Costa, D.L., and Steckel, R.H. (1997). *In* "Health and Welfare During Industrialization" (R.H. Steckel, and R. Floud, eds.). University of Chicago Press, Chicago.

Crafts, N.F.R. (1985). "British Economic Growth during the Industrial Revolution". Clarendon Press, Oxford.

Food and Agriculture Organization (1999). "The State of Food Insecurity in the World". Rome. Available: http://www.fao.org/NEWS/1999/img/SOFI99-E.PDF

Fogel, R.W. (1997). *In* "Handbook of Population and Family Economics" (M.R. Rosenzweig, and O. Stark, eds.), 1A, pp. 433–481. North-Holland, Amsterdam.

Fogel, R.W. (in press). "The Escape from Hunger and Premature Death 1700–2000: Europe, America and the Third World". The University of Chicago, Chicago.

Fogel, R.W., and Costa, D.L. (1997). *Demography* **34**, 49–66.

Fogel, R.W., Floud, R., and Harris, B. (in progress). "A treatise on technophysio evolution and consumption". Center for Population Economics, The University of Chicago, Chicago.

Maddison, A. (1982). "Phases of Capitalist Development". Oxford University Press, Oxford.

National Center for Health Statistics (2001). "Health, United States, 2001. With Urban and Rural Health Chartbook". Hyattsville, Maryland.

Shapouri, S., and Rosen, S. (1999). Agriculture Information Bulletin 754. US Department of Agriculture, Washington, DC.

Steckel, R.H. (1995). *J. Econ. Lit.* **33**, 1903–1940.

US Bureau of the Census (1976). "The Statistical History of the United States from Colonial Times to the Present". Basic Books, New York.

US Census Bureau (2000). "Historical National Population Estimates: July 1, 1900 to July 1, 1999". Available: http://www.census.gov/population/estimates/nation/popclockest.txt

US Department of Agriculture (2000). "Track Records United States Crop Production". Available: http://www.usda.gov/nass/pubs/trackrec/track00a.htm

US Department of Commerce (2000). "Current Dollar and 'Real' Gross Domestic Product". Available: http://www.bea.doc.gov/bea/dn/gdplev.xls

Waaler, H. (1984). *Acta Med. Scand.* **679**, S1–S51.

# Food production

*Vaclav Smil*

Humans have relied during the course of their evolution on a number of distinct ways to secure their food supply. In many places in the tropics the oldest strategies (foraging and shifting agriculture) had coexisted side by side with subsequent ways of food provision (pastoralism, sedentary farming) for very long periods of time (Headland and Reid, 1989). In others, China being a perfect example, the ancient means of sedentary cultivation were gradually transformed into much more productive ways of growing crops. Foraging (food gathering and hunting) dominated all hominid and most of human existence and some of its key nutritional attributes will be noted in the first section of this chapter offering a brief history of food production. In this section I will also note a number of traditional agricultural practices, as they are still very much in evidence throughout the developing world. My review of the current global food situation will focus primarily on production and consumption gaps between developed and developing countries (I prefer to label them simply rich and poor).

While looking ahead I will avoid any quantitative point forecasts, as these tend to become irrelevant almost as soon as they are published; instead, I will identify the main factors that will be driving changes in food demand during the next 50 years. Increased demand for animal foods will be a key ingredient of this change and hence I will devote a separate section to analyzing its likely growth and its consequences for the global demand for feeds. I will close by stressing the need for two critical kinds of investment in agriculture: in the maintenance of irreplaceable ecosystemic structures and services without which no agriculture can succeed, and in genetic engineering whose advances will help to eliminate malnutrition even as the population of developing countries keeps expanding.

## A brief history of food production

Every new find of hominid remains in East Africa reignites the controversy about the origin of our species, but at least one conclusion remains unchanged: we have come from a long lineage of opportunistic foragers, and for millions of years both the natural diet and the foraging strategies of hominids resembled those of their primate ancestors

The Nutrition Transition
ISBN: 0-12-153654-8

(Whiten and Widdowson, 1992). Larger brains improved the odds of their survival but to secure food, hominids relied only on their muscles and on simple stratagems as scavengers, gatherers, hunters, and fishers helped by stone implements, bows and arrows and by fibrous or leather lines and nets. Controlled use of fire needed to prepare cooked food may have come first nearly half a million years ago, but a more certain time is about 250 000 years ago (Goudsblom, 1992).

Childe's (1951) idea of Neolithic Revolution has been one of the most unfortunate caricatures of human evolution: there was no sudden shift from foraging to sedentary farming. Diminishing returns in gathering and hunting led to a gradual extension of incipient cultivation present in many foraging societies, and foraging and agriculture commonly coexisted for very long periods of time (Smil, 1994). Similarly, there were no abrupt changes in the way most traditional agricultures produced food; some places experienced prolonged stagnation, or even declines, in overall food output, others have undergone gradual intensification of crop cultivation that has resulted in higher yields and more secure food supplies. Even then, traditional farming was able to produce only monotonous diets and it remained highly vulnerable to environmental stresses. Only modern agriculture, highly intensive and fossil fuel-based, has been able to produce enormous surpluses of food in all affluent nations and to raise most of the world's populous developing countries at least close to, and for most of the Chinese even well above, subsistence minima.

## Foraging societies

The great diversity of the preserved archaeological record makes it impossible to offer any simple generalizations concerning prehistoric diets. Modern studies of foraging societies that have survived in extreme environments (tropical rain forest, semideserts) into the 20th century have provided very limited insight into the lives of prehistoric foragers in more equable climates and more fertile areas. Moreover, these societies have often been affected by contacts with pastoralists, farmers or overseas migrants. Given the unimpressive physical endowment of early humans and the absence of effective weapons, it is most likely that our ancestors were initially much better scavengers than hunters (Blumenschine and Cavallo, 1992). Large predators often left behind partially eaten carcasses and this meat, or at least the nutritious bone marrow, could be reached by enterprising early humans before it was devoured by vultures and hyenas.

Fishing, collecting of shellfish, and near-shore hunting of sea mammals provided diet unusually rich in proteins and made it possible to live in semipermanent, and even permanent, settlements (Price, 1991). In contrast, both gathering and hunting were surprisingly unrewarding in species-rich tropical forests where energy-rich seeds are a very small portion of total plant mass and are mostly inaccessible in high canopies, as are most animals, which are also relatively small and highly mobile. Grasslands and open woodlands offered much better opportunities for both collecting and hunting. Many highly nutritious seeds and nuts were easy to reach, and patches of large starchy roots and tubers provided particularly high energy returns. So did the hunting of many grasslands herbivores which were often killed without any weapons, by driving the herds over precipices. This hunting was intensive enough to explain the disappearance of most large herbivores from preagricultural landscapes (Alroy, 2001).

There is no doubt that all preagricultural societies were omnivorous and that although they collected and killed a large variety of plant and animal species only a few principal foodstuffs usually dominated their diets. Preference for seeds and nuts among gatherers was inevitable; they are easy to collect, and they combine high energy content (13–26 MJ/kg) with relatively high protein shares (commonly above 10%). Wild grass seeds have as much food energy as cultivated grains (15 MJ/kg), and nuts have energy densities up to 75% higher. All wild meat is an excellent source of protein (>20%), but the flesh of small and agile animals (e.g., hares or monkeys) contains very little fat (<10%) and hence has very low energy density (5–6 MJ/kg). Consequently, there has been a widespread hunting preference for such large and relatively fatty species, such as mammoths and bisons (containing 10–12 MJ/kg). Even so, except for maritime hunters of fatty fish (salmon) and mammals (whales, seals), lipids usually supplied no more than 20% of food energy in preagricultural societies.

The extremes of daily intakes of animal protein among the remaining foraging populations studied after 1950 range from more than 300 g/capita among Inuit feeding on whales, seals, fish, and caribou to less than 20 g a day for foragers in arid African environments subsisting mainly on nuts and tubers (Smil, 1994). Eaton and Konner (1997) used nutrient analyses of wild plant and animal foods eaten by recent gatherers and hunters in order to estimate the dominant composition of prevailing preagricultural diets. They concluded that compared to the typical recent US intakes they were more than twice as rich in fiber, potassium, and calcium, but contained less than one-third of today's sodium consumption.

Prehistoric survival modes and diets were extremely diverse but this fact has not prevented some anthropologists making inadmissible generalizations. Undoubtedly, for some groups the total foraging effort was low, only a few hours a day, and this fact, confirmed by some modern field surveys, led to the portrayal of foragers as "the original affluent society" (Sahlins, 1972). This conclusion, based on very limited and highly debatable evidence, ignored the reality of much of the hard, and often dangerous, work in foraging and the frequency with which environmental stresses repeatedly affected most foraging societies. Seasonal food shortages in fluctuating climates necessitated the eating of unpalatable plant tissues and led to weight loss, low fertility, high infant mortalities, infanticide and often to devastating famines (Smil, 1994).

## Traditional agricultures

In comparison to foraging, traditional farming nearly always required higher inputs of human energy (and later also of animal labor), but it could support higher population densities and provide a more reliable food supply. Whereas foraging (except for maritime hunting) could support no more than a few people per 100 hectares (ha) of territory used for gathering and hunting, early traditional agricultures managed to support at least one person/ha of arable land (Fig. 3.1). By the end of the 19th century China's nationwide mean was above five people/ha, and double cropping of rice and wheat in the most fertile areas could yield enough to feed 12–15 people/ha (Smil, 1994).

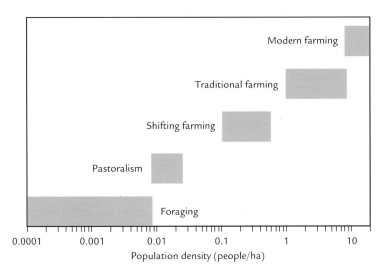

**Figure 3.1**  Comparison of carrying capacities of the principal modes of human food production showing that farming can support $10^3$–$10^4$ more people than foraging (based on Smil, 2000).

The need for higher energy inputs explains why so many foraging societies kept delaying adoption of permanent cultivation and why shifting farming – a less intensive method of cultivation alternating short (1–3 years) cropping periods with much longer (a decade or more) fallow spells – was practiced so extensively. In spite of many regional and local differences there were many fundamental similarities that persisted across the millennia of traditional farming. Above all, these agricultures were entirely renewable; photosynthetic conversion of solar radiation produced food for people, feed for animals, recyclable wastes for the replenishment of soil fertility, as well as wood (often turned into charcoal) for smelting metals needed to make simple farm tools. But the renewability of traditional farming was no guarantee of its sustainability. In many regions poor agronomic practices gradually depleted soil fertility or caused excessive soil erosion or desertification. These changes brought lower yields or even the abandonment of cultivation. But in most regions traditional farming progressed from extensive to relatively, or even highly, intensive modes of cultivation.

Except for small-scale cultivation of tubers (above all cassava) in the tropics and the Inca's reliance on potatoes, all of the Old World's traditional agricultures, as well as plowless Mesoamerican societies, shared their dependence on cereal grains. Cereal cultivation was supplemented by legumes, tubers and oil, fiber and, in some agricultures, also feed crops. After the domestication of draft animals the traditional crop cycles always started with plowing. Primitive wooden implements were used for millennia before the introduction of metal moldboard plows, 2000 years ago in China, but only some 17 centuries later in Europe. Plowing was followed by harrowing and by manual seeding. Harvesting also remained manual (sickles, scythes) until the introduction of grain reapers before the middle of the 19th century. Wheat cultivars had diffused worldwide from the Near East, rice from Southeast Asia, corn from Mesoamerica and millets from China.

Continuous primacy of grains in crop cultivation is due to the combination of their relatively high yields (two or three times higher than legume harvests), good nutritional value (high in filling, easily digestible carbohydrates, moderately rich in proteins), relatively high energy density at maturity (at 13–15 MJ/kg roughly five times higher than for tubers), and low moisture content (<14%) suitable for long-term storage. Dominance of a particular species has been largely a matter of environmental conditions and taste preferences. Without understanding the nutritional rationale for their actions all traditional agricultures combined the cultivation of cereal and legume grains thus assuring complete amino acid supply in largely vegetarian diets. The Chinese planted soybeans, beans, peas, and peanuts to supplement millets, wheat and rice. In India protein from lentils, peas, and chickpeas enriched wheat and rice. In Europe the preferred combinations included peas and beans with wheats, barley, oats, and rye, in West Africa peanuts and cowpeas with millets, and in the New World corn and beans.

The principal means of agricultural intensification included more widespread and more efficient use of draft animals, increasing fertilization and regular crop rotations, more frequent irrigation in arid regions, and multicropping in the places where climate could support more than a single crop per year. The use of draft animals (horses, mules, oxen, water buffaloes, camels, donkeys) eliminated the most exhaustive field work and it also sped up considerably many farmyard tasks (threshing, oil pressing), improved the quality of plowing (and later also of seeding), allowed for drawing of water from deeper wells for irrigation. The introduction of collar harness, invented in China about two millennia ago, iron horseshoes, and heavier animal breeds made field work more efficient (Smil, 1994). Feeding larger numbers of these animals eventually required further intensification to produce requisite feed crops.

Irrigation and fertilization moderated, if not altogether removed, the two key constraints on crop productivity, shortages of water and nutrients. Unaided gravity irrigation could not work on plains and in river valleys with minimal stream gradients; the invention and introduction of a variety of simple mechanical, animal- and people-driven water-lifting devices (mostly in the Middle East and China) solved this challenge (Molenaar, 1956). Fertilization involved recycling of crop residues and increasingly intensive applications of animal and human wastes. Extensive practices used no manure, whereas peak manuring rates in the 19th century Netherlands and in the most productive provinces in China surpassed 20 t/ha. Green manuring, cultivation of leguminous cover crops (clovers, vetches) which were then plowed under, was widely used in Europe ever since ancient Greece and Rome, and it has also been widely employed in east Asia (Smil, 2001). Even so, nutrient deficiencies commonly limited traditional crop productivity.

Growing of a greater variety of crops lowered the risk of total harvest failure, discouraged the establishment of persistent pests, reduced erosion, and maintained better soil properties. Crop rotations were chosen to fit climatic and soil conditions and dietary preferences. In poor societies they could substantially improve food self-sufficiency and food security at the local level. Traditional varieties of crops and their rotation schemes were enormous. For example, Buck's (1937) survey of Chinese farming counted nearly 550 different cropping systems in 168 localities. The adoption of new crops – most notably the post-1500 introductions of such New World staples as corn and potatoes and such versatile vegetables as tomatoes and peppers – had an enormous impact on food production throughout the world. In spite of these innovations preindustrial agricultures brought only very limited improvements in average harvests. For example, European wheat yields, except in the Netherlands and the UK, did not begin to rise decisively before the last decade of the 19th century (Smil, 1994).

Traditional farming also provided no more than basic subsistence diets for most of the people. Even during fairly prosperous times typical peasant diets, although more than adequate in terms of total food energy, were highly monotonous and not very palatable. In large parts of Europe bread (mostly dark, and in northern regions with little or no wheat flour), coarse grains (oats, barley, buckwheat), turnips, cabbage, and later potatoes, were the everyday staples. Typical rural Asian diets were, if anything, even more dominated by rice or coarse grain (millet, buckwheat). In many cases traditional peasant diets also contained less animal protein than did the earlier intakes with higher consumption of wild animals, birds, and aquatic species. This qualitative decline was not offset by a more equitable availability of basic foodstuffs: major consumption inequalities, both regional and socioeconomic, persisted until the 19th century. The majority of people in all traditional farming society had to live on food supplies that were below the level required for a healthy and vigorous life and different kinds of malnutrition were common.

Documentary and anthropometric evidence does not demonstrate any consistent upward trend in per capita food supply across the millennia of traditional farming. Regardless of the historical period, environmental setting and prevailing mode of cropping and intensification, no traditional agriculture could consistently produce enough food to eliminate extensive malnutrition. More importantly, no preindustrial agriculture could prevent recurrent famines. Droughts and floods were the most common natural triggers, and as a recent study demonstrates these natural disasters often represented the worst imaginable climatic teleconnections arising from the El Niño-Southern Oscillation (ENSO) whose effects are felt far beyond the Pacific realm (Davis, 2001). The combined (and never to be accurately quantified) toll of large-scale famines that repeatedly swept late 19th century India and China, and that also severely affected parts of Africa and Brazil, amounted to tens of millions of casualties.

In China in the 1920s peasants recalled an average of three crop failures brought by such disasters within their lifetime that were serious enough to cause famines (Buck, 1937). Some famines were so devastating that they remained in collective memory for generations and led to major social, economic and agronomic changes: the famous collapse of *Phytophthora*-infested Irish potato crops between 1845 and 1852, or the great Indian drought-induced famine of 1876–79. The world's most devastating famine, in China between 1958 and 1961, was only secondarily a matter of drought; the primary causes lie in the delusionary Maoist policies (Smil, 1999a).

## Modern farming

New energy sources and three intertwined strands of innovation explain most of the success of modern farming. In contrast to traditional agricultures, nonrenewable fossil fuels and electricity are essential inputs in modern farming. They are needed to build and operate agriculture machinery whose nearly universal adoption mechanized virtually all field and crop-processing tasks. The second key innovation is the use of fossil energies and electricity to extract and synthesize fertilizers and pesticides. The third key advance was to develop and diffuse new crop varieties responsive to higher inputs of water and nutrients. These innovations brought higher and more reliable yields, they displaced draft animals in all rich countries and greatly reduced their importance in the poor ones. The replacement of muscles by internal combustion engines and electric motors and the substitution of organic recycling by inorganic fertilizers have drastically cut labor needs in agriculture and led to huge declines in rural populations and to the worldwide rise of urbanization. For example, in the US rural labor fell from more than 60% of the total workforce in 1850 to less than 40% in 1900, 15% in 1950, and a mere 2% since 1975 (US Bureau of the Census, 1975).

Fertilizers made the earliest, and also the greatest, difference. The use of chemically treated phosphates became common after the discoveries of new rock deposits in Florida in 1888, and in Morocco in 1913. After 1850 nitrogen from Chilean nitrates, supplemented later by the recovery of ammonium sulfate from coking ovens, provided the first inorganic alternative to organic recycling. The nitrogen barrier was finally broken by the invention of ammonia synthesis from its elements by Fritz Haber and the subsequent rapid commercialization of the process by Carl Bosch (Smil, 2001). This invention allowed, for the first time in history, to optimize nitrogen inputs on large scale.

Modern civilization is now critically dependent on the Haber–Bosch synthesis of ammonia. Recent global applications of nitrogen fertilizers to field crops – and also to permanent grasslands and tree (orchard, palm) and shrub (coffee, tea) plantations – have been in excess of 80 million tonnes (Mt) N/year, mostly in the form of urea (IFA, 2001; Fig. 3.2). The process currently provides the means of survival for about 40% of the world's population. Only half as many people as are alive today could be supplied

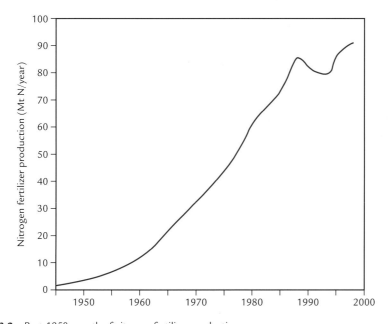

**Figure 3.2** Post-1950 growth of nitrogen fertilizer production.

by traditional cultivation lacking any synthetic fertilizers and producing very basic, and overwhelmingly vegetarian, diets; and prefertilizer farming could provide today's average diets to only about 40% of the existing population (Smil, 2001). Western nations, using most of their crop production for feed, could easily reduce their dependence on synthetic nitrogen by lowering their high meat consumption. Populous poor countries, where all but a small share of grain is eaten directly, do not have that option. Most notably, synthetic nitrogen provides about 75% of all inputs in China. With some 75% of the country's protein supplied by crops, more than half of all nitrogen in China's food comes from synthetic fertilizers.

In addition to nitrogen the world's crops now receive also close to 15 Mt of phosphorus, and about 18 Mt of potassium a year (IFA, 2001). This massive use of fertilizers has been accompanied by the expanding use of herbicides used to control weeds, and pesticides to lessen insect and fungal infestations. Pesticide use has often been much maligned and many of these chemicals, especially following improper applications, undoubtedly leave undesirable residues in harvested products, but their use has helped to reduce the still excessively large preharvest losses.

Farming mechanization was first accomplished in the US and Canada. Its most obvious consequence was the precipitous decline in agricultural labor requirements. For example, in 1850 an average hectare of the US wheat needed about 100 hours of labor; by 1900 the rate was less than 40 hours/ha, and 50 years later it sank below 2 hours/ha (US Bureau of the Census, 1975). Until the 1950s agricultural mechanization proceeded much more slowly in Europe, and in the populous countries of Asia and Latin America it really started only during the 1960s. Today's agriculture operates with more than 26 million tractors of which about 7 million are in developing countries (FAO, 2001). Mechanization also completely transformed crop processing tasks (threshing, oil pressing, etc.) and fuel and electric pumps greatly extended field irrigation. The global extent of crop irrigation more than quintupled between 1900 and 2000, from less than 50 to more than 270 million hectares, or from less than 5% to about 19% of the world's harvested cropland (FAO, 2001). Half of this area is irrigated with pumped water, and about 70% is in Asia.

The key attribute common to all new high-yielding varieties (HYV) is their higher harvest index, that is the redistribution of photosynthate from stalks and stems to harvested grain or roots. Straw:grain ratio of wheat or rice was commonly above 2:1 in traditional cultivars, whereas today's typical ratio is just 1:1 (Smil, 1999b). HYVs receiving adequate fertilization, irrigation, and protection against pests did responded with much increased yields. This combination of new agronomic practices, introduced during the 1960s, became widely known as the Green Revolution and the term is not a misnomer as the gains rose very rapidly after the introduction of these rewarding, but energy-intensive, measures. Higher reliance on intensively cultivated grain monocultures, narrowing of the genetic base in cropping and environmental impacts of agricultural chemicals have been the most discussed worrisome consequence of this innovation, but all of these concerns can be addressed by better agronomic practices (Smil, 2000).

Aggregate achievements of modern farming have been impressive. Between 1900 and 2000 the world's cultivated area expanded by about one-third, but the global crop

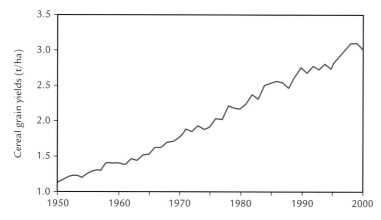

**Figure 3.3**   Post-1950 growth of average cereal grain yields epitomizing the rising productivity of modern farming (plotted from data in FAO, 2001).

harvest rose nearly sixfold. This was because of a more than fourfold increase of average crop yields made possible by a more than 80-fold increase of energy inputs to field farming (Smil, 2000). But even though the global mean harvest of all cereals more than doubled between 1950 and 2000 (Fig. 3.3), there are still large gaps between average yields and best (not record) harvests (FAO, 2001). Global corn harvest averages just over 4 t/ha but farmers in Iowa are bringing in close to 10 t/ha. Average wheat yield (spring and winter varieties) is 2.7 t/ha but even national averages in the UK, the Netherlands or Denmark Western are more than 8 t/ha today. Extensive diffusion of HYV of rice raised the global mean yield to almost 4 t/ha, whereas Japan or China's Jiangsu average in excess of 6 t/ha.

   Higher cereal and tuber yields freed more agricultural land for nonstaple species, above all for oil and sugar crops. Higher cereal yields have also allowed for more and more efficient animal feeding in rich countries where the abundance of meat and dairy products has made high-protein diets much more affordable. HYVs also raised the food output of many developing countries above subsistence minima. However, a substantial gap still divides the typical agricultural performances of rich and poor countries, and, given the far greater social inequalities in the latter group, this production disparity translates readily into continuing large-scale presence of malnutrition in scores of African, Asian, and Latin American countries.

# Current food production and supply

A word of caution first: only a minority of food production and consumption figures readily accessible in FAO databases and widely used in assessments of global food availability and needs is derived from the best available national statistics which may themselves contain many inaccuracies even when prepared by the most advanced statistical services of developed countries. Although some of the developing countries (notably China and India) have massive statistical bureaucracies and issue a great number of regular reports many of their numbers are known to be highly inaccurate.

For example, for many years Chinese official statistics listed less than 100 million hectares (Mha) as the total of the country's cultivated land (about 95 Mha until 2000) although many people in Beijing bureaucracy and some foreign experts knew that total was vastly undervalued. China now admits to having 130 Mha of cultivated land (National Bureau of Statistics, 2000) and the best remote sensing studies based on classified US information indicate 140, or even 150 Mha (Smil, 1999c). This change means, of course, that every official yield figure for the past 20 years is inaccurate. And, obviously, countries with protracted civil wars (several in Africa, Colombia) or with a disintegrating central government (Indonesia) are in no position to collect and publish any reliable agricultural statistics. Given these realities it is not surprising that most of the numbers for most of the developing nations that appear in FAO databases are just the best expert estimates made in the organization's Rome headquarters (FAO, 2001).

These realities mean that both exaggerations and underestimates are common and that often the resulting numbers may not be accurate reflections of the actual situation but are best used in order to derive fair approximations of the current state of agricultural affairs. It should also be noted that according to the FAO developed countries numbered 1.3 billion people in the year 2000, the developing ones 4.7 billion, a division slightly different from that used by the UN's population experts (UN, 2001). These realities should be kept in mind when considering the following brief review of current food output and availability.

## Global food production

Today's food producers fall mostly into four uneven categories. Several thousand large agribusiness companies, most of them in North America and Europe, control extensive areas of food and feed crops and highly concentrated meat production in giant feedlots. Their production goes directly to large-scale food processors or is destined for export. Several million highly mechanized family-owned farms in affluent countries rely on intensive practices to achieve high crop and animal productivities. Tens of millions of the most successful farmers in the most productive agricultural regions of many developing countries (e.g., China's Jiangsu and Guangdong or India's Punjab) use generally high levels of the best locally available inputs in order to produce food beyond their family's and region's need. And hundreds of millions of subsistence peasants, either landless or cultivating small amounts of often inferior land, use inadequate inputs, or no modern means of production at all, to grow barely enough food for their own families.

Cereal grains continue to dominate the global crop harvest. Their annual output is now just above 2 billion tonnes. Developing countries produce nearly 60% of all grain, with twice as much rice as wheat (about 570 vs. 270 Mt in 2000), but in per capita terms their output (about 260 kg/year) is only about 40% of the developed countries mean (660 kg/year). Most of the poor world's grain (more than 85%) is eaten directly, whereas most of the rich world's grain (more than 60% during the late 1990s) is fed to animals. Consequently, actual per capita supply of processed food cereals is still about 25% higher in developing countries (165 vs. 130 kg/year), reflecting simpler diets dominated by grain staples. Not surprisingly, rich countries enjoy even higher per capita disparities in production of nonstaple crops, with the differences being particularly large for sugar (30 vs. 15 kg/year) and meat (almost 80 vs. 25 kg).

Per capita consumption of legumes has been declining for several generations in every country where pulses previously played a critical nutritional role. Only India's annual per capita consumption of legumes remains above 10 kg/year (FAO, 2001). In contrast, no other crop diffusion in agricultural history has been as rapid and as economically far-reaching as the cultivation of soybeans for feed. US soybean plantings rose from a few thousand hectares in the early 1930s to more than 20 Mha since the early 1970s, and they now produce more than 50 Mt/year. Brazilian soybean production rose even faster, from a negligible total in the early 1960s to more than 20 Mt by the early 1990s. These two countries now produce two-thirds of the global soybean harvest, virtually all of it for animal feed.

Rising affluence combined with concerns about healthy diets has resulted in a steady growth of fruit production. Global fruit output has tripled since 1950, but this does not convey the unprecedented variety of fruits, including many tropical imports as well as winter shipments of subtropical and temperate species from the southern hemisphere, that are now available virtually year-round in all rich countries. The trend of rising fruit production recently has been most obvious in rapidly modernizing China where fruit harvests (now also increasingly for export) rose more than 10-fold (from less than 7 to more than 70 Mt) between 1980 and 2000 (National Bureau of Statistics, 2000).

With global annual output of nearly 500 Mt cow's milk is the most important animal food. Annual output of all kinds of milk amounts to about 570 Mt. Per capita availabilities of dairy products are large in North America and Western Europe (in excess of 250 kg/year) and negligible in traditionally nonmilking societies of East Asia. Pork, with about 80 Mt/year and rising, is by far the most important meat worldwide, with China and the US slaughtering the largest number of animals. Total meat output, including poultry, is now over 200 Mt a year, prorating to almost 80 kg/capita in rich countries and to about 25 kg/capita in the poor world. Poultry production (near 60 Mt/year) is now ahead of the combined beef and veal output and it will continue to rise. Consumption of hen eggs is now at more than 40 Mt a year, and recent rapid growth of aquaculture (its combined freshwater and marine output is now close to 30 Mt a year, equal to nearly a quarter of ocean catch) has put cultured fish, crustaceans, and mollusks ahead of mutton.

After a period of decline and stagnation the global marine catch began rising once more during the mid-1990s and is now close to 100 Mt/year but major increases are highly unlikely. A conservative assessment of the global marine potential concluded that by 1996 the world ocean was being fully fished, with about 60% of some 200 major marine fish resources being either overexploited or at the peak of their sustainable harvest (FAO, 1997). Consequently, if long-term marine catches were to be kept at around 100 Mt a year then 50 years from now the population growth would cut per capita fish supply by more than half compared to the late 1990s level. The importance of this harvest is due to its nutritional quality. During the late 1990s the world's average per capita supply of some 14 kg of marine species contained only a few percent of all available food energy, but it supplied about one-sixth of all animal protein. More importantly, aquatic species provide more than a third of animal protein to at least 200 million people, mostly in east and southeast Asia (FAO, 2001).

## Food supply

The world's recent edible crop harvests prorate to about 4700 kcal/day per capita, but nearly half of the cereal production, worth about 1700 kcal/day, is fed to animals, and postharvest crop losses amount to some 600 kcal/day (Smil, 2000). This leaves about 2400 kcal/day of plant food and with some 400 kcal/day from animal foods (including aquatic products) the average per capita availability adds up to roughly 2800 kcal/day, well above a generous estimate of average needs of 2200 kcal/capita. Similarly, the world's mean daily protein supply of 75 g/capita is well above the needed minimum. An egalitarian global civilization would thus have no problems with adequate nutrition. Equitable distribution of available food among the planet's more than 6 billion people would provide enough protein even if the global food harvests were to be some 10% lower than they are today.

In the real world these adequate global means hide, as do other global averages, large inter- and intranational differences. All Western nations enjoy uniformly high per capita food availabilities averaging about 3200 kcal/day. Their mean per capita supply of dietary protein is about 100 g/day, including about 55 g from animal foods. No elaborate calculations are needed to conclude that the average per capita food supply is more than adequate in all affluent countries. Because the actual requirements of mostly sedentary populations are no more than 2000–2200 kcal/day it is no exaggeration to label the resulting food surpluses (at least 1000–1200 kcal/day and up to 1600 kcal/day) as obscene.

After all, even when leaving aside the large energy and protein losses in animal feeding, at least 30% of all food available at the retail level in Western societies is wasted! Average Western diets in general, and the North American one in particular, also contain excessive amount of lipids, which now supply 30–40% of all food energy compared to the average of less than 20% in developing countries and to shares below 15% in the poorest societies (FAO, 2001). Surfeits of food energy and lipids are the two key nutritional factors implicated in the increase of obesity and diabetes and in a high frequency of cardiovascular disease (see Chapters 9–11). Fortification of many foodstuffs (from flour to juices) with vitamins and minerals and a fashionable use of dietary supplements (including recurrent megadose manias) by increasingly health-conscious segments of the aging population would suggest that there are very few micronutrient deficiencies. This is, unfortunately, not true as clinical and biochemical studies in the US show that intakes of calcium, iron, and zinc are not adequate in some groups (Pennington, 1996).

Given the obviously high incidence of overweight and obesity it is not surprising that hunger and malnutrition in affluent nations have received so little attention, but their extent is far from negligible (Riches, 1997). Poppendieck's (1997) estimates that 22–30 million Americans cannot afford to buy enough food to maintain good health have been questioned, but even the most conservative estimates acknowledge that 10–20 million poor Americans could not feed themselves adequately without assistance, and that far from all of them are actually receiving it. The coexistence of undernutrition and widespread obesity is thus one of the most peculiar features of America's current nutritional situation.

Japan, which is highly dependent on food imports, is the only high-income country with per capita food supply below 3000 kcal/day (the rate has been steady at about 2900 kcal/day for nearly two decades). Specific features of the country's food consumption include the already noted world's highest per capita intake of aquatic products, exceptionally high intakes of soybeans (eaten mostly as beancurd), and very low consumption of sugar. Average food availability in China is now almost as high as in Japan (close to 2800 kcal/day), but in spite of impressive post-1980 diversification (Fig. 3.4) its variety and quality is still much lower. Moreover, unlike in a highly egalitarian Japan, China's mean hides large differences between coastal and interior provinces.

India and Indonesia in the late 1990s were, respectively, at about 2400 and 2600 kcal/day. This would have provided adequate nutrition for everybody only if the two countries had a perfectly egalitarian access to food; in reality, highly skewed income distribution makes India the country with the largest number of undernourished people (FAO, 2000). Many sub-Saharan African countries average less than 2200 kcal/day, some even less than 2000 kcal/day, and these obviously inadequate food supplies are reflected in the world's shortest life expectancies at birth. Even when adequate in terms of total energy and protein, typical diets in most developing countries are monotonous. And, unlike in affluent nations where nearly all traces of seasonal food supply have been erased by international trade, diets in many poor countries still strongly reflect the seasonality of plant harvests or fish catches.

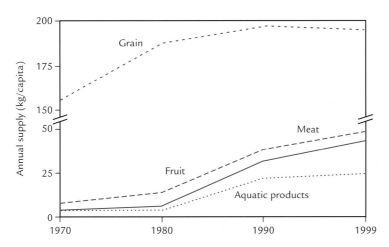

**Figure 3.4**   Dramatic changes in China's average per capita food supply brought by Deng Xiaoping's post-1980 economic reforms exemplify a rapid dietary transition in a modernizing country. Based on data from State Statistical Bureau (1980–2000); these figures exaggerate actual meat consumption (see the text for details).

## Malnutrition in the developing world

Food deficits, regardless of whether they are on national, local or individual level, or if they range from marginal to crippling, are rarely caused by absolute physical shortages. Such cases arise repeatedly only as a result of protracted civil wars (recently in Afghanistan, Angola, Ethiopia, Mozambique, Somalia, and Sudan) and temporarily as an aftermath of major natural catastrophes. Chronic undernutrition and malnutrition result from inadequate individual or group access to food that is strongly related to social status and income. This conclusion is true for both the richest as well as the poorest countries.

FAO's past estimates of the global share of undernourished people ranged from a clearly exaggerated fraction of two-thirds in the late 1940s (an overestimate caused largely by unrealistically high assumptions regarding average protein needs) to less than one-seventh in the early 1990s. The latest estimate, for the period between 1996 and 1998, adds up to 826 million undernourished people, or about 14% of the world's population at that time (FAO, 2000). As expected, the total is highly unevenly split, with 34 million undernourished people in the developed and 792 million people in the developing world. The highest shares of undernourished population (about 70% of the total) are now in Afghanistan and Somalia, whereas the rates for India and China are, respectively, about 20% and just above 10%. These shares make India the country with the largest number of undernourished people (just over 200 million, or roughly a quarter of the world's total, spread pretty much all around the country), whereas China's aggregate (mostly in the northwestern and southwestern interior provinces) is about 140 million.

There are, of course, different degrees of undernutrition, ranging from mildly underweight (with body mass index of 17–18.5) to severely underweight (with body mass index below 16; the normal healthy range is 18.5–25). The FAO (1996) also put the number of stunted children (with low height-for-age) at 215 million, underweight children (low weight-for-age) at 180 million, and wasted children (low weight-for-height) at 50 million. As there are many uncertainties regarding both the data and assumptions that go into the process of comparing food supplies and needs, all of these figures must be seen as informative estimates rather than as accurate totals. Nevertheless, there can be no doubt about the enormous human and socioeconomic toll of this nutritional deprivation. Perhaps the worst health impact arises from the well-documented effect of undernutrition on early brain development (Brown and Pollitt, 1996).

Shortages of food energy and dietary protein are not the only causes of serious malnutrition as micronutrient deficiencies are even more common. Blindness caused by shortages of vitamin A is among the most cruel consequences of inadequate diets. The xerophthalmia syndrome includes night reversible blindness caused by lack of retinol in the eye's retina, corneal ulceration and eventually irreversible loss of eyesight. In addition, low levels of vitamin are associated with higher mortality from respiratory and gastrointestinal diseases, and with their more severe course. FAO estimates that the total population at risk is well over half a billion, that there are about 40 million preschool children with vitamin A deficiency, and that perhaps half a million of them go blind annually (FAO, 1996).

Some micronutrient deficiencies have environmental origins. The World Health Organization estimated that 1.6 billion people, or more than a quarter of the world's population, have some degree of iodine deficiency (WHO, 1993). Estimates of the total number of people with goiter, the condition almost always associated with some mental impairment, are as high as 600 million (Lamberg, 1993). WHO also credits iodine deficiencies during pregnancy with at least 25 million seriously brain-damaged children and nearly six millions cretins, whose severe mental retardation is combined with hearing loss or mutism and abnormal body movements. As for the economic impact, Arcand (2000) concluded that if the sub-Saharan countries with average dietary supply below the minimum requirement in 1960 had eliminated hunger by raising the average per capita food availability to nearly 2800 kcal/day (i.e., essentially China's current mean) their per capita GDP in 1990 could have been as much as $3500 rather than the actual $800.

# Future food needs

Three key factors will drive future demand for food. By far the most important is the continuing population growth throughout the developing world. Second, is the all too obvious need to close the gap between today's inadequate food intakes that have to be endured by some 800 million people throughout the poor world and the minima compatible with healthy and productive lives. The third factor is the further improvement of the quality of diets in poor countries (given the great existing food surplus, getting rid of nutritional inadequacies throughout the rich world should not call for any increases in production). At least three principal factors will determine the eventual outcome: the level of agricultural investment and research; the extent and tempo of dietary transitions, particularly the higher consumption of animal food in today's developing countries; the success in making future food production more compatible with biospheric limits and services; and the fate of genetic engineering.

## Population growth

After decades of accelerating growth the global rate of population increase peaked at just over 2% a year during the late 1960s, and gradual declines of fertilities also speeded up the arrival of the absolute peak, at about 86 million people a year, during the latter half of the 1980s and the annual increase was down to 77 million people by the year 2000 (UN, 1998, 2001). As a result population projections issued during the 1990s had repeatedly lowered the long-term global forecasts for the next 50 years. The medium version of the 1998 revision envisaged just 8.9 billion people by the year 2050, down from 9.4 billion forecast in 1996, and 9.8 billion in the 1994 revisions (UN, 1998). And the high variant in 1998 was well below 12 billion people by the year 2050, in line with increasing indications that yet another doubling of human population to 12 billion people is unlikely (Lutz et al., 2001).

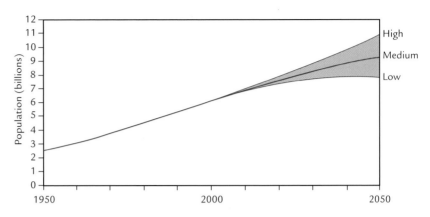

**Figure 3.5**   The UN's latest long-term projections of global population growth (UN, 2001).

But the latest UN (2001) projection raised its medium 2050 forecast to 9.3 billion (Fig. 3.5). The difference of some 400 million people above the 1998 forecast is explained largely by the assumption of somewhat higher fertilities for the 16 developing countries whose fertility has not, so far, shown any sustained decline. There is a different kind of uncertainty concerning the rich world's population. Without substantial immigration it would start declining as a whole within a few years and by the year 2050 it would be barely above one billion, 20% below its current total (as already noted, UNO's and FAO's definitions of developed and developing populations are not identical: they differ by about 100 million people). With continued immigration it would be more or less stable, reaching 1.8 billion in 50 years. Even then many European nations and Japan would experience substantial population declines. Russia's case is particularly noteworthy, as it now appears that there is little chance of reversing its population decline brought on by economic deprivation, social disintegration and exceptionally high rates of alcoholism. As a result, Russia may have 30 million fewer people by the year 2050. By that time the US population will, most likely, approach 340 million.

Inherent uncertainties of long-range forecasting aside, there is no doubt that virtually all the net population increase of the next two generations will take place in today's developing world, and that the global population of 2050 will, most likely, be 50% larger than it is today. Moreover, most of the additional population growth of some 2.8–3.2 billion people will be concentrated in nations whose agricultural resources, although absolutely large, are already relatively limited. Brazil is the only modernizing populous country (i.e., with more than 100 million people) with abundant reserves of arable land and water (Fig. 3.6). Fifty years from now India, after adding nearly 600 million people, would have a population more than 50% larger than today and would be, with just over 1.5 billion, the world's most populous country, with China a very close second. Three African and two Asian countries would add more than 100 million people each: Nigeria, Pakistan, Indonesia, Congo, and Ethiopia. As a group these nations would have to increase their food harvests by two-thirds merely to maintain their existing, and in many respects inadequate, diets.

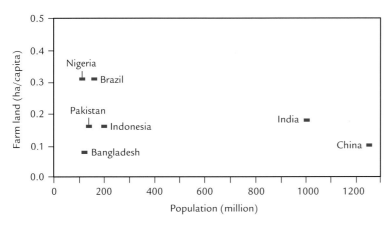

**Figure 3.6** Brazil and Nigeria are the only two developing countries with considerable reserves of potentially arable land; in all other populous modernizing countries future increases of food output will have to come from further intensification of cropping. Plotted from data in FAO (2001).

Only Congo and Nigeria have relatively low population density per hectare of cultivated farmland and large untapped agricultural potential. At the same time, the late 20th-century record of these two countries makes it hard to imagine that they will be the ones to mobilize their resources effectively and to evolve a civil society determined to bring widespread economic advances. China and Indonesia are already the paragons of highly intensive cropping, and India and Pakistan are close behind. But, some poorly informed and sensationalized judgments notwithstanding (Brown, 1995), there is more hope for China's farming than is the case with perhaps any other large populous country (Smil, 1995). As already noted, China has about 50% more farmland than has been officially acknowledged (which means that its actual average yields are substantially lower than reported) and it has many opportunities for increasing the productivity of its cropping (Smil, 1999c). India's situation, though undoubtedly highly challenging, appears to be more hopeful than the Indonesian or Pakistani prospect. As for Ethiopia, natural aridity affects large parts of its territory and already limits its food production capacity.

## Improved food intakes

This is a very broad category of concerns as it embraces both overall quantitative gains and specific qualitative changes; and most of the eventual demand due to these needs is also very difficult to quantify because its future levels will be determined by complex interplays of economic, political, social, and environmental factors. Nevertheless, several general conclusions are fairly solid. In those poor countries that have been peaceful and whose agriculture has not been neglected, the elimination of the worst nutritional deficiencies is not primarily a matter of higher output but rather of improved access to food for the poorest groups, and hence a matter amenable to further political and economic interventions. Countries living with years, or even decades, of conflict have no realistic hope for better nutrition without peace. Unfortunately, if the past two generations are any guide for the future then the experience of sub-Saharan Africa, nutritionally the world's worst afflicted region, offers little hope. A massive epidemic of autoimmune deficiency syndrome (AIDS) makes African recovery even more unlikely.

Most of the future demand for improved food supply that has a high likelihood of being met by increasing domestic production rather than by food aid will thus come as larger populations will be earning higher incomes in Asian and Latin American countries. Judging by the experience of every country that has undergone economic modernization, perhaps the most obvious feature of this qualitative change will be the higher demand for animal foods. This appears to be a truly universal trend as only a very small proportion of humanity voluntarily chooses strictly vegetarian diets and there is also a strong evolutionary argument in favor of omnivory.

Well-documented studies have shown that the closest primate relatives of our species – the two chimpanzee species *Pan troglodytes* and *Pan paniscus* – regularly hunt colobus monkeys and eat other small vertebrates (Stanford, 1998). Moreover, Aiello and Wheeler (1995) argue that the only way humans could accommodate larger brains without raising their average metabolic rate was by reducing the size of another metabolically expensive organ, and that, unlike liver, heart and kidneys, the gastrointestinal tract was the only such tissue whose size could be reduced by including more digestible animal foods in the regular human diet. Plant-dominated diet supplemented by meat is thus our evolutionary heritage and strict herbivory is a cultural adaptation.

Archaeological and anthropological evidence for human omnivory is undeniable and a relatively recent domestication of milking animals extended the human consumption of animal foods to include milk and dairy products from at least half a dozen mammalian species. When prorated per unit of body mass, chimpanzee meat intakes are equivalent to eating about 6–17 kg a year and this range clearly overlaps the typical per capita meat consumption of preindustrial societies. Rates near the lower end of the range (5–10 kg/capita) were common in those peasant societies where meat was eaten infrequently and consumed in larger amount only during some festive occasions; most of the pre-1980 rural China was a perfect example of this pattern of eating.

## Increased demand for animal foods

As described in the previous section, affluence changed this consumption pattern but intakes of animal foods are badly skewed in favor of high-income populations. Industrialized nations, amounting to only a fifth of the global population total, now produce a third of hen's eggs, two-fifths of all meat, and three-fifths of all poultry and cow's milk. Animal foods now supply around 30% of all food energy in North America and Europe, around 20% in those East Asian countries that have reached apparent satiation levels (Japan, Taiwan) and far below 10% in the most food-deficient countries of sub-Saharan Africa (FAO, 2001). This means, as already noted, that the daily food supply of rich nations now averages about 55 g of meat and milk protein per capita, compared to just 20 g in the developing world, and the actual gap is even larger for hundreds of millions of subsistence peasants and poor urbanites surviving on diets virtually devoid of any animal foods.

With meat and dairy intakes being up to an order of magnitude higher in affluent nations than in many poor countries this means that extending the current per capita supply means of developed countries (i.e., above 250 kg for milk and close to 80 kg for meat) to all of today's low income countries (i.e., to 4.7 billion people), as well as to the additional three to four billion people that will be added in those countries during the next two generations, would call for an impossibly large expansion of feed production. The three important questions are then as follows. Should such a goal be seen as being at least theoretically desirable? What are the chances that developing countries would move as rapidly, and as far, toward the affluent (Western) consumption pattern as their limited resources will allow? And to what extent can we improve the prevailing feeding efficiencies?

Only the first question has an easy answer. There is no need to present a massive survey of current nutritional understanding or to engage in polemics on behalf of, or against, vegetarianism, a nutritional choice that most people will not consider following voluntarily in any case, or high-level carnivory. What is abundantly clear is that humans do not need high levels of animal food intakes either to lead healthy and productive lives or to achieve average population longevities in excess of 70 years, and that no other known existential benefits are predicated on consuming at least as much meat and dairy products as the developed countries do today. Moreover, as recent experiences with some consequences of animal feeding and rearing have demonstrated (European mad cow disease and foot-and-mouth epizootic leading to large-scale slaughter of cattle and sheep, and Asian bird viruses resulting in mass killings of poultry) the scale and the very nature of meat-producing enterprises may actually be a threat to human health, or at least a costly inconvenience. In contrast to these fairly indisputable conclusions the pace and the extent of dietary transition is much harder to predict.

## Dietary patterns

No other factor will determine the future demand for animal foods as much as the degree of westernization of diets in developing countries in general, and in populous Asian nations in particular. Informed discussion of this prospect must start by acknowledging the fact that, in spite of broad similarities, there are substantial differences in meat and fat intakes among Western countries. This means that there is no generic Western diet to which the developing countries might aspire. Although all major indicators of quality of life are very similar for all of the affluent nations of Western Europe, per capita supplies of meat differ by about 40%: Norwegians get less than 60 kg/year, French almost 100 kg/year (FAO, 2001). And whereas Greeks consume less than 5 kg of butter and lard a year per capita, the Finnish mean is close to 15 kg. Such comparisons make it clear that the European pattern, although very similar in total energy and protein intakes, spans a range of distinct categories from the Mediterranean to the Scandinavian diets.

Taking such differences into account, Seckler and Rock (1995) suggested that two different patterns of food consumption should be considered when forecasting the future composition of food intakes in developing countries. They define what they call the Western model as the daily mean supply of more than 3200 kcal/capita with more than 30% of food energy coming from animal foodstuffs. But a great deal of evidence confirms that another model – what they label the Asian–Mediterranean pattern, with overall food energy availability below 3200 kcal/capita and with animal products supplying less than 25% of food energy – appears to be a more powerful attractor for many developing countries.

Food balance sheets of the last two generations show that animal food intakes in the economically most successful developing countries have not been moving rapidly toward the Western consumption pattern. Egypt and Turkey have basically the same proportion of meat in their typical diets as they had 30 years ago. Japanese meat intakes have stabilized at around 40 kg, as did the Malaysian average. Official output statistics would appear to put China into a different category and forecasts based on these numbers see China as a gargantuan meat-eating nation, but a closer look shows that the country will not move rapidly toward the Western attractor. China's official output statistics, and hence also FAO food balance sheets based on them, credit the country with per capita output of about 47 kg meat in 1999, but the *China Statistical Yearbook* puts actual per capita purchases of urban households at 25 kg (unchanged in a decade!) and the meat consumption of rural families at less than 17 kg, up from about 13 kg in 1990 (National Bureau of Statistics, 2000). This means that the eventual doubling of average nationwide per capita meat consumption would result in a rate only marginally higher than the current value claimed by official statistics.

Forecasts of China's future meat consumption have also been affected by simplistically extrapolating Taiwan's experience. The island's very high average per capita meat intake (about 80 kg) is not only the highest in Asia, it is even higher than the British mean, and its very low direct cereal consumption (less than 110 kg) is below the OECD's mean of some 130 kg (FAO, 2001). Moreover, differences of scale between the two countries (1.2 billion vs. some 20 million of people) and the still very limited purchasing power of most of China's peasants are two other factors militating against a further rapid rise of China's per capita meat consumption.

Finally, it must be noted that the total consumption of meat, although still slowly rising in the US, has been declining in Europe (for example, in Germany it is down by 15% since 1980), which means that the Western pattern is actually shifting gradually toward the alternative attractor. Consequently, there is a fairly high probability that tomorrow's developing world, although definitely demanding higher animal food intakes, will not look toward yesterday's French, Dutch, or US example. Widespread assumptions that rising disposable incomes will be readily translated into rapidly, and virtually universally, rising demand for meat may not come to pass. Whatever its actual level may be, lower than anticipated demand for animal foods would be much easier to meet, especially once a concerted commitment is made to improve the efficiency of feeding as much as practicable. But whatever the pace and the extent of coming dietary changes may be, the increasing carnivory could have a much lower demand on agricultural resources and could also result in much reduced environmental impacts if we were to feed the animals much more efficiently.

## Feeding efficiencies

Better management of grasslands, and some of their inevitable, but undesirable, expansion in Latin America, Africa, and Asia (as nearly all new grazing land will be created through deforestation) will supply only a small fraction of future increases in meat and milk production and more than 90% of additional output of animal foods will have to come from growing more concentrate feeds, above all corn and soybeans, in direct competition with food crops. This trend has been one of the most obvious features of the 20th-century cropping. In 1900 just over 10% of the global grain harvest was consumed by animals; by 1950 the share surpassed 20% and now it is approaching 50%, with national shares ranging from nearly 70% in the USA to less than 5% in India.

But future feeding requirements are not irrevocably determined by a given demand for animal protein. As these proteins are all of the highest quality they are mutually substitutable and long-term dietary shifts can reduce the relative, or even absolute, consumption of one kind of animal food while greatly increasing the demand for another. For example, in 1950 chicken made up less than 10% of average US per capita meat consumption, but in 2000 its share was about one-third (USDA, 1950–2001). Consequently, a future combination of animal foodstuffs that is inherently more efficient to produce can lead to substantial feed savings in comparison to the prevailing consumption pattern.

Milk is by far the most efficient animal food. Highly productive animals need just 1–1.1 kg of concentrate feed per kg of milk. They convert more than 30% of the total metabolizable feed energy, and 30–40% of feed protein to milk protein. Eggs come second (current best practices need less than 3 kg of feed per kg of eggs), and chicken third. Large-scale broiler production requires fewer than 5 units of concentrate feed per unit of edible tissue and feed proteins are converted into meat proteins with efficiency averaging 20%, twice as high as in pigs. Pigs grown for their lean meat can turn more than 20% of metabolizable energy into edible tissues and they need about 7.5 units of concentrate per kg of meat; pigs are also the most efficient convertors of feed energy into edible lipids which give meat its satisfying palatability.

Conversion efficiencies for beef clearly indicate the extravagant cost of that meat; feedlot-fed animals need at least 20 kg of corn and soybeans for each kg of meat, and only 5% of all fed protein is converted into protein in beef. Obviously, only those animals that do not require any concentrates, i.e., raised completely by grazing, or consuming crop-processing residues such as brans and oilseed cakes, that is digesting biomass that cannot be used by nonruminant species, can be seen as efficient users of agricultural resources. Consequently, it is difficult to imagine a less-desirable change of dietary habits than the global expansion of hamburger empires.

Aquacultured herbivorous fishes are better convertors of feed than pork or chicken. Conversion ratios (kg of feed per kg of live weight) for semi-intensively bred carp in warm waters are 1.4–1.8, and for catfish 1.4–1.6. As a smaller share of fish total mass is wasted in comparison with mammalian or bird carcasses, herbivorous fish need fewer than 2.5 kg of concentrate feed per unit of edible weight, and their protein conversion efficiency is as good as chicken (Smil, 2000). Salmon are even better protein convertors, but these carnivores need fish oils and proteins and their feeding actually results in a net protein loss. Use of concentrate feed in aquaculture of herbivorous species is thus an excellent way of increasing global availability of animal protein and the FAO believes that this rapidly growing enterprise has excellent prospects.

# Investing in agriculture

For most people the idea of investing in agriculture conjures the images of extending credit to farmers or building new irrigation schemes but the most important investments needed to assure high agricultural productivity are in maintaining viable agroecosystems. Although modern agriculture has eliminated many environmental limits and insulated itself from many environmental interferences through fertilization, irrigation, use of pesticides and breeding of better cultivars, crop production remains embedded within the dynamic complexities of the living biosphere and depends critically on reliable provision of many natural services and on the maintenance of essential ecosystem structures. These necessities range from having sufficiently friable soils containing large amounts of organic matter and protected against excessive erosion to promoting practices that will minimize nutrient losses from fertilizer applications and increase water use efficiencies in irrigation as much as practicable.

Achieving these goals is a matter of complex management that can be effective only when we use the best understanding of how agroecosystems operate. For example, the first necessity (maintaining desirable soil structure) requires the use of appropriate tillage methods (including minimum tillage practices), recycling of crop residues and animal wastes, regular crop rotations, and where possible also planting of leguminous cover crops (Agassi, 1995). Without these measures soil bacteria and invertebrates could not thrive, high organic matter content able to maintain soil structure would decline, soil would not be able to hold moisture and would be prone to erosion losses that would eventually lower its productivity. Similarly, reducing nutrient losses requires measures ranging from repeated soil and plant testing and split applications of fertilizers to selecting appropriate cultivars and regular planting of cover crops (Smil, 2001). These practices require a great deal of understanding and ongoing personal commitment by individual farmers but most of them now rest on fairly well-understood principles.

In contrast, new methods of more productive farming will require further intensification of agricultural research and technical innovation. Not surprisingly, many observers of the current agricultural situation argue for substantially increased public support of basic and applied agricultural research (Pinstrup-Andersen, 2001), and there is no shortage of studies to show the efficacy of this approach. For example, Huang and Rozelle (1996) showed that innovation accounted for almost all of the growth in agricultural productivity in China during the latter half of the 1980s and in the early 1990s. Avery (1997) stressed that only further intensification of crop production can save the remaining tropical rainforests, and hence most of the world's existing biodiversity, from eventual destruction. Virtually every assessment of future agricultural needs prepared by the FAO or by specialized crop research centers (International Maize and Wheat Improvement Center, International Rice Research Institute) notes that returns to public investments in agricultural research and extension are very high and urges that future funding should be increased. In spite of this well-proven reality research funding remains inadequate throughout the developing world.

Given this state of affairs it is even more worrisome that the developing world may not be able to take full benefit of one of the most important scientific advances of the past generation, our increasingly effective ability to confer desirable traits on plants and animals by means of genetic engineering. Of course, an argument could be made that the rich countries, with their obscene surplus of food, have really no need to use arcane techniques in order to further boost their crop and animal production. But a common view that genetic engineering is a tool of multinational companies geared toward the rich world's markets and that developing countries have no chance to benefit from biotechnology is wrong. As Wambugu (2001) argues, small-scale farmers have profited by using hybrid seeds and transgenic seeds simply add more value to these hybrids.

This is a very important point that needs constant stressing to scientifically illiterate critics. All but a few of our currently planted crops are products of extensive breeding modifications and today's world could not feed itself without using these hybrid and high-yielding cultivars. Traditional breeding has made a fundamental difference to the agricultural productivity of the 20th century; current harvests would be impossible without hybrid corn (introduced in the 1930s), HYV of rice and wheat (first released during the 1960s) and hybrid rice (developed in China during the 1970s). Hybrid corn, the planting of which began slowly in Iowa in the early 1930s, has transformed US corn harvests since World War II and is now benefiting both small- and large-scale corn producers throughout the developing world. Hybrid rice, which can boost average yields by 15–20%, has been finally adapted to tropical climates and is now being accepted throughout Asia (Virmani *et al.*, 1996).

Genetic engineering is thus only the latest, and the most powerful, tool of agricultural innovation. Admittedly, it is also a tool with considerable potential for adverse effects and unwanted complications but this reality should not be the reason for banning the effort and walking away from the prospect of immense future benefits. After all, this combination of risks and benefits is nothing unique to genetic engineering. Modern society constantly confronts such dilemmas and has found ways to deal with them. Perhaps the most apposite example is that of drug companies and the billions of users of prescription medicines who must weigh the benefits against a range of potentially even fatal side effects. Careful research and testing and responsible regulation are the answers, not a ban on the drugs. Genetic engineering alone will not solve food shortages that are now experienced by hundreds of millions of people but it could become the most powerful tool in that quest.

I will note just a few of the recent bioengineering advances whose potential for producing larger and better harvests or more desirable animals is self-evident.

Broader-leafed rice can deprive weeds of sunlight, thus reducing the need for applying herbicides or for laborious weeding. Rice with higher vitamin A and iron content can be the most cost-effective, as well as the most practical, way to end two of the most persistent micronutrient deficiencies in rice-eating countries. Millions of poor tropical families cultivating sweet potatoes in their fields and kitchen gardens would benefit from a transgenic cultivar resistant to feathery mottle virus which can reduce the yields by up to 80% (Wambugu, 2001). And, to give perhaps the most impressive example from animal farming, transgenic pigs able to produce phytase (the enzyme needed to digest phytate phosphorus in their feed) in their saliva will void manure with phosphorus content reduced by up to 75% (Goloran *et al.*, 2001). This impressive achievement will reduce one of the principal causes of aquatic eutrophication, algal growth and fish kills in affected waters.

Seeing genetic engineering as the solution to the world's food problems would be naïve. Refusing to proceed with careful research and regulated applications might be one of the most shortsighted human choices ever made as the technique has potential not only for increased and improved food production but also for enhanced environmental protection. Well-conceived bioengineering research, together with the stress on environmentally sound farming and higher efficiency in the use of all farm inputs, should be one of the key ingredients with which to build greater food security for tomorrow's developing world.

# References

Agassi, M. (ed.) (1995). "Soil Erosion, Conservation and Rehabilitation". Marcel Dekker, New York.

Aiello, L.C., and Wheeler, P. (1995). The expensive-tissue hypothesis. *Curr. Anthropol.* **36**, 199–221.

Alroy, J. (2001). A multispecies overkill simulation of the end-Pleistocene megafauna. *Science* **292**, 1893–1896.

Arcand, J.L. (2000). "Malnutrition and Growth: The Efficiency Cost of Hunger". FAO, Rome.

Avery, D.T. (1997). "Agricultural Research: The Most Vital Investment for People and the Environment". Senate Agriculture Committee's Hearing on Agricultural Research. US Senate, Washington DC.

Blumenschine, R.J., and Cavallo, J.A. (1992). Scavenging and human evolution. *Sci. Am.* **267**(4), 90–95.

Brown, L. (1995). "Who Will Feed China?" W.W. Norton, New York.

Brown, J.L., and Pollitt, E. (1996). Malnutrition, poverty and intellectual development. *Sci. Am.* **274**(2), 38–43.

Buck, J.L. (1937). "Land Utilization in China". Nanking University, Nanking.

Childe, V.G. (1951). "Man Makes Himself". C.A. Watts, London.

Davis, M. (2001). "Late Victorian Holocausts, El Niño Famines and the Making of the Third World". Verso, London.

Eaton, S.B., and Konner, M.J. (1997). Paleolithic nutrition revisited: a twelve-year retrospective on its nature and implications. *Eur. J. Clin. Nutr.* **51**, 207–216.

FAO (1996). "The Sixth World Food Survey". FAO, Rome.

FAO (1997). "The State of World Fisheries and Aquaculture". FAO, Rome.

FAO (2000). "The State of Food Insecurity in the World 2000". FAO, Rome. http://www.fao.org/DOCREP/X8200/X8200E00.HTM

FAO (2001). "FAOSTAT Database". FAO, Rome. http://apps.fao.org

Goloran, S.P., *et al.* (2001). Pigs expressing salivary phytase produce low-phosphorus manure. *Nature Biotechnol.* **19**, 741–745.

Goudsblom, J. (1992). "Fire and Civilization". Allen Lane, London.

Headland, T.N., and Reid, L.A. (1989). Hunter–gatherers and their neighbors from prehistory to the present. *Curr. Anthropol.* **30**, 43–66.

Huang, J., and Rozelle, S. (1996). Technological change: rediscovering the engine of productivity growth in China's agricultural economy. *J. Dev. Econ.* **49**, 337–369.

International Fertilizer Industry Association (2001). "World Fertilizer Consumption". IFA, Paris. http://www.fertilizer.org/ifa/statistics/

Lamberg, B.A. (1993). Iodine deficiency disorders and endemic goitre. *Eur. J. Clin. Nutr.* **47**, 1–8.

Lutz, W., Sanderson, W., and Scherbor, S. (2001). The end of world population growth. *Nature* **412**, 543–545.

Molenaar, A. (1956). "Water Lifting Devices". FAO, Rome.

National Bureau of Statistics (2000). "China Statistical Yearbook". China Statistics Press, Beijing.

Pennington, J.A.T. (1996). Intakes of minerals from diets and foods: is there a need for concern? *J. Nutr.* **126**, 2304S–2308S.

Pinstrup-Andersen, P. (2001). Feeding the world in the new millennium. *Environment* **43**, 22–30.

Poppendieck, J. (1997). The USA: hunger in the land of plenty. *In* "First World Hunger" (G. Riches, ed.), pp. 134–164. St Martin Press, New York.

Price, T.D. (1991). The Mesolithic of Northern Europe. *Annu. Rev. Anthropol.* **20**, 211–233.

Riches, G. (ed.) (1997). "First World Hunger". St Martin Press, New York.

Sahlins, M. (1972). "Stone Age Economics". Aldine, Chicago.

Seckler, D., and Rock, M. (1995). "World Population Growth and Food Demand to 2050". Winrock International Institute for Agricultural Development, Morrilton, AK.

Smil, V. (1994). "Energy in World History". Westview, Boulder, CO.

Smil, V. (1995). Who will feed China? *China Quarterly* **143**, 801–813.

Smil, V. (1999a). China's great famine: 40 years later. *BMJ* **319**, 1619–1621.

Smil, V. (1999b). Crop residues: agriculture's largest harvest. *BioScience* **49**, 299–308.

Smil, V. (1999c). China's agricultural land. *China Quarterly* **158**, 414–429.

Smil, V. (2000). "Feeding the World: Challenge for the 21st Century". MIT Press, Cambridge, MA.

Smil, V. (2001). "Enriching the Earth: Fritz Haber, Carl Bosch and the Transformation of World Agriculture". MIT Press, Cambridge, MA.

Stanford, C.B. (1998). "Chimpanzee and Red Colobus". Harvard University Press, Cambridge, MA.

United Nations (1998). "World Population Prospects: The 1998 Revision". UN, New York.

United Nations (2001). "World Population Prospects: The 2000 Revision". UN, New York. http://www.un.org/esa/population/wpp2000.htm

US Bureau of the Census (1975). "Historical Statistics of the United States: Colonial Times to 1970", pp. 510–512. USGPO, Washington, DC.

US Department of Agriculture (USDA) (1950–2001). "Agricultural Yearbook". USDA, Washington, DC. http://www.usda.gov/nass/pubs/agstats.htm

Virmani, S.S., Siddiq, E.A., and Muralidharan, K. (eds.) (1996). "Advances in Hybrid Rice Technology". IRRI, Los Banos.

Wambugu, F. (2001). Why Africa needs agricultural biotech. *Nature* **400**, 15–16.

Whiten, A., and Widdowson, E.M. (eds.) (1992). "Foraging Strategies and Natural Diet of Monkeys, Apes and Humans". Clarendon Press, Oxford.

WHO (1993). "Global Prevalence of Iodine Deficiency Disorders". WHO, Geneva.

# Can the challenges of poverty, sustainable consumption and good health governance be addressed in an era of globalization?

4

*Tim Lang*

The nutrition transition has taken different characteristics in various developing countries, cultures, and historical eras. Huge policy challenges arise. Is the nutrition transition inevitable? Can its patterns be altered? What policies minimize its adverse health outcomes most effectively? This chapter, while perhaps adding further complexity to an already difficult issue, outlines four policy elements that ought to inform and be part of the debate about the nutrition transition.

The first element relates to the interaction between food and nutrition and the environment – the issue of sustainable consumption. The second is social inequality – the extent of poverty and food insecurity. The third is governance, the notion that, if human policy "frames" nutrition, then human forces should themselves be shaped to do this equitably, responsibly, and effectively. The English word "governance" refers not just to what governments do, but also to the actions of other powerful social forces, such as private business.

The last element is culture, a key and often a missing component in the nutrition transition debate. Food culture is the "pull" in the transformation of tastes, just as marketing and corporate reach are the "push".

The Nutrition Transition
ISBN: 0-12-153654-8

# Globalization and the nutrition transition

A distinction must be made between the nutrition transition and the wider socioeconomic process of globalization, which refers to the process by which goods, people, and ideas spread throughout the world. The subject has been the source of much excitement in sociological and political circles recently, to which the topic of food can add a suitably gentle corrective. Globalization of food is, of course, nothing new. Plants have moved and been moved around the globe for centuries. Today, many are grown

**Table 4.1** Top economic countries and corporations, 2001 (from Davidson, 2001)

| The richest player ranking | Ranking by country or corporation[a] | Country or corporation | Food role[b] | GDP or revenue 1999 (millions of US$) |
|---|---|---|---|---|
| 1 | 1 | United States | | 9 152 098 |
| 2 | 2 | Japan | | 4 346 922 |
| 3 | 3 | Germany | | 2 111 940 |
| 4 | 4 | United Kingdom | | 1 441 787 |
| 5 | 5 | France | | 1 432 323 |
| 6 | 6 | Italy | | 1 170 971 |
| 7 | 7 | China | | 989 465 |
| 8 | 8 | Brazil | | 751 505 |
| 9 | 9 | Canada | | 634 898 |
| 10 | 10 | Spain | | 595 927 |
| 23 | **1** | **General Motors** | | **176 558** |
| 25 | **2** | **Wal-Mart Stores** | Retailer | **166 809** |
| 26 | **3** | **Exxon Mobil** | | **163 881** |
| 27 | **4** | **Ford Motor** | | **162 558** |
| 28 | **5** | **Daimler-Chrysler** | | **159 986** |
| 32 | 27 | Indonesia | | 142 511 |
| 33 | 28 | Saudi Arabia | | 139 383 |
| 34 | 29 | South Africa | | 131 127 |
| 38 | **6** | **Mitsui** | | **118 555** |
| 39 | **7** | **Mitsubishi** | | **117 766** |
| 40 | **8** | **Toyota Motor** | | **115 671** |
| 41 | 33 | Portugal | | 113 716 |
| 42 | **9** | **General Electric** | | **111 630** |
| 44 | **10** | **Itochu** | | **109 069** |
| 45 | **11** | **Royal Dutch/Shell Group** | Retailer | **105 366** |
| 46 | 35 | Venezuela, RB | | 102 222 |
| 47 | 36 | Israel | | 100 840 |
| 48 | **12** | **Sumitomo** | | **95 701** |
| 57 | **17** | **BP Amoco** | Retailer | **83 566** |
| 72 | **29** | **Philip Morris** | Processor and tobacco | **61 751** |
| 75 | 44 | Pakistan | | 58 154 |
| 88 | **41** | **Nestlé** | Processor | **49 694** |
| 97 | **46** | **Metro** | Retailer | **46 664** |
| 99 | 52 | Bangladesh | | 45 961 |
| 100 | **48** | **Tokyo Electric Power** | | **45 728** |

[a] Countries are indicated in normal type; company rankings are shown in bold.
[b] All countries produce food; only those corporations with direct food interests are noted in this column.

far from their site of original cultivation. The same has happened to animals: cows, poultry, pigs, sheep, and goats. What is new about current globalization is its pace, scale, and extent, primarily fueled by government and private market forces.

Table 4.1 combines World Bank figures of national Gross Domestic Product (GDP) (World Bank, 2001) with estimates of corporate turnover from the Fortune 500 (Fortune, 2001). Produced by CAFOD, an international aid agency (Davidson, 2001), it seeks to measure relative economic "punch". Of the richest 100, 48 are companies and 52 are countries. When ordered, one notes that Wal-Mart (26th), a retailer, had revenues greater than the GDP of Indonesia (32nd), Saudi Arabia (33rd) or South Africa (34th). Phillip Morris (72nd), a tobacco company which in 1998 was also the world's largest food company, had a turnover greater than the GDP of Pakistan (75th). Nestlé (88th) had a turnover greater than the GDP of Bangladesh (99th).

The diverse reach of modern food corporations is considerable. Food companies are in discrete markets, mostly either in production or trading of raw commodities – such as Cargill, the world's largest grain trader, a private corporation – or in value-adding industries such as food processing. Table 4.2 provides a picture of the world's largest food global corporations. These are key framers of the food system.

# Food policy

Food policy poses special challenges to public policy. Key features of the contemporary food system, sometimes, to the detriment of health outcomes, are a focus on profits as a primary driver, value-adding, brand image, market share and "efficiency". Meanwhile in political discourses, health issues are often combined or confounded with safety, rather than recognized as specific population-based indicators. Conflicting policies are common, particularly when government subsidies undermine food policies with a potential benefit to public health. An example can be found in policies over fish. Although nutritionists generally encourage consumption of fish, environmental considerations urge if not caution then reduction. Whereas 5% of humanity consumes

**Table 4.2** Largest food corporations, by turnover, 1998 (from FT 500, *Financial Times*, 28 January 1999, excepting Cargill, website: www.cargill.com)

|  | Sales | Profits | Chief products | Employees |
|---|---|---|---|---|
|  | (US$ billion) |  |  |  |
| Philip Morris | 56.11 | 6.31 | Tobacco, cereals, beverages | 152 000 |
| Cargill | 51.00 | 4.68 | Cereals, seeds, oils, beverages | 80 600 |
| Unilever | 50.06 | 7.94 | Oils, dairy, beverages, meals | 287 000 |
| Nestlé | 49.96 | 4.11 | Beverages, cereals, infant food | 225 808 |
| Pepsico | 20.92 | 1.49 | Beverages, snacks | 142 000 |
| Sara Lee | 20.01 | −0.53 | Meat and bakery | 139 000 |
| Coca-Cola | 18.87 | 4.13 | Beverages, foods | 29 500 |
| McDonalds | 11.41 | 1.64 | Restaurants | 267 000 |

**Table 4.3** Some features of the 20th century food revolution

| Sector | Feature | Example | Comment |
| --- | --- | --- | --- |
| Agriculture | Labor efficiency | Decline of animal power, replacement by fossil power | Decline in farms, rise in size of holdings |
| Processing | Value-adding | Sugar and fruit extract added to fermented milk | "New adulterations" |
| Distribution | Creation of entire new sector in modern food supply chains | Chill systems of storage | More long-distance food transport |
| Retail | Transfer of sales force from direct customer contact | Electronic Point of Sale (EPOS) systems using laser scanners of "barcodes" | Key to supermarket efficiency and logistics control |
| Catering | Bought-in ready-made ingredients | Soups, gravy mixes | De-skilling of cooking |
| Marketing | Search for new niche markets by use of advertising | Low calorie drinks using artificial sweeteners | Coexistence of niche and mass markets; market fragmentation |

45% of all meat and fish, the poorest 20% consumes only 5%. North American cod banks are severely depleted and subject to fishing bans, and according to the FAO, 69% of world fish stocks are in a "dire condition". The FAO sees the problem as the world "having too many vessels or excessive harvesting power in a growing number of fisheries," yet governments are subsidizing the fish industry an annual $14–20 bn, equivalent to 25% of sector's revenues (World Trade Organization, 1999).

Food production has changed dramatically over the 20th century. New products, processes (both on and off the land), distribution (supply chain management), and marketing (e.g., advertising) have had major impacts on health, environment, and culture. A spiral has occurred in which changing supply chain features have both fed and reacted to changing aspirations and food culture. Table 4.3 gives illustrations of some key features.

The food economy unfolding worldwide has some features in common. It is characterized by:

- Value-adding – the pursuit of "difference", i.e., a feature (e.g., packaging, taste, image) to differentiate between one product and another;
- Company mergers and acquisitions leading to high levels of concentration in the food economy;
- Quality, which may be defined cosmetically (by how the food looks or can be sold);
- Brand value – name and marketability are to market success;
- The search for new markets – or "new" to the dominant Western food companies, who desire to open previously untapped markets such as the former Soviet Union, China and India;
- Trader power – with complex supply chains, there appears to be a rule whereby whoever dominates the relationship between primary producers and processors, on the one hand, and end consumers, on the other, is sovereign;

| **Table 4.4  Some policy options** | |
|---|---|
| **Fragmented policy** | **Systemic solutions** |
| Intensification | Diversification |
| Cost externalization | Cost internalization |
| Marginalization of health | Health central to economics |
| Food miles | More local food |
| Productionism | Sustainability |
| Individual health | Ecological public health |
| Integrated policy | Technical fixes |
| Short term | Long term |
| Consumerism | Citizenship |
| Health focus mainly on food safety | Policy linkage between safety, nutrition and sustainable food supply |

- A two-tier food economy characterized by large transnational corporations with enormous power on the one hand, and a plethora of small and medium-sized enterprises restricted to local or subnational markets on the other;
- Social fragmentation – the coexistence of over- and underconsumption (see Table 4.4).

# Food inequalities

Many health disparities are the result of differences in diet availability and intake. History suggests that food insecurity is not inevitable and that maldistribution of food is a classic illustration of the social determination of health. In both war and peace, equitable public policy can decrease infant mortality and increase overall human health. That the toll of diet-related inequalities is so sobering is a political challenge. There is, of course, some good news but 800 million children globally are undernourished and an estimated two billion people show the effects of poor diet (UNICEF, 2000). Deficiencies of both macro- and micronutrients are well documented, as is the fact that women, children, and older people are at greatest risk.

A self-perpetuating cycle of health and income inequalities reflects inequalities in housing and education, leading to greater exposure to environmental hazards such as unsafe food, and contaminated air and water. Such life hazards are associated with rapid urbanization, which can reduce rather than enhance the range of good dietary ingredients and increase the likelihood of ill-health through pollution and accidents, which in turn reduces the opportunities for income and education of children. It is the task of public policy to break such negative cycles.

From the end of World War II, food policy on inequalities was fractured by a clash of analyses about the way forward. On one side stood those arguing for policies of national or possibly regional self-reliance. On the other stood those arguing for greater flow of trade and cross-border food security.

A key thinker in the 1940s was John Boyd Orr, who became the first Secretary General of the Food and Agriculture Organization (FAO) when it was created in 1946 (Orr, 1966). He tried to bridge the two policy camps, arguing that those that could grow food, should and those that could not, should be fed by others. The problem was that countries that needed to import food had to export hard goods, commodities, or other commercial crops to generate foreign exchange. Boyd Orr argued that countries should set "targets for tomorrow". In today's parlance, he argued for multilevel governance, a combination of local, national, and international targets that should work to the common good for health (Orr, 1943). The approach is worth rehearsing, not just for its historical significance, but because it attempted, over half a century ago, to address some problems in food policy that still exist today. In relation to countries such as the UK, i.e., with pockets of real deprivation amidst wealth, Boyd Orr argued as follows.

- Countries should set targets within a new global system and foster intergovernmental cooperation to help each other over good times and bad, to ease out booms and slumps in production.
- Targets should be based on nutrition and agricultural science.
- Targets should be set to achieve health. Premature death from undernutrition was inexcusable; investment in better food would yield health and economic gains and savings.
- Agriculture should be supported to produce more. Agriculturally rich countries, such as the UK, ought to emulate the advanced agricultural economies such as the USA where targets had been set to raise production of fruit and vegetables (up by 75%), milk (up by 39%), eggs (up by 23%), etc.
- Industry should be geared to produce tools to enable agricultural productivity to rise, e.g., new buildings, tractors, equipment.
- Trade should be encouraged to meet the new markets. Trade would ease the overproductive capacity of some world areas and match them with underconsumption in other areas.
- International cooperation would have to follow the (proposed) UN Conference on Food and Agriculture.
- New organizations would have to be created such as a new International Food and Agricultural Commission, National Food Boards to monitor supplies, Agricultural Marketing Boards, Commodity Boards.

This was visionary indeed and was the position Boyd Orr argued with passion in the post-war reconstruction period. But this mixed approach to food policy – part market, part state action – which was rejected by some at the time, was marginalized entirely by the 1980s. Retrospectively, the 1974 World Food Summit may be seen as the high water mark of the appeal of state-led, national policies of self-reliance. The new neo-liberal orthodoxy from the 1980s replaced this central role of the State with an emphasis on market-driven growth. In the process, the definition of food security was altered in two important ways.

Firstly, a new focus had emerged from researchers who placed more stress on subnational or local and domestic food security. They argued that countries might have an overall sufficiency of supply, when at the household or local level, there could be deficiencies; what was needed, argued the researchers, was attention to the microlevel. Four core foci emerged (Lang *et al.*, 2001):

- **sufficiency** of food for an active healthy life;
- **access** to food and entitlement to produce, purchase or exchange food;
- **security** in the sense of the balance between vulnerability, risk and insurance;
- **time** and the variability in experiencing chronic, transitory, and cyclical food insecurity.

Accompanying this focus on the micro- and household level of food security, were new macroeconomic frameworks for achieving food adequacy. According to the new position, economic goals should aim for sufficient purchasing power to ensure that citizens ate adequately. Considerations of national or regional food security would be rejected. What mattered was not how much food a nation, state or locality produced but whether the people could afford to purchase their needs on the open market. If they could not, the market needed to be opened to imports and at the same time income generation within economies needed to be maximized. This import–export model triumphed at the 1994 General Agreement on Tariffs and Trade (GATT).

If the pursuit of food self-reliance was killed in the 1980s, the GATT buried it. However, as often happens in public policy, when a policy regime celebrates its triumph, a replacement or opposition can already be waiting in the wings. This has happened with the import–export neoliberal approach. Largely driven initially by environmental considerations, the 1990s saw the increasing articulation of new models. One might be termed appropriate localism. This position suggests that meeting environmental goals of sustainability by producing more diverse foods locally, both empowers people and protects their capacity to feed themselves (Pretty, 1998). Another position is associated with the work of Nobel Laureate Amartya Sen, who with Jean Dreze, has articulated a view that people experience hunger when a political culture denies them "entitlement" (Sen, 1981a, 2000). Social legitimacy is a precursor to adequate food, but social legitimacy can be made or broken by policy choices.

The amazing gap between rich and poor within and between societies is well documented. There are 1.2 billion people living on US$1 per day (UNDP, 2000). Meanwhile, the top 200 billionaires doubled their wealth in 1994–98 and just three of their number have more wealth than the combined Gross National Product (GNP) of all least developed countries, a total of 600 million people (UNDP, 1999). Michael Jordan, a US athlete, was paid US$20 million for endorsing Nike trainers, more than the entire workforce was paid for making them (Klein, 2000). Although our focus here is on the nutrition transition experienced by developing or recently developed countries, it is important to remember that even in rich countries, policies can determine the variation in rates of diet-related health inequalities. In the European Union, for instance, rates of diet-related ill-health vary considerably (Lang, 1999a). The UK has the worst indices and, despite being wealthy, has a disproportionate share of European Union low income (Societe Francais de Santé Publique, 2000). In the period 1979–97, inequalities in income and health widened due to macroeconomic policy choices under the Conservative Government. According to the New Labour government's own health inquiry, the poorest decile in the UK experienced both real and relative income decline (Acheson, 1998). As in other countries with far lower incomes, the UK's lower socioeconomic groups have a greater incidence of premature and low birthweight babies, heart disease, stroke, and some cancers in adults. Risk factors including lack of breast feeding, smoking, physical inactivity, obesity, hypertension, and poor diet are clustered in lower socioeconomic groups (James *et al.*, 1997).

## Sustainable consumption: constraint on consumerism?

Over the last decades of the 20th century evidence mounted about the deleterious effect of contemporary food and agricultural policies. These include:

- pollution and chemical contamination from pesticide (over-)use (Conway and Pretty, 1991);
- falling water tables from over-irrigation and intensive crop production (de Moor, 1998);
- drinking water quality (McMichael, 1999);
- loss of biodiversity (Gardner, 1996);
- degraded soil (Oldeman *et al.*, 1991; McMichael, 2001);
- wasteful use of land and sea (World Resources Institute, 1993).

There is now considerable concern in agricultural policy on whether the earth's food infrastructure can feed populations. The Worldwatch Institute has pointed to evidence of slowing of yield increases, declining crop diversity, declining fish stocks, and the impact of climate change (Gardner and Halweil, 2000). The challenge of meeting sustainability goals is not just a matter for ecology, but also society. Key trends include urbanization, rising meat consumption and civil wars, which upset agricultural capacities. The growing debate about sustainable consumption raises additional long-term questions about the "pull" exerted by consumerism. What are the implications of continued changing consumer demands for more meat, fish and use of nonrenewable resources, such as in packaging?

A foretaste of what could follow in the wake of the nutrition transition, if developing countries adopt the entire Western intensive approach to food production and consumption exemplified by hygienic packaging, can be appreciated by looking at what the "advanced" economies do. The global packaging industry is worth an annual $100 billion and in some developed countries, packaging accounts for between 10% and 50% of end food costs. The USA's packaging industry manufactures 32 billon kilograms of plastic food packaging each year, and its population of 280 million people throws away 60 million plastic bottles each day, less than 3% are recycled. If the USA is a world leader in such waste, the UK with a population of 60 million also manages to use 15 million plastic bottles per day, of which less than 3% are recycled. Where does this waste go? The choice is either to bury it in landfills or to recycle it.

The European Union has now set the ambitious goal of recovering 50% of all plastic waste and of recycling half of that. But the recycling currently means that shiploads of plastic waste are taken to China for sorting by cheap labor (Vidal, 2001). Such solutions are probably unsustainable. That what is required is more than palliatives, but rather a structural rethink, is given further weight by the enormity of carbon emissions. The UK's food, drink, and tobacco industries produce 4.5 million tons (Mt) of carbon a year, and also deposit 6 Mt of waste in landfill sites each year (DETR, 1998). A policy debate about the relative health value of packaging is urgently required.

A similar challenge for health is raised by the rapid urbanization of global populations. In policy terms, the questions are: firstly, how are the populations of cities to be fed? Secondly, who is to do it? In 1900, approximately 5% of the world's people lived in cities with populations greater than 100 000. By the 1990s, an estimated 45% – more than 2.5 billion people – lived in large urban centers. And by 2025, that proportion is likely to be 61% of the world's population (Howson *et al.*, 1998). This is likely to be accompanied by a considerable growth of the urban poor. As the population in cities continues to expand into the 21st century, the demand for food to feed urban people will grow. The FAO estimates that in a city of 10 million people, 6000 tonnes of food may need to be imported on a daily basis (FAO, 1998). By the year 2025, there will be a huge increase in the numbers of people in the south living in cities. Between 1950 and 1990, the world's towns and cities grew twice as fast as rural areas (World Bank, 1999). In 1950, only two cities had more than 8 million inhabitants, London and New York (Harrison, 1992). It is estimated that over the next 20 years, 93% of urban growth will take place, whereas the majority of the population in the continents of Africa and Asia will remain in the rural areas.

Urbanization poses a special challenge for building a sustainable route to development. If just one feature associated with the nutrition transition – meat consumption – were to be replaced by a greater emphasis on increasing availability and consumption of vegetables and fruits, patterns of production would have to be markedly different. To reduce the use of nonrenewable energy via transportation, more local cultivation would be desirable. The UN Habitat 2 conference in 1996 concluded that urban or peri-urban agriculture will have to make a come-back, after decades of declining policy focus (UNDP, 1996). In fact, for half a century, the emphasis in global food policy, and certainly in the Western model of agriculture, has been specialization and intensification. Despite this policy marginalization, in 1993 15–20% of world food was produced in urban or peri-urban areas and was worth US$500 million (WHO-E, 1999).

In cities such as Kathmandu where 37% of urban gardeners already grow all the vegetables consumed, and Hong Kong, where 45% of demand for vegetables is supplied from 5–6% of the land mass, a practical alternative to long-distance food exists. The new global movement of urban agriculture (Pretty, 1998), which tends to be encouraged on ecological and community self-reliance grounds, is beginning to receive public health encouragement. The WHO European Region, concerned about diet-related diseases, has recently produced an ambitious and far-sighted policy document (WHO-E, 1999). This notes that up to 80% of Siberian or Asian cities are already involved in urban agriculture, and that in 1997 in Poland, for example, 500 000 tonnes of vegetables and fruits (one-sixth of the national consumption) were produced on 8000 council "employees" gardens. In Georgia, home-produced food accounted for 28% of income and in Bulgaria in 1998, 47% of people were self-sufficient in vegetables and fruit and 90% of urban families make preserves for winter (WHO-E, 1999).

To orthodox Western food economists, a policy emphasis on local urban or peri-urban food smacks of an irrational return to a mythical halcyon past. But the case for thinking through the connection between *what* is produced, grown, processed, and consumed and *how* this happens sits at the heart of the new food policy challenge. The issue is not just quantity but quality. An illustration is the huge amount of nonrenewable energy (fossil fuels) used in transporting food increasingly long distances, as the food supply chain intensifies, concentrates, and specializes. To neoliberals, that a developing country could produce, for example, dessert apples and export them to the UK would be a good thing. The fact that the UK has a good climate and could grow its own is secondary. In 1993, 685 000 GJ (equivalent to 14 million liters of fuel) was used to transport 417 207 tonnes of imported apples (Garnett, 1999). Four out of five pears and two out of three apples are now imported into the UK (Hoskins and Lobstein, 1998). In 1995, by foods such as these, the UK was a net importer of "ghost hectares"; in other words, its food needs were produced on 4.1 million hectares of other countries' land, as well as its own (MacLaren *et al.*, 1998).

In the period 1975–91/93, food transported on UK roads increased by 30% and the distance traveled by the UK's total food supply increased by approximately 60% (Hoskins and Lobstein, 1998). The distance traveled for shopping in general rose by 60% in that period, and travel by car more than doubled. With the citing of food shops (supermarkets) in ever larger stores, consumers had to use cars to get their food. So the net result is that the "modern", "efficient" food economy externalized environmental costs (Raven and Lang, 1995). The western model of food shopping is not appropriate as a sustainable consumption paradigm, yet that is the cultural dimension behind the nutritional transition – a change of lifestyle with consequences for ecological as well as human health.

# Food governance

Since the 1994 GATT, the developing world has fractured with some developing countries benefiting, while others do not. Sub-Saharan Africa, in particular, has been a net loser. Dissent about the new global institutions of governance symbolized by the GATT's creation of the World Trade Organization surfaced at the WTO talks in Seattle, USA, in December 1999, with demonstrations following in Washington DC, Melbourne, Gothenborg, Prague, and Genoa. Although much interest has focused on wider political and economic issues, there are important considerations for the issue of the nutrition transition and the food–health connection. Two considerations are central: firstly, whether the neoliberal model enshrined in the GATT is appropriate for the ecological and human health challenges of the 21st century and, secondly, whether, health issues are adequately championed in global governance.

## New models for old

As was outlined above in the discussion on Boyd Orr, the dominant model for food policy dates back to the post World War II period. The model centered on an analysis that

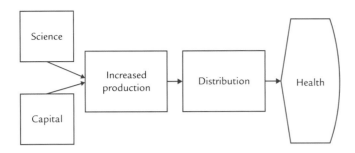

**Figure 4.1**   Food's impact on health – the mid 20th century model.

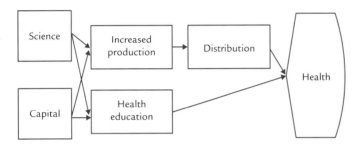

**Figure 4.2**   Food's impact on health – the mid to late 20th century model.

underproduction was the primary policy failure. If science could only unleash nature's productive capacity and if capital investment could be suitably made, then farming could increase output and nutritional deficiencies could be alleviated. As long as there was efficient distribution and a welfare safety net to "catch" failures in personal income, then improved public health would surely be the outcome. The model is schematically represented in Fig. 4.1. By the 1980s, with rising evidence of degenerative diseases, another "box" was inserted into the package in the form of health education (Fig. 4.2).

The problem with this approach was that it made a number of assumptions which events proved to be unwarranted. Firstly, it assumed that increased supply would improve health when in fact rising incomes, urbanization, and changed nature of supply allowed (or arguably encouraged) the rise of degenerative diseases such as coronary heart disease, the diet-related cancers, diabetes, and obesity – all the diseases associated with and highlighted in the nutrition transition.

Secondly, the model assumed that the era of contagion was over when in fact the opening up of food systems removed barriers to the spreading of diseases. Thus, if food traveled across continents and if processors and retailers purchase globally, new opportunities and routes for cross-contamination and spreading of diseases were created. Key causes of disease include *Salmonella, Campylobacter, Escherichia coli,* and new ones such as bovine spongiform encephalophathy (BSE).

Thirdly, changes in the nature of production and distribution opened new chances for diseases to spread further and faster. Tourism, for instance, turns more than 600 million people each year into disease carriers.

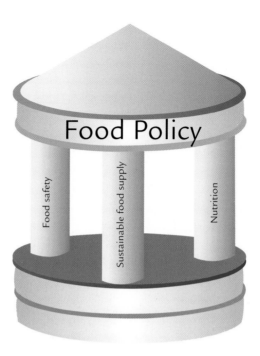

**Figure 4.3**  WHO European Region model for food and health policy (reproduced from WHO Regional Committee for Europe, 2000, with permission).

Fourthly, the model assumed that the "old" banes of food policy, such as adulteration and contamination, would be consigned to the history books when in fact they have changed. Some forms of contamination and adulteration have been successfully controlled whereas new ones such as contamination from pesticides, additives, and nitrates have been introduced or greatly enhanced.

What is now required is a much more complex and multidimensional model. The 51 member states of the WHO European Region in 2000 agreed to a new simple model (Fig. 4.3). This suggests that to meet health goals, public policy should give equal emphasis to building three pillars: nutrition, food safety, and sustainable food supply. Unless they are equal, the roof – health – under which all humans can shelter would tilt and not last. This model is highly appropriate to present this new message, being simple and intelligible. But it can be argued that in reality, the model ought to be more multifactoral; there should be many more pillars and understanding required needs to include many sciences. Figure 4.4 shows a more appropriate model, even though this might be hard to sell to politicians, who famously are both busy and need to be "sold" simple messages.

If public policy is to be built on a comprehensive rather than a partial analysis, it should integrate the goals of achieving individual, population, and ecological health.

## Institutions

When the General Agreement on Tariffs and Trade (GATT) was signed by over 100 countries in 1994, it was to have profound direct and indirect implications for public health in

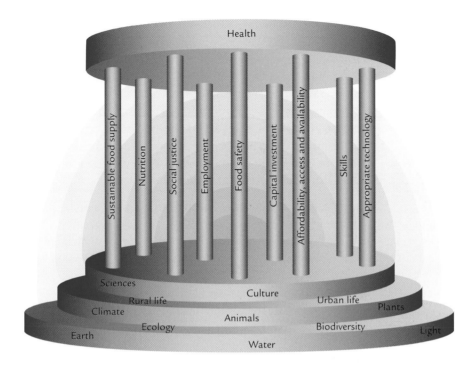

**Figure 4.4** Food's impact on health: the complex model (from Waltner-Troews and Lang, 2000) with permission.

general, and for food and agriculture in particular. It created the immensely powerful World Trade Organization (WTO) which not only monitors trade rules but runs a system of arbitration which is *de facto* a new jurisprudence. This mattered for public health for a number of reasons.

The institutions through which public health has expressed its views in the post-war period have been quietly marginalized (Labonte, 1998). A new system of world governance, much commented on by its non-governmental organization (NGO) critics, is emerging in parallel to, and more powerful than, the formerly more democratic institutions of the United Nations (Navarro, 1999). The WTO (or the World Bank) is more significant in framing the conditions for public health than the WHO (Banerji, 1999). The WHO is informed by a World Health Assembly, yet there is no parallel citizen's voice for the WTO. Economically, there is no contest as to which is more significant, the UN system or the new trade system.

The GATT is a key, if not the key, structure in the architecture of the new era of globalization. Within the many hundreds of pages of the full GATT agreement, public health barely registers, except when implied as a threat to free trade. A fear that health is a fig-leaf for protectionism stalks the neoliberal halls, whereas to proponents of public health, the notion of "protection", like prevention, carries positive rather than negative connotations. In the GATT's Agreement on Agriculture much effort was put into ensuring that national governments cannot set food standards or restrict entry of foods unless they have "sound scientific" justification. This seems reasonable, although in practice subject to subjective interpretation and commercial pressures.

Research conducted in 1991–93, before the 1994 GATT was signed, suggested that Codex was not in a fit democratic state to carry public confidence about its processes (Avery *et al.*, 1993). Codex is a large system of around 20 committees, which has many participants at meetings around the world. These working parties are usually hosted by rich countries and meet over two years and make recommendations to the bi-annual full meeting of the Codex Commission. Over the full 1991–93 cycle of meetings there were a total of 2758 participants. Codex is theoretically a meeting of governments but the study found that nearly a quarter of participants were from large international companies – the same for whose products were being set standards. Reviewing a full two-year cycle of Codex meetings, the *Cracking the Codex* study found that:

- 104 countries participated, as did over 100 of the largest multinational food and agrochemical companies;
- The vast majority (96%) of nongovernmental participants represented industry;
- There were 26 representatives from public interest groups compared to 662 industry representatives;
- Nestlé, the largest food company in the world, sent over 30 representatives to all Codex committee meetings combined, more than most countries;
- Most representation came from rich, Northern countries: over 60% came from Europe and North America with the poor countries of the South dramatically under represented – only 7% from Africa and 10% from Latin America;
- Of the participants on the working group on standards for food additives and contaminants, 39% represented Transnational Corporations (TNCs) or industry federations, including 61 representatives from the largest food and agrochemical companies in the world;
- Of the 374 participants on the committee on pesticide residue levels, 75 represented multinational agrochemical and food corporations, 34 from the world's top 20 agrochemical companies; only 80 participants represented the interests of developing countries;
- The USA sent more representatives to Codex than any other country (50% of them representing industry) and almost twice as many as the entire continent of Africa.

Following the publication of this report and despite requests to "clean up" this inadequacy, the GATT secretariat declined to act. In subsequent years, officials and companies became sensitive to these criticisms, which have been pursued by the consumers' movement. Some countries now hold tripartite national premeetings with industry, consumers, and government officials before going to Codex meetings. However, this left practice at the Codex meetings themselves unchanged. One review in 1997 concluded that little has changed (McCrea, 1997). At the 1997 Codex food labeling committee, for instance, the US delegation comprised eight government officials, three from NGOs and ten from industry. Reform is now, happily, beginning, but why so late?

Particularly sensitive is the issue of scientific judgment. The GATT stipulated that disputes would be arbitrated on grounds of "sound science", yet consumer groups argue that science is not the only salient feature, nor indeed is science quite the straightforward arbiter it is assumed to be. Whose is the research? Who funded it? Is it publicly available? What questions framed the analysis? The argument between the USA and the

EU over hormone use in meat fattening illustrates the sensitivity of the issue. Since the early 1980s, the EU has implemented a ban on the use of hormones. This was contested by the US, keen to sell its beef in Europe's rich markets. The dispute was referred to Codex and the long-awaited WTO decision was announced in early 1998. Both the US and EU claimed vindication of their positions (EC, 1998; USTR, 1998). The EU's Scientific Committee on Veterinary Measures then argued that further studies suggested scientific evidence warranting a continued ban (European Commission, 1999).

The food trade issue is now particularly sensitive. For the last few years there has been a steady stream of high profile cases where food-exporting nations fight over the right to export surpluses to each other and to markets they deem their own. There have been wars over lamb between Australia and New Zealand and the USA (International Centre for Trade and Sustainable Development, 1999); over beef hormones between the EU and USA; over genetically modified foods between the USA and many countries but especially the EU. The notion that food security stems from growing most of one's food within one's country (what used to be called self-reliance) is being eroded by the notion that security stems from being able to purchase food on the open world markets (WHO-Europe, 1995).

Food security is a concern for most developing country governments whereas rich countries are more troubled by consumer-driven food safety issues. As the WHO Regional Office for Europe's (1999) Food and Nutrition Plan recognizes, from a public health perspective, both are important and both reflect changes in methods of production and distribution and in the food system (Tansey and Worsley, 1995; Lang, 1997). The Norwegian Government was rare among rich nations in openly criticizing the drift of the new GATT talks. It should know. Its citizens voted in the early 1990s against joining the EU, in part from hostility to the Common Agricultural Policy undermining the national nutrition and food policy in place since 1976 (Royal Norwegian Ministry of Agriculture, 1976). Yet Norway by signing onto the 1994 GATT began to erode exactly the very same national policy.

In a paper prepared in June 1999, Norway laid down a clear policy challenge: food security is too important to be left to the vagaries of trade (Royal Ministry of Agriculture, 1999). Under the Plan of Action agreed at the 1996 World Food Summit, as at the earlier 1992 International Conference on Nutrition, Governments agreed they have a moral responsibility to ensure their citizens have adequate food, are free from hunger and achieve food security (World Food Summit, 1996). The GATT perspective favors the market approach to food security. Tacitly, it argues that the cheapest food is best. The new public health perspective suggests that the West's food revolution has intensified food production such that when food is cheap, other costs are being externalized onto the environment (Lang, 1999b). In this intellectual context, Norway's position was pioneering. It argued that the new Round should agree on rules to safeguard national food security. When wheat or maize prices can rise by 50% in just two years, as happened in 1993–95, reliance on being able to buy one's food in the world marketplace is a form of security only open to the affluent. (Norway, as a small population with immense oil wealth is ironically one such country.) What are the poor to do in such circumstances: tighten their belts? As Sen (1981b, 1997) and others have shown, hunger follows poor purchasing power and is not necessarily a function of food availability.

The new WTO structures are designed to facilitate cross-border economic activity and to reduce national control over capital flows, competition and even cultural control. In the age of the internet, information knows few boundaries yet vast new corporations are emerging which dominate almost everything humans do or consume. The irony about the new GATT is that it is based upon the free trade model of globalization just when evidence about its negative effects is mounting up. According to the tenth annual UN Human Development Report, the richest 20% of the world now account for 86% of world GDP, while the poorest 20% have just 1% (UNDP, 1999); 200 of the world's richest people have doubled their net worth in the last four years. The richest three people in the world have assets greater than the combined Gross National Product of all the least developed countries in the world, 600 million people. There is little chance of health for all in such a socially divided world.

Another reason for public health involvement in trade talks and debate concerns the work of public health monitoring itself. Public health action has to be based on a good understanding of the real world. Perspective is in order. Postwar development has brought astonishing gains for billions of people, but equally, as the *Human Development Report* documents, the scale of contemporary inequality and poor healthcare defies sanity. The *Human Development Report* itself came into existence because a decade ago, UN administrators, social scientists, and politicians were critical of the convention of measuring development through indicators such as Gross Domestic or National Product. They disguise intranational inequalities and fail to convey the quality of life issues. The Human Development Index was created to fill this gap. The *Human Development Report* shows that 80 countries have incomes lower today than a decade ago; 1.3 billion people, over a fifth of humanity, exist on less than US$1 per day. However it is measured, the gap between the richest and poorest is widening. In 1960, the gap between the richest fifth and the poorest fifth was 30:1. In 1990 it was 60:1. In 1997 it was 74:1 (UNDP, 1999). In this context, it is clear that epidemiologists as much as physicians and health activists have to ask themselves how their work does or does not confront this obscene accrual of wealth and power. And does the nutrition transition call for new health indicators? Almost certainly, yes!

The *Human Development Report*, however, argued that globalization is unstoppable and that all good people can do is try to give it "development with a human face". It is true that proponents of unfettered free trade are more defensive than in 1987–94. Faced by growing opposition and the sheer weight of evidence of harm, the architects of inequalities in health now plead that we should still trust them and that (their version of) growth must continue by a different path (Wolf, 1999). Inequalities may be bad, they admit, but now is the time to target resources on the poor. We should ignore, they imply, the accrual of power by the rich as they are the motor force of the new global economy.

## Conclusion

The nutrition transition raises immensely important challenges for food policy. This chapter argues that these need to be accompanied by sensitivity to other challenges raised by contemporary globalization.

**Table 4.5** Different Food and Health Policy Frameworks: fragmented or systemic solutions?

| Fragmented approach | Systemic approach |
|---|---|
| Food policy focus on productionism & consumerism | Food policy seeks sustainability & citizenship |
| Marketing appeal to individual health | Population approach to public health |
| Reliance on technical fixes (drugs, functional foods, etc.) | Diet-based approach to preventive health |
| Marginalization of health from supply chain thinking | Health central to economics |
| Separation of safety and nutrition | Policy linkage between safety, nutrition and sustainable food supply |
| Intensification | Diversification |
| Health costs externalized | Health costs internalized |
| Poor links between global, regional, national and local governance | Multilevel governance |
| Competing frameworks within government and corporate sector | Integrated policy across government and food supply chain |

There is a strong case for action on food and health. Interventions much cited in the literature, such as the North Karelia experiment in Finland, are often rooted in an era of more interventionist government action. Finland produced a 55% decline in male mortality due to coronary heart disease in the period 1972–92. So even in the contemporary policy climate, interventions can work. As has been illustrated by Thailand, which engineered a decline in childhood malnutrition from 50% in 1982 to 10% by 1996. The key, according to the Commission on the Nutrition Challenges of the 21st Century (2000) reporting to the UN, is a combination of political will, health planning, and community focus.

The good news is that awareness of health as a central element of development is growing. Pressure to enable the new ecological public health approach is building up. Policy options and the implications of choices are becoming clear, but much more coordinated thinking, research, and health action is needed if enormous changes such as the nutrition transition are to be steered in positive rather than negative directions.

Table 4.5 summarizes some of the policy goals that need to be reviewed and analyzed more clearly and carefully. The case argued here is that unless such issues are included in the discourse about the nutrition transition, there is a danger the transition will be seen as immutable and inevitable. The context presented here reminds us that the nutrition transition is not an isolated phenomenon. Economic, political and cultural transitions accompany, facilitate and frame the nutrition transition. It is an indicator of a wider restructuring of society and lifestyle, part driven by strong forces, part pulled by aspirations, immensely complex.

Now that so much is known about the nutrition transition, the challenge is to widen debate to include what to do about it. There are strong forces who argue that the transition is unimportant, a policy deviation, a side-show in the onward march of social progress, a matter for consumer choice. They argue that it is beyond governance. One strand of modern thinking on governance agrees with this analysis, arguing that the state and public thinking are too diffuse or weak to act on mega-trends such as the nutrition transition. We know better. The history of public health suggests that there have always been such siren voices. Good people, armed with evidence, informed governments like Thailand's or Finland's and together with progressive forces in the food supply chain acted with imagination and persistence to improve public health. The nutrition transition is an awesome challenge. It requires new alliances, new political will and new thinking. And since when were public health challenges easy?

# References

Acheson, D. (1998). "Report of the Independent Inquiry into Inequalities in Health". The Stationery Office, London.

Avery, N., Drake, M., and Lang, T. (1993). "Cracking the Codex: a report on the Codex Alimentarius Commission". National Food Alliance, London.

Banerji, D. (1999). A fundamental shift in the approach to international health by WHO, UNICEF, and the World Bank: Instances of the practice of "intellectual facism" and totalitarianism in some Asian countries. *Int. J. Health Serv.* **29**, 227–259.

Boyd Orr, J. (1943). "Food and the People – Target for Tomorrow", no. 3, pp. 41–55. Pilot Press, London.

Boyd Orr, J. (1966). "As I Recall". Macgibbon & Kee, London.

Commission on the Nutrition Challenges of the 21st Century (2000). Ending malnutrition by 2020: An agenda for change in the millennium. Final Report to the ACC/SCN. *Food Nutr. Bull.* **21** Suppl 3, p. 19.

Conway, G., and Pretty, J. (1991). "Unwelcome Harvest: Agriculture and Pollution". Earthscan, London.

Davidson, J. (2001). "The Richest 100 Economic Players". CAFOD, London.

de Moor, A.P.G. (1998). "Subsidizing Unsustainable Development", S5.1–S5.5. Institute for Research on Public Expenditure & Earth Council, The Hague.

DETR (1998). "Sustainable Business". Consultation paper on sustainable development and business in the UK. Dept of the Environment, Transport and the Regions, London.

EC (1998). Hormone meat: WTO judgement on EU ban just one step in a long process – Consumer protection will be upheld! Brussels: Commission of European Communities, Directorate-General XXIV, Background Note from DG XXIV, 16 January.

European Commission (1999). Hormone meat: more evidence of risks. *Directorate General of Agriculture. Newsletter*, 12 May. European Commission DG VI, Brussels.

FAO (1998). "The State of Food and Agriculture". Food Agriculture Organisation, Rome.

Fortune (2001). "Fortune Global 500". Forbes, New York. http://www.fortune.com

Gardner, G. (1996). "Shrinking Fields: Cropland Loss in a World of Eight Billion". Worldwatch Paper 131, Worldwatch Institute, Washington, DC.

Gardner, G., and Halweil, B. (2000). "Underfed and Overfed: The Global Epidemic of Malnutrition". Worldwatch paper 150. Worldwatch Institute, Washington, DC.

Garnett, T. (1999). "City Harvest". Sustainable Agriculture, Food and Environment (SAFE) Alliance, London.

Harrison, P. (1992). "The Third Revolution: Environment, Population and a Sustainable World". I B Tauris 169, New York.

Hoskins, G., and Lobstein, T. (1998). "Food Facts", no. 3. Sustainable Agriculture, Food and Environment (SAFE) Alliance, London.

Howson, C., Fineberg, H., and Bloom, B. (1998). The pursuit of global health: the relevance of engagement for developed countries. *Lancet* **351**, 586–590.

International Centre for Trade and Sustainable Development (1999). Australia, New Zealand Cry Fowl Over U.S. Lamb Decision. *Bridges Weekly Trade News Digest* **3**, 27.

James, W.P.T., Nelson, M., Ralph, A., and Leather, S. (1997). The contribution of nutrition to inequalities in health. *BMJ* **314**, 1545–1549.

Klein, N. (2000). "No Logo". HarperCollins, London.

Labonte, R. (1998). Healthy public policy and the World Trade Organisation: a proposal for an international health presence in future world trade/investment talks. *Health Promotion Int.* **13**, 245–255.

Lang, T. (1997). The public health impact of globalisation of food trade. *In* "Diet, Nutrition and Chronic Disease: Lessons from Contrasting Worlds" (S. Shetty, and K. McPherson, eds.), pp. 173–186. Wiley, London.

Lang, T. (1999a). Food and nutrition. *In* "Priorities for Public Health Action in the European Union" (O. Weil, M. McKee, M. Brodin, and D. Oberle, eds.), pp. 138–156. European Commission, Brussels.

Lang, T. (1999b). Food as a public health issue. *In* "Perspectives in Public Health" (S. Griffiths and D. Hunter, eds.), pp. 47–58. Radcliffe Medical Press, Oxford.

Lang, T., Dowler, E., Caraher, M., and Barling, D. (2001). "Is Food a Global Public Good for Health?: Food Security and the Challenge to Governance". Report to World Health Organisation. Centre for Food Policy, London, unpublished.

McCrea, D. (1997). Codex Alimentarius – in the consumer interest? *Consumer Policy Rev.* **7**(4), 132–138.

MacLaren, D., Bullock, S., and Yousuf, N. (1998). "Tomorrow's World: Britains Share in a Sustainable Future". Earthscan, London.

McMichael, A.J. (1999). From hazard to habitat: rethinking environment and health. *Epidemiology* **10**(4), 1–5.

McMichael, A.J. (2001). "Human Frontiers, Environments and Disease". Cambridge University Press, Cambridge.

Navarro, V. (1999). Health and equity in the world in the era of "globalisation". *Int. J. Health Serv.* **29**, 215–226.

Oldeman, L.R., *et al.* (1991). "World Map of the Status of Human-Induced Soil Degradation". Wageningen, Netherlands and Nairobi: International Soil Reference and Information Centre, and UN Environment Programme, Wageningen, Netherlands and Nairobi.

Pretty, J. (1998). "The Living Land". Earthscan, London.

Raven, H., and Lang, T. (1995). "Off Our Trolleys?: Supermarkets and the Hypermarket Economy". Institute of Public Policy Research, London.

Royal Ministry of Agriculture (1999). "Food Security and the Role of Domestic Agricultural Food Production". Royal Ministry of Agriculture, Oslo.

Royal Norwegian Ministry of Agriculture (1976). "On Norwegian Nutrition and Food Policy". Report no. 32 to the Storting (1975–76). Royal Ministry of Agriculture, Oslo.

Sen, A. (1981a). "Poverty and Famines: An Essay on Entitlement and Deprivation". International Labour Organisation, Geneva.

Sen, A. (1981b). "Poverty and Famines". Clarendon Press, Oxford.

Sen, A. (1997). "Inequality Re-examined". Oxford University Press, Oxford.

Sen, A. (2000). "The Ends and Means of Sustainability", key note address, International Conference on Transition to Sustainability, InterAcademy Panel on International Issues, Tokyo, May.

Societe Francais de Santé Publique (2000). "Health and Human Nutrition: Elements for Action". Working Paper of the French Presidency. European Commission, Brussels.

Tansey, G., and Worsley, T. (1995). "The Food System". Earthscan, London.

UNDP (1996). "Urban Agriculture: Food, Jobs and Sustainable Cities", Vol. 1, United Nations Development Programme, New York.

UNDP (1999). "Human Development Report 1999". Oxford University Press/United Nations Development Programme, New York.

UNDP (2000). "Human Development Report 2000". Oxford University Press/United Nations Development Programme, New York.

UNICEF (2000). "State of the World's Children". United Nations' Children Fund, New York.

USTR (1998). "EC Hormone Ban Relating to Meat Imports Violates SPS Agreement According to Appellate Body". Office of the US Trade Representative, Washington, DC.

Vidal, J. (2001). Banana world of packaging. *The Guardian* 24 August, G2, p. 7.

Waltner-Troews, D., and Lang, T. (2000). A new conceptual base for food and agriculture: the emerging model of links between agriculture, food, health, environment and society. *Global Change Human Health* **1**, 116–130.

WHO-E (1999). "Urban Agriculture". World Health Organisation European Regional Office, Nutrition Department, Copenhagen.

WHO-Europe (1995). Nutrition Policy in WHO European Member States. Progress report following the 1992 International Conference on Nutrition. June. WHO-Europe, Copenhagen.

WHO Regional Office for Europe (1999). Draft Food and Nutrition Action Plan. World Health Organisation Regional Office for Europe, Copenhagen.

Wolf, M. (1999). A world divided. *Financial Times* 14 July, p. 16.

World Bank (1999). World Development Report 1999–2000. World Bank, New York.

World Bank (2001). "2001 World Development Indicators Database". World Bank, New York; (accessed on 4/11/2001) http://www.worldbank.org/data/databytopic/GDP.pdf

World Food Summit (1996). Rome, Objective 7.4.

World Health Organisation Regional Committee for Europe (2000). "Resolution: The Impact of Food and Nutrition on Public Health: The Case for a Food and Nutrition Policy and an Action Plan for the European Region of WHO, 2000–2005". Fiftieth session, Copenhagen, 11–14 September, EUR/RC50/R8, 14 September. World Health Organisation, Copenhagen.

World Resources Institute (1993). "World Resouces 1992–93". WRI and Oxford University Press, Washington, DC.

WTO (1999). "Trade and Environment Bulletin". 30 July.

# Demographic trends

*Hania Zlotnik*[1]

Over the past four centuries the population of the world has increased tenfold, rising from about 580 million persons in 1600 to slightly over six billion in 2000 (Biraben, 1979; United Nations, 2001a). Most of that growth occurred during the 20th century when the population nearly quadrupled (Fig. 5.1). Thus, whereas it took three centuries – from 1600 to 1900 – for the population to increase from 0.6 billion to 1.6 billion, between 1900 and 2000 a further 4.4 billion persons were added to the world population. Such rapid population growth, unprecedented in human history, resulted largely from the major reductions of mortality that occurred during the 20th century. Between 1900 and 2000, life expectancy at the world level nearly doubled, reaching 65.5 years by the end of the century. Almost universally mortality reductions preceded changes in fertility. In populations where mortality had been traditionally high, women had to bear large numbers of children to ensure that enough of them survived to adulthood. As mortality declined, populations did not immediately adjust their fertility levels to match the reduced risks of death. As a result, populations grew rapidly when high fertility persisted even as mortality declined.

The more developed countries of today were the first to experience sustained declines of mortality. Starting in the 18th century, better hygiene and improving standards of living contributed to reduce mortality rates in those countries. Between 1750 and 1850, for instance, life expectancy in a number of European countries increased from 25 years to 35 years (Vallin, 1989) and during the 19th century, as mortality reductions accelerated, a widespread fertility decline began as well. Although even for Europe the data available on fertility trends over the 19th century are partial, it would appear that fertility in the continent declined from about 5–5.5 births per woman in the early part of the 19th century to about four children per woman in the early part of the 20th century (Clark, 1968).

The process whereby reductions of mortality are followed by reductions of fertility sufficient to ensure that overall population growth remains low is known as the demographic transition. During the 20th century, most developing countries embarked on the demographic transition. Indeed, with the discovery of antibiotics and other means

---

[1] The views and opinions expressed in this chapter are those of the author and do not necessarily represent those of the United Nations.

The Nutrition Transition
ISBN: 0-12-153654-8

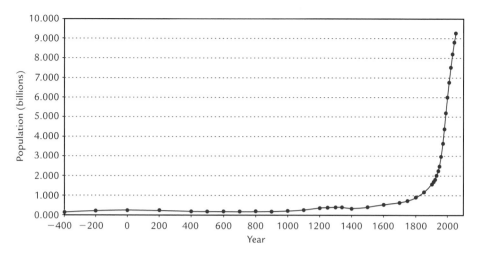

**Figure 5.1**  Long-term population increase, 400 BC to 2000 AD.

to combat the spread of the infectious diseases endemic in developing countries, rapid reductions of mortality were achieved in those countries after 1945–1950. As in the more developed countries earlier, the continuation of high fertility as mortality declined gave rise to very rapid population growth, but fertility reductions in the developing world have been occurring more rapidly than in the more developed countries. The availability of modern contraceptives has facilitated such developments. By the end of the 20th century, most developing countries had initiated the transition to lower fertility. According to United Nations (2001a) estimates, by 1995–2000 only 16 developing countries had not yet shown signs of a fertility reduction and they comprised just 3% of the world's population.

Not only did the 20th century witness a rapid rise of population but, in addition, it saw the distribution of the population between rural and urban areas change dramatically. Indeed, although the existence of populous cities with urban attributes dates back several centuries if not millennia depending on the region under consideration, the vast majority of the world's population has lived in rural settings during most of human history. Even as late as 1800, only 5% of the world population lived in urban areas and by 1900 that proportion had increased to just over 13% (United Nations, 1980). But over the course of the 20th century the proportion urban more than tripled, reaching 47% by 2000 (Fig. 5.2). The process of widespread urbanization started earlier in the more developed regions than in the developing world. Already by 1900 one out of every four inhabitants of more developed countries was an urban dweller whereas in the developing world the equivalent proportion was one in fifteen. Although levels of urbanization have risen markedly in developing countries, by 2000 less-developed regions are still about half as urbanized as more-developed regions. Thus, whereas 76% of the population of the latter lives in cities, just 40% of the population of less-developed countries is made of urban dwellers.

This chapter describes in more detail the evolution of the size and growth of the world population and the dynamics of the process of urbanization in the major regions

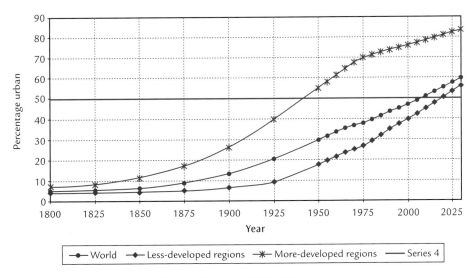

**Figure 5.2**   Percentage of population in urban areas, 1800–2030.

of the world since 1950. It also discusses future prospects and their implications. The data presented were derived from the 2000 Revision of estimates and projections of national populations prepared by the United Nations Population Division (United Nations, 2001a,b) and from the 1999 Revision of World Urbanization Prospects (United Nations, 2001c). To ensure consistency between the two sets of data, estimates and projections of the urban and rural populations were derived using the national populations produced by the 2000 Revision and the proportions residing in urban areas as estimated and projected by the 1999 Revision of World Urbanization Prospects.

# Population growth

After remaining at very low levels during most of human history, the average annual rate of population growth for the world began to accelerate at about 1700, when mortality in Europe started to decline steadily. Nevertheless, the rate of population growth did not rise above 0.5% per year until the first half of the 19th century and remained well below 1% per year until 1925 (Fig. 5.3). After piercing the 1% barrier in the late 1920s, World War II made the growth rate drop again below 1% per year during the 1940s, but the 1950s witnessed an unprecedented resurgence of growth fueled both by rising fertility in the more developed countries that experienced a "baby boom" after the war and by high fertility and declining mortality in developing countries. As mortality reductions in the developing world accelerated, so did population growth, with the result that during 1965–1970 the population of the world grew at more than 2% per year, a rate that, if sustained, would have led to a doubling of the world's population in just 34 years. However, the late 1960s also marked the point where fertility in a number of developing countries began to show a clear tendency to decline. As Fig. 5.4 shows, reductions in fertility became more clear cut during the 1970s and

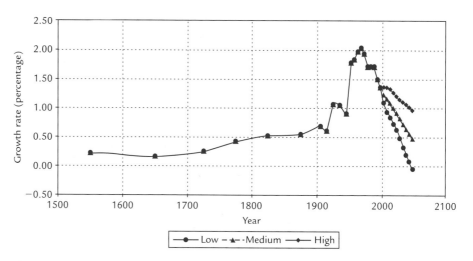

**Figure 5.3** Average annual growth rate of the world population, 1500–2050.

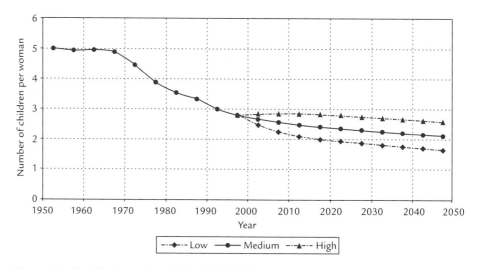

**Figure 5.4** Total fertility at the world level, 1950–2050.

a declining trend set in. It is estimated that between 1960–1965 and 1995–2000, total fertility at the world level, that is, the average number of children women would have if they were subject during their whole reproductive lives to the fertility of each period, declined from 5 children per woman to 3 children per woman. Largely as a result of that reduction, the population growth rate declined from just above 2% per year in 1965–1970 to 1.35% per year in 1995–2000. Although this reduction has been sizable, the growth rate for 1995–2000 is still well above the levels prevailing during the first half of the 20th century and, if sustained, would produce a doubling of the world population in 51 years.

Today, the potential for continued population growth at the world level remains high, not only because further reductions of mortality are expected but also because many developing countries still experience moderate to high fertility levels and have, in addition, young populations where the numbers of future parents already surpass those belonging to previous generations. The term "population momentum" is used to denote the tendency of young populations to continue growing even when fertility declines significantly. To understand the mechanics of population momentum imagine a population with three generations: grandparents, parents and children. As the population moves from one period to the next, children become parents, parents become grandparents and the original grandparents die. For the population to stop growing, the number of children that parents have in a period must equal the number of grandparents who die. If the population starts by having more children than parents and more parents than grandparents, when the children become parents their offspring will surpass the number of grandparents who die even if the new parents have only the children necessary to replace themselves. That difference will result in population growth.

What then are the prospects for future population growth? Population projections prepared by the United Nations (2001a,b) indicate that the world population will continue to rise over the next few decades but, because the rate at which population grows is expected to continue declining, there is considerable uncertainty regarding the size that the world population may attain in the future. In the United Nations projections future population growth is the result of assumptions made about the paths that fertility and mortality will take in the future at the country level. For the majority of countries, mortality is assumed to decline steadily between 2000 and 2050, the exception being the 45 countries highly affected by the HIV/AIDS epidemic for some of which mortality levels stagnate or even increase over the medium-term future because of AIDS. Only one mortality path is projected for each country and that path is combined with each of three different paths for future fertility to produce three projection variants known as the low, the medium and the high.

Assumptions about future fertility are made separately for three different categories of countries. The first is constituted of countries whose fertility in 1995–2000 was estimated to be below replacement level, that is, the level of fertility that would ensure that each woman has a daughter who survives to reproductive age. In countries with low mortality replacement-level fertility is about 2.1 children per woman. For countries that already have fertility below replacement level, future fertility is projected to remain below replacement level during most of the 2000–2050 period and to reach in 2045–2050 the total fertility level attained by the cohort of women born in the early 1960s[2]. The second category of countries includes all those where the transition to low fertility has started but where fertility is still above replacement level. For those countries, fertility is assumed to reach replacement level (2.1 children per woman) on or before 2045–2050 and to remain at replacement level once it is reached. Lastly, for the third category of countries, those in which the transition to low fertility has not yet started, total fertility is assumed to decline at a rate of one child per decade starting in 2005 and no fertility change is assumed before that date. Given the high current

---

[2] For countries lacking cohort data, the total fertility in 2045–2050 is set at 1.7 children per woman if total fertility in 1995–2000 is below 1.5 children per woman and at 1.9 children per woman otherwise.

levels of fertility that countries in this category have, most of them are projected to have fertility above replacement level in 2045–2050. This set of assumptions underlies the medium projection variant. Low and high variants are produced by letting fertility be approximately 0.5 children below or above, respectively, that of the medium variant[3].

The assumptions about future fertility are based on an analysis of past fertility trends. Although, as mentioned above, most countries have already embarked on the transition to low fertility, as of 1995–2000 there was still considerable heterogeneity among countries in terms of the stage of the transition that they had reached. Using their 1995–2000 total fertility levels and information on past trends, countries were classified according to the stage of the transition they were in. As Table 5.1 indicates, in 2000 about 20% of the world population lived in the 43 countries that had experienced an early transition to low fertility, the large majority of which (35) are located in Europe. The group also includes Australia, Canada, Georgia, Japan, New Zealand, and the United States, as well as Argentina and Uruguay, the only two countries that experienced an early transition but whose fertility has remained well above replacement level. In contrast, all other early-transition countries have been experiencing below-replacement fertility levels, levels that have been maintained for at least a decade or two in most cases. It is this persistence of below-replacement fertility in the more-developed countries that provides the rationale for keeping future fertility below-replacement level for all countries that have a current fertility lower than 2.1 children for women. Table 5.1 shows that in addition to the early-transition countries there are 23 countries, accounting for about a quarter of the world population, whose fertility is also below-replacement level, the largest of which is China. For these countries as well, fertility is kept below replacement level during the projection period in the medium variant.

A further 52 countries are already fairly advanced in the transition to low fertility, with total fertility levels ranging from 2.1 children per woman to 4 children per woman. In the medium variant most of these countries are assumed to continue experiencing a decline of fertility but only until the level of 2.1 children per woman is reached. No further reductions of fertility are assumed thereafter. Because this group of countries accounts for nearly 40% of today's population, assumptions about their future fertility have an important impact on long-term prospects for population growth and, given the experience of developed countries where below-replacement fertility is the rule, the issue of whether some of the intermediate fertility countries may reach below-replacement fertility in the future and maintain it thereafter is beginning to be considered. For some of the countries in this group, however, evidence regarding fertility trends in the recent past has shown that reductions have not been as fast as previously expected and suggest that stagnation of fertility levels may occur in the future. This is the case of populous countries such as Bangladesh and Egypt.

Lastly, there are still 69 countries with fertility levels above 4 children per woman. Among them, 16 have not yet shown signs of embarking on the transition to low

---

[3] In countries with fertility below replacement level, the low variant has a fertility 0.4 children per woman below the medium and the high variant has a fertility 0.4 children above the medium.

**Table 5.1** Distribution of countries according to the stage they have reached in the transition to low fertility by major area, 1995–2000

| Major area | No transition | Decline but TF still > 5 | Decline to 4 < TF ≤ 5 | Decline to 3 < TF ≤ 4 | Decline to 2.1 < TF ≤ 3 | Decline to TF ≤ 2.1 | Early transition, with 2.1 < TF < 3 | Early transition with "baby boom", TF < 2.1 | Total |
|---|---|---|---|---|---|---|---|---|---|
| *Number of countries* | | | | | | | | | |
| Africa | 15 | 21 | 8 | 6 | 2 | 1 | 0 | 0 | 53 |
| Asia | 1 | 10 | 3 | 11 | 11 | 12 | 0 | 2 | 50 |
| Europe | 0 | 0 | 0 | 0 | 1 | 3 | 0 | 35 | 39 |
| Latin America and the Caribbean | 0 | 0 | 7 | 3 | 14 | 7 | 2 | 0 | 33 |
| Northern America | 0 | 0 | 0 | 0 | 0 | 0 | 0 | 2 | 2 |
| Oceania | 0 | 1 | 3 | 2 | 2 | 0 | 0 | 2 | 10 |
| World | 16 | 32 | 21 | 22 | 30 | 23 | 2 | 41 | 187 |
| *Percentage of population in each major area* | | | | | | | | | |
| Africa | 20.7 | 43.2 | 12.4 | 22.3 | 1.3 | 0.1 | 0.0 | 0.0 | 100.0 |
| Asia | 0.5 | 6.3 | 0.8 | 37.9 | 10.9 | 39.9 | 0.0 | 3.6 | 100.0 |
| Europe | 0.0 | 0.0 | 0.0 | 0.0 | 0.4 | 0.9 | 0.0 | 98.7 | 100.0 |
| Latin America and the Caribbean | 0.0 | 0.0 | 8.7 | 3.7 | 76.4 | 3.4 | 7.8 | 0.0 | 100.0 |
| Northern America | 0.0 | 0.0 | 0.0 | 0.0 | 0.0 | 0.0 | 0.0 | 100.0 | 100.0 |
| Oceania | 0.0 | 1.5 | 17.2 | 3.2 | 1.5 | 0.0 | 0.0 | 76.5 | 100.0 |
| World | 3.0 | 9.5 | 2.9 | 26.3 | 13.4 | 24.6 | 0.7 | 19.6 | 100.0 |

Source: United Nations (2001a). TF, total fertility, the average number of children a woman would have over her reproductive life if subject to the fertility rates of a given period, 1995–2000 in this case.

fertility and a further 32 have fertility levels above 5 children per woman. Together, these two subsets of countries account for one-eighth of the world population. Even if these high-fertility countries proceed with the transition to low fertility at the average pace at which developing countries whose fertility has declined in the past 40 years achieved reductions, their populations will grow very rapidly. In fact, 12 of the 16 countries where the fertility transition has not yet started are projected to have a total fertility higher than 2.1 children per woman in 2045–2050, and the populations of all 16 countries combined are expected to grow at an average annual rate of nearly 2.8% during 2000–2050. In consequence, their share of the world population is expected to rise from 3% in 2000 to nearly 8% in 2050.

The heterogeneity characterizing countries both with respect to current fertility levels and in terms of expected future trends, results in trends at the world level that reflect a slowing down of the fertility decline in the medium variant, a more rapid reduction of future fertility in the low variant, and a slight rise followed by the stagnation of fertility levels in the high variant (Fig. 5.4 and Table 5.2). In the medium variant, total fertility declines from 2.82 children per woman in 1995–2000 to 2.15 children per woman in 2045–2050, thus remaining above replacement level during the whole projection period. In the low variant, total fertility drops below replacement level in 2015–2020 and continues to decline so that by 2045–2050 it has reached 1.68 children per woman. In the high variant, fertility remains between 2.8 and 2.9 children per woman until 2025 and then declines slightly to reach 2.62 children per woman in 2045–2050. In all projection variants, fertility is lower in more developed regions than in less developed regions, but the tendency is for the fertility levels of those two groups to converge. Thus, whereas in 1995–2000 the difference in fertility levels between the more developed and the less developed regions is of approximately 1.5 children per woman – 1.57 children per woman vs. 3.1 children per woman, respectively – by 2045–2050 the largest difference is found in the high variant and amounts to just about 0.3 children per woman. That is, in all projection variants the fertility of less-developed regions declines significantly, whereas that of more-developed regions remains almost constant in the low variant and increases in the medium and high variants.

Among the countries in less-developed regions, those classified as least developed countries by the United Nations[4] have, as a group, high levels of fertility (5.5 children per woman in 1995–2000). Although their fertility is expected to decline markedly during the next 50 years, by 2045–2050 the medium variant still has them exhibiting a total fertility of 2.5 children per woman, considerably above replacement level. In the high variant their fertility surpasses 3 children per woman and only in the low

[4] The least-developed countries, as defined by the United Nations General Assembly in 1998, include 48 countries: Afghanistan, Angola, Bangladesh, Benin, Bhutan, Burkina Faso, Burundi, Cambodia, Cape Verde, Central African Republic, Chad, Comoros, Democratic Republic of the Congo, Djibouti, Equatorial Guinea, Eritrea, Ethiopia, Gambia, Guinea, Guinea-Bissau, Haiti, Kiribati, Lao People's Democratic Republic, Lesotho, Liberia, Madagascar, Malawi, Maldives, Mali, Mauritania, Mozambique, Myanmar, Nepal, Niger, Rwanda, Samoa, São Tomé and Príncipe, Sierra Leone, Solomon Islands, Somalia, Sudan, Togo, Tuvalu, Uganda, United Republic of Tanzania, Vanuatu, Yemen and Zambia. These countries are also included in the less developed regions.

**Table 5.2** Total fertility estimates and projected values for the world, major areas and regions, 1950–1955 to 2045–2050

| Major area | 1950–1955 | 1975–1980 | 1995–2000 | 2000–2005 | | | 2020–2025 | | | 2045–2050 | | |
|---|---|---|---|---|---|---|---|---|---|---|---|---|
| | | | | Low | Medium | High | Low | Medium | High | Low | Medium | High |
| World | 5.01 | 3.90 | 2.82 | 2.49 | 2.68 | 2.87 | 1.96 | 2.39 | 2.83 | 1.68 | 2.15 | 2.62 |
| More-developed regions | 2.84 | 1.91 | 1.57 | 1.44 | 1.50 | 1.58 | 1.40 | 1.65 | 1.92 | 1.52 | 1.92 | 2.33 |
| Less-developed regions | 6.16 | 4.62 | 3.10 | 2.70 | 2.92 | 3.13 | 2.03 | 2.49 | 2.95 | 1.70 | 2.17 | 2.65 |
| Least-developed countries | 6.60 | 6.40 | 5.47 | 4.91 | 5.24 | 5.47 | 3.40 | 3.90 | 4.40 | 2.02 | 2.51 | 3.02 |
| Africa | 6.71 | 6.56 | 5.27 | 4.65 | 4.97 | 5.21 | 3.17 | 3.64 | 4.10 | 1.91 | 2.39 | 2.88 |
| Asia | 5.88 | 4.17 | 2.70 | 2.35 | 2.54 | 2.74 | 1.73 | 2.19 | 2.64 | 1.60 | 2.08 | 2.56 |
| Latin America and the Caribbean | 5.89 | 4.49 | 2.69 | 2.26 | 2.50 | 2.73 | 1.67 | 2.16 | 2.65 | 1.60 | 2.10 | 2.59 |
| Northern America | 3.47 | 1.78 | 2.00 | 1.76 | 1.90 | 2.09 | 1.61 | 1.93 | 2.32 | 1.68 | 2.08 | 2.48 |
| Europe | 2.66 | 1.97 | 1.41 | 1.31 | 1.34 | 1.38 | 1.26 | 1.47 | 1.69 | 1.41 | 1.81 | 2.20 |
| Oceania | 3.87 | 2.78 | 2.41 | 2.27 | 2.39 | 2.50 | 1.98 | 2.26 | 2.57 | 1.61 | 2.06 | 2.50 |

Source: United Nations (2001a).

variant do they reach replacement-level fertility. Countries in this group not only have lagged behind other countries in the transition to low fertility but are also characterized by higher mortality levels, especially since many of them are highly affected by the HIV/AIDS epidemic. Given the other social and economic constraints they face, the likelihood that they may progress rapidly through the demographic transition seems low. Even the moderate reductions of fertility projected under the medium variant may be hard to achieve.

Most of the least-developed countries are located in Africa. Among all major areas of the world, Africa has today the highest fertility: 5.3 children per woman, nearly double the level in Asia or Latin America and the Caribbean. As Table 5.2 shows, although fertility in Africa has already declined with respect to the higher levels prevalent in the late 1970s, most of the continent is still at the early stages of the transition to lower fertility and both the medium and high variants assume that it will take the best part of the next 50 years for fertility in Africa to reach levels similar to those of Asia or Latin America today.

At the other end of the spectrum, Europe is experiencing very low levels of fertility, levels that are unprecedented in human history and that, if continued, will lead to a significant reduction of the population. According to past estimates, Europe's fertility has been under replacement level since the 1970s and it is not expected to rise above replacement level in the near future. In fact, further fertility reductions are projected in all variants for the period 2000–2005 and only a small increase in fertility is projected by 2020–2025 in the medium and high variants. The rising fertility trend is maintained in both projection variants thereafter so that by 2045–2050, total fertility in Europe is projected to be 1.8 children per woman in the medium variant and 2.2 children per woman in the high variant. Only the low variant keeps total fertility in Europe declining steadily until 2025 and allows for a very small recuperation by 2050. Similar trends are followed by the fertility of Northern America, although the range of variation is smaller since fertility in that area has not fallen to the low levels observed in Europe. As for Asia, Latin America and the Caribbean, and Oceania, the low and medium variants project steady declines of fertility, whereas the high variant projects slight increases or a virtual stagnation of fertility levels until 2050.

Assumptions about future fertility are a key determinant of future population growth especially since they vary from one projection variant to the other. However, declining mortality also makes a significant contribution to population increases. Only one set of assumptions on future mortality trends is used to produce the various projection variants. Table 5.3 presents selected past estimates of life expectancy at birth and the assumed levels for that parameter in the future. At the world level, life expectancy increased from 46.5 years in 1950–1955 to 65 years in 1995–2000, a gain of 40%. Large reductions of mortality have been possible in the past because the interventions to control infectious and parasitic diseases are well known and of moderate cost. However, as infectious diseases come under control, the main causes of death shift to diseases that are harder to treat and that demand more costly interventions. Consequently, the higher the life expectancy already achieved, the more difficult it is to increase it further and some deceleration of the improvements of life expectancy is expected as higher levels are attained. In the case of the projected

**Table 5.3** Estimated and projected life expectancy at birth and mortality decline index, world and major areas, 1950–1955 to 2045–2050

| Major area | Life expectancy at birth (in years) | | | | | | Mortality decline index[a] | | |
|---|---|---|---|---|---|---|---|---|---|
| | 1950–1955 | 1975–1980 | 1995–2000 | 2000–2005 | 2020–2025 | 2045–2050 | 1950–1955 to 1995–2000 | 1995–2000 to 2025–2030 | 1995–2000 to 2045–2050 |
| World | 46.5 | 59.8 | 65.0 | 66.0 | 71.3 | 76.0 | 54 | 32 | 48 |
| More-developed regions | 66.2 | 72.3 | 74.9 | 75.6 | 79.3 | 82.1 | 61 | 39 | 55 |
| Less-developed regions | 41.0 | 56.8 | 62.9 | 64.1 | 69.7 | 75.0 | 56 | 32 | 48 |
| Least-developed countries | 35.5 | 45.3 | 50.3 | 51.4 | 60.6 | 69.7 | 33 | 33 | 51 |
| Africa | 37.8 | 48.3 | 51.4 | 51.3 | 59.6 | 69.5 | 32 | 29 | 50 |
| Asia | 41.3 | 58.4 | 65.8 | 67.4 | 73.0 | 77.1 | 62 | 37 | 51 |
| Latin America and the Caribbean | 51.4 | 63.0 | 69.3 | 70.4 | 74.3 | 77.8 | 62 | 31 | 45 |
| Northern America | 68.9 | 73.4 | 76.7 | 77.7 | 80.7 | 82.7 | 68 | 39 | 53 |
| Europe | 65.7 | 71.5 | 73.2 | 73.7 | 77.7 | 80.8 | 51 | 35 | 51 |
| Oceania | 60.9 | 67.7 | 73.5 | 74.4 | 77.6 | 80.6 | 65 | 34 | 49 |

Source: United Nations (2001a).

[a] The mortality decline index represents the increase in life expectancy actually attained as a percentage of the maximum possible increase over the period indicated, taking as maximum life expectancy that for Japan.

levels for the world population, it is expected that life expectancy will rise to 76 years in 2045–2050, an increase of 17% with respect to the level attained in 1995–2000.

To make comparisons between periods and among major areas on the basis of a more comparable metric, a mortality decline index was calculated by expressing the increase of life expectancy actually attained over a period as a percentage of the largest potential increase in life expectancy measured as the difference between the life expectancy in Japan (the country with the highest life expectancy) and the level a particular region had attained by the beginning of the period under consideration. Table 5.3 shows the values of the mortality decline index for three periods: 1950–1955 to 1995–2000; 1995–2000 to 2025–2030; and 1995–2000 to 2045–2050. Over the first period, which encompasses the second half of the 20th century, the index indicates that more-developed regions were somewhat more successful in reducing mortality in relative terms than less-developed regions, although less-developed regions recorded a greater absolute gain in life expectancy than more developed regions (22 years vs. 9 years). By 1995–2000, however, less developed regions still had a significantly lower life expectancy than more-developed regions: 63 years vs. 75 years. Among the less-developed regions, the least-developed countries made very small relative gains in life expectancy, achieving just 33% of the potential increase. By 1995–2000 their life expectancy still stood at a low 50 years. Once more, Africa experienced gains similar to those of the least-developed countries, achieving 32% of the potential rise in life expectancy by 1995–2000. The impact of the HIV/AIDS epidemic is largely responsible for the low gains made by Africa and the least-developed countries. In comparison, most of the other major areas fared better, achieving at least 62% of the potential rise in life expectancy. Only Europe recorded a lower overall increase, at 51% of the potential maximum, largely because of the stagnation or even the increases in mortality that have been experienced by Eastern European countries and, in particular, by the Russian Federation and other successor states of the former Soviet Union. In fact, Eastern Europe as a whole achieved only 24% of the potential rise in life expectancy between 1950–1955 and 1995–2000, with its life expectancy increasing by just 4 years over the period, from 64 years to 68 years.

For the future, relative gains in life expectancy are expected to be slightly lower over the next fifty years than over the past fifty, with most of the major areas achieving just about 50% of the potential maximum gain. More-developed regions are expected to make somewhat greater relative gains than less-developed regions, and the least-developed countries are expected to record fairly low relative gains by 2025–2030 but to improve their performance thereafter so that by the end of the projection period they are expected to attain 51% of the potential maximum increase in life expectancy. Yet, by 2045–2050 the least-developed countries are still expected to lag behind the rest of the developing world in terms of life expectancy (see Table 5.3). The low levels of the mortality index expected for the least-developed countries and for Africa by 2025–2030 are largely the result of the HIV/AIDS epidemic whose impact is projected to be greatest over the next two decades. Over the long run, however, current projections assume that HIV prevalence will decline significantly so that the disease has a smaller effect in dampening gains in life expectancy after 2030.

**Table 5.4** Life expectancy at birth in the 45 countries highly affected by the HIV/AIDS epidemic projected with and without AIDS, 1990–2020

|  | 1990–1995 | 1995–2000 | 2000–2005 | 2005–2010 | 2010–2015 | 2015–2020 |
|---|---|---|---|---|---|---|
| With AIDS | 56.4 | 56.9 | 57.5 | 58.8 | 60.4 | 62.1 |
| Without AIDS | 57.7 | 59.8 | 61.7 | 63.5 | 65.2 | 66.7 |
| Absolute difference | 1.3 | 2.9 | 4.3 | 4.7 | 4.8 | 4.6 |
| Percentage difference | 2.4 | 5.2 | 7.4 | 8.1 | 7.9 | 7.4 |

Source: United Nations (2001a).

In fact, as Table 5.4 shows, when the 45 countries highly affected[5] by the disease are taken as a whole, their life expectancy is expected to rise slowly between 2000 and 2020 even when the impact of HIV/AIDS is taken into account. Only when life expectancy with AIDS is compared with the one that would have been expected in the absence of the disease do its dire effects become evident. Thus, between 2000 and 2015 AIDS is likely to reduce life expectancy in the 45 most affected countries by about 8 years. Although this reduction will result in lower population growth in the highly affected countries than would have been expected without AIDS, outright reductions of population brought about by AIDS are generally not expected because most of the highly affected countries have and are expected to maintain moderate to high fertility levels relative to those of other countries.

In fact, as already shown in Fig. 5.3, the projected growth rates for the population of the world, though generally expected to decline over the next fifty years, are likely to remain well above the level they maintained before 1750. Furthermore, it is important to underscore that, whereas sustained low growth in the past was the result of high fertility coupled with very high mortality, in the future lower growth will most likely be universally attained by a combination of low fertility and low mortality. All the projection variants discussed above reflect this view. Even in the high variant, fertility remains at moderate to low levels which lead to substantial population growth only because they are higher than the level necessary for the long-term replacement of the population under conditions of low mortality. As Table 5.5 indicates, the high variant produces a world population of nearly 11 billion by 2050. However, the growth rates plotted in Fig. 5.3 suggest that the high variant may not represent the most likely path for future population growth at the world level since they show a marked change of trend with respect to the growth rates observed recently. Those for the medium and low variants appear to be more consistent with recent trends, at least over the next 10 or 20 years. Yet, whereas the medium variant produces a steadily increasing

---

[5] The 45 highly affected countries are, in Africa: Angola, Benin, Botswana, Burkina Faso, Burundi, Cameroon, Central African Republic, Chad, Congo, Côte d'Ivoire, Democratic Republic of the Congo, Djibouti, Eritrea, Ethiopia, Gabon, Gambia, Ghana, Guinea-Bissau, Kenya, Lesotho, Liberia, Malawi, Mali, Mozambique, Namibia, Nigeria, Rwanda, Sierra Leone, South Africa, Swaziland, Togo, Uganda, United Republic of Tanzania, Zambia and Zimbabwe. In Asia: Cambodia, India, Thailand and Myanmar. In Latin America and the Caribbean: Bahamas, Brazil, the Dominican Republic, Guyana, Haiti and Honduras. Except for Brazil and India, they all had an HIV prevalence among persons aged 15–49 of 1.9% or higher in 1999.

**Table 5.5** Estimated and projected population by major area, development grouping and projection variant, 1950–2050 (in millions)

| Major area | 1950 | 1975 | 2000 | 2025 | | | 2050 | | |
|---|---|---|---|---|---|---|---|---|---|
| | | | | Low | Medium | High | Low | Medium | High |
| World | 2519 | 4066 | 6057 | 7470 | 7937 | 8391 | 7866 | 9322 | 10 934 |
| More-developed regions | 814 | 1048 | 1191 | 1187 | 1219 | 1257 | 1075 | 1181 | 1309 |
| Less-developed regions | 1706 | 3017 | 4865 | 6283 | 6718 | 7135 | 6791 | 8141 | 9625 |
| Least-developed countries | 197 | 348 | 658 | 1112 | 1186 | 1255 | 1545 | 1830 | 2130 |
| Africa | 221 | 406 | 794 | 1275 | 1358 | 1434 | 1694 | 2000 | 2320 |
| Asia | 1399 | 2397 | 3672 | 4474 | 4777 | 5068 | 4527 | 5428 | 6430 |
| Latin America and the Caribbean | 167 | 322 | 519 | 644 | 695 | 746 | 657 | 806 | 975 |
| Northern America | 172 | 243 | 314 | 369 | 384 | 404 | 389 | 438 | 502 |
| Europe | 548 | 676 | 727 | 669 | 684 | 698 | 556 | 603 | 654 |
| Oceania | 13 | 21 | 31 | 39 | 40 | 41 | 42 | 47 | 53 |

Source: United Nations (2001a).

**Table 5.6** Estimated and projected average annual population growth rates, for the world and major areas, by projection variant, 1950–2050

| Major area | 1950–1975 | 1975–2000 | 1995–2000 | 2000–2025 | | | 2025–2050 | | |
|---|---|---|---|---|---|---|---|---|---|
| | | | | Low | Medium | High | Low | Medium | High |
| World | 1.91 | 1.59 | 1.35 | 0.84 | 1.08 | 1.30 | 0.21 | 0.64 | 1.06 |
| More-developed regions | 1.01 | 0.51 | 0.30 | −0.02 | 0.09 | 0.21 | −0.39 | −0.13 | 0.16 |
| Less-developed regions | 2.28 | 1.91 | 1.62 | 1.02 | 1.29 | 1.53 | 0.31 | 0.77 | 1.20 |
| Least-developed countries | 2.26 | 2.55 | 2.50 | 2.10 | 2.36 | 2.58 | 1.32 | 1.73 | 2.12 |
| Africa | 2.44 | 2.68 | 2.41 | 1.90 | 2.15 | 2.37 | 1.14 | 1.55 | 1.92 |
| Asia | 2.15 | 1.71 | 1.41 | 0.79 | 1.05 | 1.29 | 0.05 | 0.51 | 0.95 |
| Latin America and the Caribbean | 2.62 | 1.91 | 1.56 | 0.86 | 1.17 | 1.45 | 0.08 | 0.59 | 1.07 |
| Northern America | 1.40 | 1.02 | 1.04 | 0.64 | 0.80 | 1.01 | 0.22 | 0.53 | 0.87 |
| Europe | 0.84 | 0.29 | −0.04 | −0.33 | −0.25 | −0.17 | −0.74 | −0.50 | −0.26 |
| Oceania | 2.09 | 1.44 | 1.37 | 0.96 | 1.09 | 1.22 | 0.36 | 0.66 | 0.96 |

Source: United Nations (2001a).

population that reaches 9.3 billion by 2050, the low variant leads eventually to negative population growth (by 2045–2050) and produces a significantly lower population (7.9 billion in 2050).

The implications of the different projection variants for future population growth are even more diverse at the level of development groups and major areas. Because of the diversity of past fertility and mortality levels, the populations of major areas are already growing at very different rates. Thus, whereas Africa's population is increasing at 2.4% per year, Europe's is decreasing at a rate of −0.04% (Table 5.6). The populations of Asia, Latin America and the Caribbean, and Oceania are still increasing at robust rates of 1.4% per year or higher, and even Northern America's population is growing at a rate slightly above 1% per year, largely as a result of its moderately high fertility and net population gains through international migration. Owing to these varied experiences, population growth in the less-developed regions is nearly four times faster than in the more developed regions, and that differential is expected to become more accentuated in the future. Thus, during 2000–2025, less-developed regions are expected to grow 14 times faster than the more-developed regions in the medium variant and 7 times faster in the high variant, and according to the low variant, the population of more-developed regions will decline slowly, whereas that of less-developed regions will grow at a rate slightly above 1% per year. During 2025–2050, further reductions in growth rates for the more- and the less-developed regions are expected in all projection variants, but the differentials between them remain large. In the low and medium variants in particular, the population of more-developed regions is projected to decline during that period, whereas very substantial population increases are expected in the less-developed regions.

With regard to major areas, only Europe is expected to experience a reduction of the population in all the projection variants and Africa is expected to experience rapid population growth no matter which variant is considered. Differences between the variants become more marked the further one moves into the future so that by 2025–2050, the growth rates yielded by the high variant tend to be nearly 1% higher than those produced by the low variant. Consequently, while in the low variant most major areas are expected to experience rates of growth that approach zero, in the high variant the rates of growth are closer to 1%. The exceptions are Africa whose growth rate in the low variant is close to 1% and in the high is close to 2%, and Europe whose rate of decline in the low variant is −0.74% and in the high variant is −0.26%.

The marked differences in expected growth rates for the major areas result in a redistribution of the population among them. The population of more developed regions, which is expected to be between 1.1 billion and 1.3 billion in 2050, will not be very different from that of today (1.2 billion), but there will be a redistribution of the population between the two major areas in the developed world. Thus, whereas the population of Europe is expected to decline from the 0.73 billion of 2000 to between 0.56 billion and 0.65 billion, that of Northern America will likely increase from 0.3 billion to somewhere between 0.4 billion and 0.5 billion. In the developing world, in contrast, large population increases are expected according to all projection variants. The population of the less-developed regions is expected to rise from 4.9 billion persons in 2000 to somewhere in the range of 6.8 billion to 9.6 billion, with the medium variant producing 8.1 billion. Among the major areas in the developing world, Africa is projected to record the largest relative increase, with its population doubling or tripling depending on the projection variant. Thus, its population passes from 0.8 billion in 2000 to 2 billion in 2050 according to the medium variant and might rise as high as 2.3 billion according to the high variant. The populations of Asia and Latin America and the Caribbean increase by about 50% according to the medium variant, so that the population of Asia passes from 3.7 billion in 2000 to 5.4 billion in 2050, and that of Latin America and the Caribbean rises from 0.5 billion in 2000 to

**Table 5.7** Percentage distribution of the estimated and projected population of the world and major areas, by projection variant, 1950–2050

| Major area | 1950 | 1975 | 2000 | 2050 Low | 2050 Medium | 2050 High |
|---|---|---|---|---|---|---|
| World | 100.0 | 100.0 | 100.0 | 100.0 | 100.0 | 100.0 |
| More-developed regions | 32.3 | 25.8 | 19.7 | 13.7 | 12.7 | 12.0 |
| Less-developed regions | 67.7 | 74.2 | 80.3 | 86.3 | 87.3 | 88.0 |
| Least-developed countries | 7.8 | 8.6 | 10.9 | 19.6 | 19.6 | 19.5 |
| Africa | 8.8 | 10.0 | 13.1 | 21.5 | 21.5 | 21.2 |
| Asia | 55.5 | 58.9 | 60.6 | 57.5 | 58.2 | 58.8 |
| Latin America and the Caribbean | 6.6 | 7.9 | 8.6 | 8.4 | 8.6 | 8.9 |
| Northern America | 6.8 | 6.0 | 5.2 | 5.0 | 4.7 | 4.6 |
| Europe | 21.8 | 16.6 | 12.0 | 7.1 | 6.5 | 6.0 |
| Oceania | 0.5 | 0.5 | 0.5 | 0.5 | 0.5 | 0.5 |

Source: United Nations (2001a).

0.8 billion in 2050. For Asia the low and high variants produce populations that are lower or higher by nearly 1 billion from that yielded by the medium variant. In the case of Latin America and the Caribbean, the equivalent difference is of the order of 150 million.

The changes in projected population size imply that by 2050 there will be a greater concentration of the population in the less-developed regions (Table 5.7). Thus, whereas in 2000 nearly 80% of the world's population lived in the less-developed regions, by 2050 that proportion will rise to between 86 and 88%. Furthermore, among the major areas in the developing world a marked increase in the proportion living in Africa is expected: from 13% in 2000 to more than 21% in 2050. In contrast, the percentage living in Asia will decline slightly, from 61% to between 57 and 58%, and Europe's share will decline markedly from 12% in 2000 to between 6 and 7% in 2050.

The further concentration of the population in the less-developed regions will not be accompanied by an increasing concentration in a few countries, although most of the populous countries of the world will be developing countries. As Table 5.8 indicates, 21 countries accounted in 1950 for three-quarters of the world's population and 10 among them were located in the more-developed regions. By 2000, 24 countries were needed to account for the same proportion of the world's inhabitants, but just eight were developed countries. By 2050, 29 countries are expected to account for 75% of the world population according to the medium variant with just five belonging to the more-developed regions. Furthermore, over the next fifty years India will likely displace China as the most populous country of the world and China's share of the population will decline considerably, passing from 21% in 2000 to 16% in 2050 according to the medium variant. Indeed, given the size of China's population and the fact that China's fertility is projected to remain below replacement level after 2000 in the medium variant, China is expected to experience the largest population

**Table 5.8** Countries accounting for 75% of the world population by order of population size, 1950, 2000, and 2050, medium variant

| Country | Population in 1950 (000) | Cumulated percentage |
|---|---|---|
| 1 China | 554 760 | 22 |
| 2 India | 357 561 | 36 |
| 3 United States | 157 813 | 42 |
| 4 Russian Federation | 102 702 | 47 |
| 5 Japan | 83 625 | 50 |
| 6 Indonesia | 79 538 | 53 |
| 7 Germany | 68 376 | 56 |
| 8 Brazil | 53 975 | 58 |
| 9 United Kingdom | 50 616 | 60 |
| 10 Italy | 47 104 | 62 |
| 11 France | 41 829 | 63 |
| 12 Bangladesh | 41 783 | 65 |
| 13 Pakistan | 39 659 | 67 |
| 14 Ukraine | 37 298 | 68 |
| 15 Nigeria | 29 790 | 69 |
| 16 Spain | 28 009 | 70 |
| 17 Mexico | 27 737 | 72 |
| 18 Vietnam | 27 367 | 73 |
| 19 Poland | 24 824 | 74 |
| 20 Egypt | 21 834 | 74 |
| 21 Turkey | 20 809 | 75 |

| Country | Population in 2000 (000) | Cumulated percentage |
|---|---|---|
| 1 China | 1 275 133 | 21 |
| 2 India | 1 008 937 | 38 |
| 3 United States | 283 230 | 42 |
| 4 Indonesia | 212 092 | 46 |
| 5 Brazil | 170 406 | 49 |
| 6 Russian Federation | 145 491 | 51 |
| 7 Pakistan | 141 256 | 53 |
| 8 Bangladesh | 137 439 | 56 |
| 9 Japan | 127 096 | 58 |
| 10 Nigeria | 113 862 | 60 |
| 11 Mexico | 98 872 | 61 |
| 12 Germany | 82 017 | 63 |
| 13 Vietnam | 78 137 | 64 |
| 14 Philippines | 75 653 | 65 |
| 15 Iran (Islamic Republic of) | 70 330 | 66 |
| 16 Egypt | 67 884 | 67 |
| 17 Turkey | 66 668 | 69 |
| 18 Ethiopia | 62 908 | 70 |
| 19 Thailand | 62 806 | 71 |
| 20 United Kingdom | 59 415 | 72 |
| 21 France | 59 238 | 73 |
| 22 Italy | 57 530 | 74 |
| 23 Dem. Rep. of the Congo | 50 948 | 74 |
| 24 Ukraine | 49 568 | 75 |

| Country | Population in 2050 (000) | Cumulated percentage |
|---|---|---|
| 1 India | 1 572 055 | 17 |
| 2 China | 1 462 058 | 33 |
| 3 United States | 397 063 | 37 |
| 4 Pakistan | 344 170 | 40 |
| 5 Indonesia | 311 335 | 44 |
| 6 Nigeria | 278 788 | 47 |
| 7 Bangladesh | 265 432 | 50 |
| 8 Brazil | 247 244 | 52 |
| 9 Dem. Rep. of the Congo | 203 527 | 55 |
| 10 Ethiopia | 186 452 | 57 |
| 11 Mexico | 146 651 | 58 |
| 12 Philippines | 128 383 | 59 |
| 13 Vietnam | 123 782 | 61 |
| 14 Iran (Islamic Republic of) | 121 424 | 62 |
| 15 Egypt | 113 840 | 63 |
| 16 Japan | 109 220 | 64 |
| 17 Russian Federation | 104 258 | 66 |
| 18 Yemen | 102 379 | 67 |
| 19 Uganda | 101 524 | 68 |
| 20 Turkey | 98 818 | 69 |
| 21 United Rep. of Tanzania | 82 740 | 70 |
| 22 Thailand | 82 491 | 71 |
| 23 Afghanistan | 72 267 | 71 |
| 24 Colombia | 70 862 | 72 |
| 25 Germany | 70 805 | 73 |
| 26 Myanmar | 68 546 | 74 |
| 27 Sudan | 63 530 | 74 |
| 28 France | 61 832 | 75 |
| 29 Saudi Arabia | 59 683 | 76 |

Source: United Nations (2001a).

**Table 5.9** Countries experiencing the largest reductions or the largest increases of population in 2000–2005 and 2045–2050, medium variant

| Country or area | Population change in 2000–2005 (thousands) | Country or area | Population change in 2045–2050 (thousands) |
|---|---|---|---|
| *Reductions* | | | |
| 1 Russian Federation | −4571.3 | China | −18 874.0 |
| 2 Ukraine | −2269.8 | Russian Federation | −4370.8 |
| 3 Bulgaria | −379.7 | Japan | −3255.4 |
| 4 Italy | −365.0 | Italy | −2166.9 |
| 5 Kazakhstan | −296.6 | Ukraine | −1937.2 |
| 6 Romania | −287.4 | Germany | −1867.6 |
| 7 Hungary | −247.0 | Spain | −1521.0 |
| 8 Belarus | −203.0 | Poland | −799.5 |
| 9 Poland | −178.5 | United Kingdom | −742.3 |
| 10 Germany | −156.8 | Republic of Korea | −638.3 |
| 11 Georgia | −137.8 | Romania | −538.1 |
| 12 Yugoslavia | −77.7 | France | −508.7 |
| 13 Estonia | −77.2 | Cuba | −331.1 |
| 14 Latvia | −67.2 | Bulgaria | −303.9 |
| 15 Sweden | −57.1 | Kazakhstan | −285.4 |
| *Increases* | | | |
| 1 India | 79 644 | India | 31 805 |
| 2 China | 46 231 | Pakistan | 17 273 |
| 3 Pakistan | 19 090 | Dem. Rep. of the Congo | 15 646 |
| 4 Nigeria | 15 860 | Nigeria | 14 824 |
| 5 Bangladesh | 15 113 | Ethiopia | 14 586 |
| 6 Indonesia | 13 246 | Yemen | 11 808 |
| 7 United States | 12 834 | Uganda | 9306 |
| 8 Brazil | 10 680 | Bangladesh | 9161 |
| 9 Dem. Rep. of the Congo | 9258 | United States | 9137 |
| 10 Ethiopia | 8055 | Niger | 5828 |
| 11 Philippines | 7352 | Indonesia | 5376 |
| 12 Mexico | 7267 | Angola | 5349 |
| 13 Egypt | 5922 | Afghanistan | 4990 |
| 14 Vietnam | 5260 | Somalia | 4250 |
| 15 Iran (Islamic Republic of) | 5036 | United Rep. of Tanzania | 4185 |

Source: United Nations (2001a).

reductions: during 2045–2050 alone its population is projected to decrease by nearly 19 million persons. At that time, 64 countries or areas are projected to experience negative rates of growth and therefore reductions of the population, up from the 27 expected to do so during 2000–2005. Table 5.9 shows the 15 countries expected to experience the largest reductions in population in 2000–2005 and 2045–2050. Note that, whereas the list for the earlier period includes mostly European countries and some of the successor states of the former Soviet Union, that for 2045–2050 also includes several countries from Eastern Asia (China, Japan, and the Republic of Korea) as well as Cuba.

Table 5.9 also shows the countries expected to record the largest increases of population in 2000–2005 and 2045–2050: they are mostly located in the developing world. India heads the list in both periods, although its population increment is expected to drop by more than half between the two periods. Only one developed country, the United States, is expected to experience large population increments partly as a result of the high numbers of immigrants projected to move to that country. In 2000–2005, countries from nearly all major areas are among those expected to experience large population increases, including two from Latin America (Brazil and Mexico) and three from sub-Saharan Africa (the Democratic Republic of Congo, Ethiopia, and Nigeria). By 2045–2050, in contrast, the countries with the highest population increases in absolute terms are most likely to be in sub-Saharan Africa (8 out of 15) or in the Indian subcontinent (Bangladesh, India, and Pakistan). Furthermore, the largest increments in 2045–2050 are generally considerably smaller than those expected in 2000–2005. That is, as a result of the projected long-term reduction of fertility, expected population increments are expected to decline markedly even in the most populous countries over the next 50 years.

To complete the picture, let us consider the countries that are expected to experience the highest and the lowest rates of population growth during 2000–2050 (Table 5.10). The fastest growing countries tend to have relatively small populations that are projected to grow at sustained rates well above 2% per year over the period. As a result, their populations will increase dramatically, tripling in most cases but becoming five times larger than in 2000 in the cases of Liberia, Niger, and Yemen. The most populous country in this group, the Democratic Republic of Congo, is expected to see its population quadruple by 2050, rising from 51 million in 2000 to 204 million. Most of the countries with rapidly growing populations are among those that have not yet shown clear signs of embarking on the fertility transition or those whose fertility is still high. Even with the fairly large fertility reductions projected for the future, their fertility levels remain above those of other countries and have the potential of leading to very rapid and sustained growth if mortality levels keep on declining as projected.

At the other end of the distribution, the countries expected to experience the lowest rates of growth are among those whose populations are expected to decline during the projection period. Expected rates of population decline, even for the most rapidly declining populations, are considerably more moderate in absolute terms than the highest rates of population growth expected. Consequently, they lead in most cases to moderate reductions of population size over the next fifty years. Only two countries, Bulgaria and Estonia are expected to see their populations reduced by about half during 2000–2050. In most countries with rapidly declining populations the overall reductions over that period are expected to be in the range of 20–30%. The population of the Russian Federation, for instance, is projected to decline by about 28%, from 145 million in 2000 to 104 million in 2050. Sustained low fertility combined with mortality levels that are expected to decline more slowly than in other developed countries contribute to this outcome.

These results underscore the increasing heterogeneity of population dynamics that has been plain for the past century and that is expected to continue well into the

**Table 5.10** Countries with the highest and lowest expected rates of growth during 2000–2050 (medium variant)

| Country or area | Population (thousands) | | Growth rate (percentage) |
|---|---|---|---|
| | 2000 | 2050 | |
| *Highest growth rate* | | | |
| 1 Yemen | 18 349 | 102 379 | 3.44 |
| 2 Liberia | 2913 | 14 370 | 3.19 |
| 3 Niger | 10 832 | 51 872 | 3.13 |
| 4 Somalia | 8778 | 40 936 | 3.08 |
| 5 Uganda | 23 300 | 101 524 | 2.94 |
| 6 Angola | 13 134 | 53 328 | 2.80 |
| 7 Burkina Faso | 11 535 | 46 304 | 2.78 |
| 8 Dem. Rep. of the Congo | 50 948 | 203 527 | 2.77 |
| 9 Occupied Palestinian Terr. | 3191 | 11 821 | 2.62 |
| 10 Mali | 11 351 | 41 724 | 2.60 |
| 11 Congo | 3018 | 10 744 | 2.54 |
| 12 Chad | 7885 | 27 732 | 2.52 |
| 13 Oman | 2538 | 8751 | 2.48 |
| 14 Afghanistan | 21 765 | 72 267 | 2.40 |
| 15 Solomon Islands | 447 | 1458 | 2.36 |
| *Lowest growth rate* | | | |
| 1 Estonia | 1393 | 752 | −1.23 |
| 2 Bulgaria | 7949 | 4531 | −1.12 |
| 3 Ukraine | 49 568 | 29 959 | −1.01 |
| 4 Georgia | 5262 | 3219 | −0.98 |
| 5 Guyana | 761 | 504 | −0.82 |
| 6 Russian Federation | 145 491 | 104 258 | −0.67 |
| 7 Latvia | 2421 | 1744 | −0.66 |
| 8 Italy | 57 530 | 42 962 | −0.58 |
| 9 Hungary | 9968 | 7486 | −0.57 |
| 10 Slovenia | 1988 | 1527 | −0.53 |
| 11 Switzerland | 7170 | 5607 | −0.49 |
| 12 Spain | 39 910 | 31 282 | −0.49 |
| 13 Gibraltar | 27 | 21 | −0.49 |
| 14 Austria | 8080 | 6452 | −0.45 |
| 15 Lithuania | 3696 | 2989 | −0.42 |

Source: United Nations (2001a).

21st century as countries undergo the demographic transition to low mortality and low fertility at different paces and facing different obstacles. Countries that have lagged behind in the transition to low fertility also tend to be those where mortality levels remain high. Many are already affected significantly by the HIV/AIDS epidemic and are therefore facing a more difficult task than in the past to ensure a longer life for most of their citizens. Whether they can muster the resources needed both to reduce mortality levels and to provide support for the reduction of fertility is still an open question. In the developed world, the maintenance of very low fertility levels is already producing reductions of population, especially in countries where mortality levels have stagnated or increased over the past two or three decades. In countries with economies in transition, achieving a steady reduction of mortality in future demands important changes in access to health care, the improvement of health systems, and the implementation of programs to effect behavioral change at the societal level, interventions that are both demanding and costly. In addition, several of those countries are being faced with the spread of infectious diseases, such as tuberculosis and HIV/AIDS, whose treatment is expensive and requires close supervision by health professionals. Under such conditions, it is unlikely that much effort will be expended in devising measures to promote higher fertility, especially since the evidence on their effectiveness is weak. Consequently, the likelihood of the continuation of recent trends, that is, of low fertility and only moderate gains in life expectancy, in the medium-term future is high. Lastly, varying rates of population aging will also lead to further heterogeneity among the world's population, since countries that embarked early on the transition to low fertility and those that have been experiencing below-replacement fertility will experience very marked aging whereas the populations of countries that are expected to continue growing at a rapid pace will experience a more moderate aging process. The dynamics of aging will be discussed in the next section.

# Population aging

One of the major consequences of the transition to low fertility is the aging of the population. Indeed, sustained fertility reductions lead over time to populations where the proportion of children declines while that of adults rises, especially that of adults at older ages. Following the usual definition of children as persons aged 0 to 14, elderly persons as those aged 60 years or over, and using the term adults from now on to refer only to persons aged 15 to 59, in 2000, 30% of the world's population was constituted by children, 60% by adults and 10% by elderly persons. According to the medium variant, it is expected that by 2050 the proportion of the elderly will more than double, reaching 21%, that of children will be reduced by approximately one-third, reaching also 21%, and that of adults will remain largely unchanged, at 58% (Table 5.11). This changing distribution of the population by age is brought about by major changes in the rate of growth of the populations of children and the elderly (Fig. 5.5). Thus, whereas the growth rate of children declined from about 2.5% per year in the 1950s to nearly 0.4% per year in 1995–2000 and is expected to stay below that level until 2050, the growth rate of the elderly has been consistently high, varying largely between 2% and 2.5% annually since 1960, and is expected to increase even further over the period 2000–2030 to remain above 2.5% per year before declining to 1.6% per year in 2045–2050. The expected high rates of growth of the elderly population will result in more than a threefold increase in their numbers between 2000 and 2050, from 0.6 billion to nearly 2 billion, so that whereas in 2000 there were nearly three children for every elderly person, by 2050 there will be just one child per elderly person.

Because the process of population aging started earlier in the more-developed regions than in the rest of the world, their age distribution in 2000 is similar to the one expected at the world level for 2050. Indeed, as of 2000, the more-developed regions already had as many elderly persons as the number of children, and each of those

**Table 5.11** Age composition of the population by broad age group, major area and region, medium variant, 2000 and 2050

| Major area | 2000 | | | 2050 | | |
|---|---|---|---|---|---|---|
| | 0–14 | 15–59 | 60+ | 0–14 | 15–59 | 60+ |
| *Population (thousands)* | | | | | | |
| World | 1815 | 3636 | 606 | 1955 | 5404 | 1964 |
| More-developed regions | 218 | 742 | 231 | 183 | 603 | 395 |
| Less-developed regions | 1597 | 2894 | 374 | 1771 | 4801 | 1569 |
| Least-developed countries | 284 | 342 | 32 | 533 | 1123 | 173 |
| Africa | 338 | 415 | 40 | 559 | 1236 | 205 |
| Asia | 1111 | 2240 | 322 | 1061 | 3141 | 1227 |
| Latin America and the Caribbean | 164 | 314 | 41 | 161 | 463 | 181 |
| Northern America | 67 | 196 | 51 | 80 | 238 | 119 |
| Europe | 127 | 453 | 147 | 84 | 298 | 221 |
| Oceania | 8 | 19 | 4 | 9 | 27 | 11 |
| *Percentage* | | | | | | |
| World | 30.0 | 60.0 | 10.0 | 21.0 | 58.0 | 21.1 |
| More-developed regions | 18.3 | 62.3 | 19.4 | 15.5 | 51.0 | 33.5 |
| Less-developed regions | 32.8 | 59.5 | 7.7 | 21.8 | 59.0 | 19.3 |
| Least-developed countries | 43.1 | 52.0 | 4.9 | 29.1 | 61.4 | 9.5 |
| Africa | 42.6 | 52.3 | 5.1 | 28.0 | 61.8 | 10.2 |
| Asia | 30.2 | 61.0 | 8.8 | 19.5 | 57.9 | 22.6 |
| Latin America and the Caribbean | 31.5 | 60.5 | 8.0 | 20.0 | 57.5 | 22.5 |
| Northern America | 21.5 | 62.3 | 16.2 | 18.3 | 54.5 | 27.2 |
| Europe | 17.5 | 62.3 | 20.3 | 13.9 | 49.4 | 36.6 |
| Oceania | 25.4 | 61.2 | 13.4 | 19.4 | 57.3 | 23.3 |

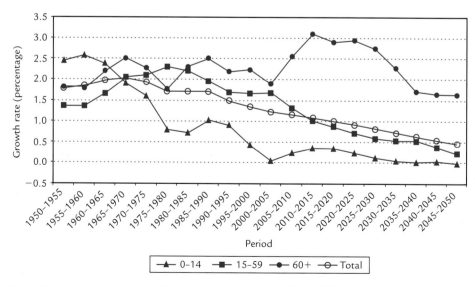

**Figure 5.5** Growth rates of the different age groups at the world level, 1950–2050.

**Table 5.12** Median age of the population for the world and major areas, by projection variant, 1950, 2000, and 2050

| Major area or region | 1950 | 2000 | 2050 High | 2050 Medium | 2050 Low |
|---|---|---|---|---|---|
| World | 23.6 | 26.5 | 31.9 | 36.2 | 41.5 |
| More-developed regions | 28.6 | 37.4 | 42.2 | 46.4 | 50.3 |
| Less-developed regions | 21.4 | 24.3 | 30.8 | 35.0 | 40.2 |
| Least-developed countries | 19.5 | 18.2 | 24.0 | 26.5 | 29.5 |
| Africa | 19.0 | 18.4 | 24.8 | 27.4 | 30.5 |
| Asia | 22.0 | 26.2 | 33.4 | 38.3 | 44.2 |
| Latin America and the Caribbean | 20.1 | 24.4 | 32.6 | 37.8 | 44.4 |
| Northern America | 29.8 | 35.6 | 36.5 | 41.0 | 45.4 |
| Europe | 29.2 | 37.7 | 45.9 | 49.5 | 52.7 |
| Oceania | 27.9 | 30.9 | 34.6 | 38.1 | 41.7 |

Source: United Nations (2001a).

groups accounted for about a fifth of the population (actually, children were less numerous than the elderly). But aging in the more-developed regions is continuing. The maintenance of low fertility over the foreseeable future produces a population in 2050 where the elderly are expected to constitute a third of the population and children will account for only one in every seven persons. In fact, because fertility has already been very low in the more-developed regions for some time, the proportion of children is not expected to decline as much (from 18% in 2000 to 15% in 2050) as the adult population (from 62% in 2000 to 51% in 2050). That is, the population of more-developed regions is already entering the advanced stages of the aging process as the population of adults itself becomes considerably older. Another way to gauge the effects of population aging is to consider the median age of the population, that is, the age that divides the population into two equal halves. For the more developed regions, the median age rose from 29 years in 1950 to 37 years in 2000 and is expected to reach 46 years in the medium variant (Table 5.12). Aging would be more pronounced if fertility were to remain even lower, so that the low variant produces a population with a median age of 50 years, but even the higher fertility of the high variant would lead to substantial further rises in the median age which would be above 42 years in 2050.

Population aging is also expected in the less-developed regions as a whole, whose median age is expected to rise from 24 years in 2000 to between 31 and 40 years in 2050, with the medium variant producing a median age of 35 years. According to the medium variant, the elderly population in the less-developed regions would increase fourfold during 2000–2050, rising from 0.4 billion to nearly 1.6 billion, whereas the number of children would remain largely unchanged, passing from 1.6 billion to 1.8 billion. By the end of the projection period the less-developed regions would still have 58% of their population in the adult ages, with about a fifth of the population in each of the other two categories. Among the less-developed regions, the group of least-developed countries is expected to experience a more moderate aging, with the median age rising from 18 years in 2000 to between 24 and 30 years by 2050 (the medium variant produces a median age of 27 years). Nevertheless, in the medium variant the elderly population of the least-developed countries increases fivefold during 2000–2050, rising from 32 million to 172 million, and its share of the population nearly doubles, passing from 4.9% to 9.5%. Yet, by 2050 the least-developed countries will still have about three children for each elderly person, approximating therefore the age distribution of the less-developed regions of today.

At the level of major areas, Europe is expected to have the most aged population by 2050, whereas Africa will have the least aged. The median age of Europe's population is expected to be between 46 and 53 years in 2050, with a medium variant value of approximately 50 years. By that time, nearly 37% of the population is expected to be aged 60 or over and slight less than half is expected to be aged 15–59. Children will account for just 14% of the population and the elderly will outnumber children nearly 3 to 1. In Africa, in contrast, the number of children is expected to be nearly double that of the elderly, and the latter will likely constitute just 10% of the population. The median age in Africa is expected to rise considerably, but starting at 18 in 2000 will at most rise to 30 years by 2050, being more likely to remain in the 20s (24 is projected under the high variant and 27 under the medium variant).

All other major areas are expected to have similar age distributions in 2050, with about 22% of the population being aged 60 or over, about 19% being children and 57% being adults aged 15–59. Northern America will have a slightly more aged population than the other major areas, with a median age of 41 years in 2050 according to the medium variant, rather than the 38 years expected for Asia, Latin America and the Caribbean, and Oceania. However, the convergence of the age distributions of Asia and Latin America and the Caribbean, in particular, to that of Northern America is the result of the very rapid aging of the populations of those two major areas. Indeed, as of 2000 both Asia and Latin America and the Caribbean had a considerably younger population than that of Northern America: their proportion of elderly persons was nearly half of that in Northern America and their median ages were about ten years lower than that of Northern America. The rapid reductions of fertility projected for Asia and Latin America and the Caribbean, which are largely based on the very substantial fertility reductions already experienced by some of the largest countries in those continents, are responsible for accelerating the aging of their population. That is, these developing regions will have less time to adapt to the economic and social implications of an aging population and need to act early to ensure that their societies are able to cope with the added demands for services, health care and social security associated with an aging population. The problem will be particularly acute in Asia, where the number of elderly persons is expected to rise fourfold during 2000–2050, so that by the end of the period Asia will have by far the largest elderly population in the world (1.2 billion), accounting for six out of every ten elderly persons in the world at that time. Furthermore, most of the elderly will be concentrated in the populous countries of Asia, especially in China (437 million), India (324 million), Indonesia (70 million), Japan (46 million), Bangladesh and Pakistan (each with 43 million). In Latin America, Brazil and Mexico will also have large populations of elderly persons: 59 million in Brazil and 36 million in Mexico. Although the more-developed countries will have more aged populations than most

**Table 5.13** Countries with the highest and the lowest median ages, 1950, 2000, and 2050, medium variant

| Country or area | 1950 | Country or area | 2000 | Country or area | 2050 |
|---|---|---|---|---|---|
| *Highest* | | | | | |
| 1 Austria | 35.80 | 1 Japan | 41.22 | Spain | 55.21 |
| 2 Channel Islands | 35.73 | 2 Italy | 40.19 | Slovenia | 54.10 |
| 3 Belgium | 35.55 | 3 Switzerland | 40.18 | Italy | 54.08 |
| 4 Germany | 35.37 | 4 Germany | 40.06 | Austria | 53.70 |
| 5 Luxembourg | 35.00 | 5 Sweden | 39.70 | Armenia | 53.45 |
| 6 United Kingdom | 34.63 | 6 Finland | 39.43 | Japan | 53.14 |
| 7 France | 34.51 | 7 Bulgaria | 39.14 | Czech Republic | 52.37 |
| 8 Sweden | 34.26 | 8 Belgium | 39.13 | Greece | 52.32 |
| 9 Switzerland | 33.33 | 9 Greece | 39.12 | Switzerland | 52.03 |
| *Lowest* | | | | | |
| 1 Occupied Palestinian Terr. | 17.19 | 1 Benin | 16.58 | Malawi | 23.71 |
| 2 Malawi | 17.12 | 2 Zambia | 16.55 | Burundi | 23.25 |
| 3 Iraq | 17.04 | 3 Burundi | 16.03 | Mali | 22.95 |
| 4 Rwanda | 16.97 | 4 Somalia | 15.97 | Liberia | 22.92 |
| 5 United Rep. of Tanzania | 16.94 | 5 Angola | 15.88 | Burkina Faso | 22.75 |
| 6 Vanuatu | 16.78 | 6 Democratic Rep. of the Congo | 15.58 | Uganda | 22.11 |
| 7 Botswana | 16.78 | 7 Burkina Faso | 15.56 | Somalia | 21.54 |
| 8 Fiji | 16.58 | 8 Uganda | 15.36 | Angola | 21.23 |
| 9 Samoa | 16.56 | 9 Niger | 15.06 | Yemen | 21.10 |
| 10 Djibouti | 16.53 | 10 Yemen | 14.97 | Niger | 20.39 |

Source: United Nations (2001a).

developing countries, the largest numbers of elderly persons will be increasingly concentrated in the developing world.

To conclude this analysis of the dynamics of population aging, let us consider the countries that have had or are expected to have the "oldest" and the "youngest" populations in the world. Table 5.13 shows the list of countries with the highest and lowest median ages in 1950, 2000, and 2050. Over the course of that century, the median age of the oldest population has been rising steadily and that trend is expected to continue, so that the highest median age will likely pass from 36 years in Austria in 1950, to 41 years in Japan in 2000 and to a remarkably high 55 years in Spain in 2050. In contrast, the median age of the youngest population declined from 1950 to 2000 as a result of reductions in mortality and the consequent increases in the proportions of surviving children. Thus, the lowest median age declined from 16.5 years in Djibouti in 1950 to a remarkably low 15 years in Yemen in 2000. However, in future, signs of population aging are expected even in countries whose fertility is expected to decline at a slower pace. Indeed, by 2050 the lowest median age is expected to be 20 years in Niger, a full five years higher than the lowest median age in 2000. For Yemen itself, the median age is expected to rise by seven years, reaching 21 years by 2050. Consequently, by the middle of this century countries will vary significantly in terms of the stage they are likely to have reached in the transition to an older population. Very young populations, such as those expected in countries like Angola, Niger, Uganda, or Yemen, to name just a few, will coexist with very aged populations, such as those of Austria, Italy, Japan, or Spain. Diversity in the dynamics of population growth is at the root of such a wide variation of outcomes and implies that the average trends observed at the world level are not necessarily representative of the experience of many of the countries of the world.

## The dynamics of urbanization

If overall population growth during the second half of the 20th century was very rapid, even more rapid was the growth of the world's urban population. It is estimated that

**Table 5.14** Population in urban and rural areas, and proportion urban, for the world and major areas, 1950–2030

| Development group | 1950 | 1975 | 2000 | 2030 |
|---|---|---|---|---|
| *Urban population (millions)* | | | | |
| World | 750 | 1542 | 2847 | 4964 |
| More-developed regions | 447 | 734 | 906 | 1017 |
| Less-developed regions | 304 | 808 | 1941 | 3948 |
| Least-developed countries | 14 | 50 | 171 | 582 |
| Africa | 32 | 102 | 301 | 805 |
| Asia | 244 | 592 | 1348 | 2638 |
| Latin America and the Caribbean | 69 | 197 | 391 | 603 |
| Northern America | 110 | 180 | 243 | 334 |
| Europe | 287 | 455 | 544 | 554 |
| Oceania | 8 | 15 | 21 | 31 |
| *Rural population (millions)* | | | | |
| World | 1769 | 2524 | 3210 | 3306 |
| More-developed regions | 367 | 314 | 286 | 200 |
| Less-developed regions | 1402 | 2209 | 2924 | 3106 |
| Least-developed countries | 183 | 298 | 487 | 732 |
| Africa | 189 | 304 | 493 | 684 |
| Asia | 1155 | 1804 | 2324 | 2312 |
| Latin America and the Caribbean | 98 | 125 | 128 | 121 |
| Northern America | 62 | 64 | 72 | 62 |
| Europe | 261 | 221 | 184 | 116 |
| Oceania | 5 | 6 | 9 | 11 |
| *Percentage urban* | | | | |
| World | 29.8 | 37.9 | 47.0 | 60.0 |
| More-developed regions | 54.9 | 70.0 | 76.0 | 83.6 |
| Less-developed regions | 17.8 | 26.8 | 39.9 | 56.0 |
| Least-developed countries | 7.1 | 14.4 | 26.0 | 44.3 |
| Africa | 14.7 | 25.2 | 37.9 | 54.0 |
| Asia | 17.4 | 24.7 | 36.7 | 53.3 |
| Latin America and the Caribbean | 41.4 | 61.2 | 75.3 | 83.3 |
| Northern America | 63.9 | 73.8 | 77.2 | 84.4 |
| Europe | 52.4 | 67.3 | 74.8 | 82.7 |
| Oceania | 61.6 | 72.2 | 70.3 | 73.5 |

Source: United Nations (2001a,c).

the number of persons living in cities rose from 0.8 billion in 1950 to nearly 2.9 billion in 2000, implying a growth rate of 2.67% per year, higher than the rate of 1.75% per year at which the world population grew over the period (Tables 5.14 and 5.15). Since the difference between these two rates determines the speed of growth of the proportion urban, between 1950 and 2000 the world population urbanized rapidly, with the proportion urban rising at a rate of 0.91% per year and passing from 30% in 1950 to 47% in 2000. Although the urbanization of the world population is expected to continue, neither the urban population nor the proportion urban is expected to grow as rapidly in the future. During 2000–2030, the world urban population is projected to increase at a rate of 1.9% per year, reaching nearly 5 billion in 1930. In addition,

**Table 5.15** Urban and rural rates of population growth and rate of urbanization for the world and major areas, 1950–2030

| Development group | 1950–2000 | 2000–2030 |
|---|---|---|
| *Urban growth rate (%)* | | |
| World | 2.67 | 1.85 |
| More-developed regions | 1.41 | 0.39 |
| Less-developed regions | 3.71 | 2.37 |
| Least-developed countries | 5.00 | 4.08 |
| Africa | 4.46 | 3.28 |
| Asia | 3.42 | 2.24 |
| Latin America and the Caribbean | 3.46 | 1.44 |
| Northern America | 1.59 | 1.07 |
| Europe | 1.28 | 0.06 |
| Oceania | 2.03 | 1.20 |
| *Rural growth rate (%)* | | |
| World | 1.19 | 0.10 |
| More-developed regions | −0.50 | −1.19 |
| Less-developed regions | 1.47 | 0.20 |
| Least-developed countries | 1.95 | 1.35 |
| Africa | 1.92 | 1.09 |
| Asia | 1.40 | −0.02 |
| Latin America and the Caribbean | 0.54 | −0.20 |
| Northern America | 0.29 | −0.48 |
| Europe | −0.70 | −1.52 |
| Oceania | 1.25 | 0.66 |
| *Rate of urbanization (%)* | | |
| World | 0.91 | 0.81 |
| More-developed regions | 0.65 | 0.32 |
| Less-developed regions | 1.61 | 1.13 |
| Least-developed countries | 2.60 | 1.78 |
| Africa | 1.90 | 1.18 |
| Asia | 1.49 | 1.24 |
| Latin America and the Caribbean | 1.20 | 0.34 |
| Northern America | 0.38 | 0.30 |
| Europe | 0.71 | 0.34 |
| Oceania | 0.27 | 0.15 |

Source: United Nations (2001c).

since the world's total population will also increase more slowly, the proportion urban is expected to rise at a robust rate of 0.83% per year so that by 2030 the population of the world will likely be 60% urban.

In contrast with the rapid rise of the urban population, the growth of the world rural population has been slowing markedly. In 1950, seven out of every ten persons on earth lived in rural areas, and they numbered 1.8 billion. Over the course of the next fifty years, rural population growth averaged 1.19% per year and the rural population nearly doubled, reaching an estimated 3.2 billion by 2000, but during 2000–2030, rural population growth is expected to be minimal so that the number of rural inhabitants will have barely risen, reaching 3.3 billion by 2030. Consequently, most of the population growth expected during 2000–2030 will be absorbed by urban areas. Since natural increase is generally lower in urban than in rural areas and is expected to decline in both, a large proportion of the 2.1 billion persons that will be added to the urban population will be rural–urban migrants or persons who become urban dwellers as urban settlements expand geographically through the transformation of rural villages into cities.

The differences in population dynamics between the more- and the less-developed regions become accentuated when one considers the process of urbanization. Whereas the rural areas still house the majority of the population of less-developed regions, cities are the place of residence of most of the population of more-developed regions (Table 5.14). Moreover, the urban population of the less-developed regions has been growing considerably faster than that of the more-developed regions and, as a result, its share of the world urban population has been rising. In 1950 the urban population of more-developed regions was greater than that of less-developed regions (447 million vs. 304 million), but by 1975 the latter had surpassed the former (808 million vs. 734 million) and the difference between the two increased rapidly thereafter. In 2000, 1.94 billion urban dwellers were estimated to live in the less-developed regions and just 0.9 billion in the more-developed regions (Table 5.14). By 2030, with 3.9 billion urban dwellers, the less-developed regions are projected to have 79% of the world urban population, four times as many urban dwellers as the more-developed regions. To sustain such rapid population growth, the urban areas of the less-developed regions have been absorbing an increasing share of the annual increment of the urban population. Thus, whereas in 1950–1955 they absorbed 55% of the annual increment of the world urban population, by 1995–2000 they were absorbing 91% and by 2025–2030 they are expected to absorb 97%. In absolute terms, the urban areas of less-developed regions grew by 52 million persons annually in 1995–2000, whereas those of more-developed regions grew by just 5 million annually. By 2025–2030 it is expected that 69 million persons will be added annually to the urban population of the less-developed regions whereas the urban areas of more-developed regions will gain just 2 million new residents every year.

Not only are the urban areas of less-developed regions absorbing most of the population growth occurring in urban areas worldwide, they are also increasingly absorbing most of the growth of the total world population. Thus, whereas in 1950–1955 the increase in the population of the urban areas of the less-developed regions accounted for 28% of the total increment to the world population, by 1995–2000 that increase accounted for 67% of the annual increment to the world population and by 2020–2025 it is expected to surpass the latter. Such an outcome is consistent with a net transfer of population from rural to urban areas in the less-developed regions, either through migration or as a result of the territorial expansion of urban settlements and the transformation of rural villages into cities.

Levels and trends of urbanization also vary considerably among the world's major areas. Europe and Northern America, being part of the developed world, exhibit high levels of urbanization (i.e., high proportions of the population living in urban areas) and slowing rates of urban population growth (Tables 5.14 and 5.15). In the developing world, Africa and Asia remain largely rural, whereas Latin America and the Caribbean considered jointly have a high proportion of their population living in cities. Oceania, which straddles the developed and the developing world, is also highly urbanized. However, high levels of urbanization do not imply equally high numbers of urban dwellers. Asia, despite having the lowest proportion urban (36.7% in 2000), has the largest number of persons living in urban areas (1.3 billion). It is followed by Europe, with 544 million urban dwellers, Latin America and the Caribbean with 391 million, and Africa with 301 million. Because of the high urban growth rates expected in Africa and Asia during 2000–2030, by 2030 those two major areas will have the largest numbers of urban dwellers in the world: 2.6 billion in Asia and 0.8 billion in Africa, although they will still be the least urbanized major areas of the world. Yet, by 2030 the level of urbanization in both Africa and Asia will have passed the 50% mark and their populations will have become more urban than rural.

Latin America and the Caribbean has been the most highly urbanized area of the developing world. In addition, between 1950 and 2000, its proportion urban grew at a rate of 1.2% per year, more rapidly than those of Europe or Northern America. Consequently, by 2000, Latin America and the Caribbean had become just as urbanized as the major areas of the developed world. Over the next thirty years, however, these three major areas are expected to experience a marked decline in the rate of urbanization since the proportion urban is already quite high (around 75%) and is expected to rise to reach values in the range of 82.6–84.4% by 2030. By that date, Latin America and the Caribbean will be the second most urbanized major area of the world (Table 5.14).

In general, the urbanization rates experienced by Europe, Northern America, and Oceania have been considerably lower than those exhibited by the major areas of the developing world. Furthermore, between 1960 and 1980 the urbanization rates in those three major areas were low or even negative as a result of the phenomenon known as "counter-urbanization" which entailed a shift in the population distribution down the urban hierarchy. Although, strictly speaking, counter-urbanization involves a redistribution of the population within the urban system and not a return of urban dwellers to rural areas, in highly urbanized countries counter-urbanization was associated with a faster aggregate growth of nonmetropolitan populations in relation to the growth of the population in metropolitan areas (Korcelli, 1984; Champion, 1998), and in some countries an increase of the rate of growth of the rural population was also noticeable. Thus, in Europe, Northern America, and Oceania, the rate of growth of the rural population increased significantly between the late 1960s and the late 1970s, although in the case of Europe the rate of rural growth remained negative. In addition, particularly low rates of urbanization were recorded in Northern America and Oceania during the same period. Although the rates of urbanization in Europe were higher than in the other major areas, by 1990–1995 they had fallen to just 0.35% per year. During 2000–2030, all three major areas are expected to experience even lower urbanization rates than during 1950–2000, ranging from 0.15% per year in Oceania to 0.34% per year in Europe (Table 5.15).

The flip side of urbanization is the reduction of rural population growth. In the major areas of the less-developed world, two types of trends are discernible. In Latin America and the Caribbean the rural growth rate has declined steadily so that by 1990–1995 it was just 0.05% per year. In contrast, in Africa and Asia, the rate of rural growth increased during the 1950s, 1960s, and even 1970s, reaching a peak in 1975–1980 in Africa (at 2.22% per year) and in 1965–1970 in Asia (at 2.18% per year). Since then, the growth rates of the rural population of Africa and Asia have been declining steadily and are expected to continue declining during 2000–2030. By 2025–2030, the rural populations of all major areas, with the exception of Africa, will be decreasing. A particularly high rate of decline is projected for the rural population of Europe (−1.69% per year in 2025–2030), followed in magnitude by those of Northern America, Asia, Latin America and the Caribbean, and Oceania, whose rates are expected to range from −0.9 to −0.1% per year. Only Africa's rural population will be increasing at a rate of 0.47% per year during 2025–2030. As a result of such trends, Africa's rural population is expected to increase by about 40% between 2000 and 2030, whereas the rural populations of other major areas will change little, except in the case of Europe where a sizable reduction of the rural population is expected (Table 5.14).

One of the major changes in the spatial distribution of the world population over the past two centuries is the concentration of large numbers of people in relatively small, highly urbanized areas known as urban agglomerations. During the 20th century, the population of certain urban agglomerations rose to levels unprecedented in human history. By 2000, 19 urban agglomerations had at least 10 million inhabitants each, implying that the population of a single one of them surpassed the total population of countries such as Belgium, Hungary, or Sweden. Understandably, such populous agglomerations have become known as mega-cities. But despite their size and importance, mega-cities still account for a relatively small share of the world population. In 2000 the population of the 19 mega-cities constituted 4.3% of the world population and by 2015 the projected population of the 23 mega-cities that will exist then will account for 5.2% of the world population. In fact, most urban dwellers live in cities with fewer than 500 000 inhabitants and those cities are expected to account for a rising share of the urban population (Table 5.16). In both the more-developed and the less-developed regions, the proportion of persons living in cities with fewer than 500 000 inhabitants has been rising, reaching 40.5% in the more-developed regions and 19.4% in the less-developed regions by 2000. Because that trend is expected to continue, by 2015 a quarter of the world population is expected to live in cities with at most 500 000 inhabitants. In the highly urbanized more-developed regions, such small cities have accounted for the largest proportion of the population since 1975 and

**Table 5.16** Distribution of the world population and that of more- and less-developed regions by type of settlement and size of urban settlement, 1975, 2000, and 2015

| Development grouping | Type of settlement and number of inhabitants of urban settlement | Percentage distribution | | | Growth rate (%) | |
|---|---|---|---|---|---|---|
| | | 1975 | 2000 | 2015 | 1975–2000 | 2000–2015 |
| World | 10 million or more | 1.7 | 4.3 | 5.2 | 5.4 | 2.4 |
| | 5 million to 10 million | 3.1 | 2.6 | 3.5 | 0.8 | 3.1 |
| | 1 million to 5 million | 8.0 | 11.6 | 14.1 | 3.1 | 2.4 |
| | 500 000 to 1 million | 4.3 | 5.0 | 5.2 | 2.2 | 1.4 |
| | Fewer than 500 000 | 20.8 | 23.5 | 25.4 | 2.1 | 1.6 |
| | Rural areas | 62.1 | 53.0 | 46.6 | 1.0 | 0.3 |
| | Total population | 100.0 | 100.0 | 100.0 | 1.6 | 1.1 |
| More-developed regions | 10 million or more | 3.4 | 5.7 | 5.7 | 2.5 | 0.2 |
| | 5 million to 10 million | 5.9 | 3.8 | 4.2 | −1.3 | 0.8 |
| | 1 million to 5 million | 13.9 | 18.5 | 20.6 | 1.6 | 0.9 |
| | 500 000 to 1 million | 6.6 | 7.6 | 7.9 | 1.1 | 0.4 |
| | Fewer than 500 000 | 40.2 | 40.5 | 41.4 | 0.5 | 0.3 |
| | Rural areas | 30.0 | 24.0 | 20.3 | −0.4 | −1.0 |
| | Total population | 100.0 | 100.0 | 100.0 | 0.5 | 0.1 |
| Less-developed regions | 10 million or more | 1.1 | 4.0 | 5.1 | 7.1 | 3.0 |
| | 5 million to 10 million | 2.1 | 2.3 | 3.3 | 2.1 | 3.9 |
| | 1 million to 5 million | 6.0 | 10.0 | 12.7 | 3.9 | 3.0 |
| | 500 000 to 1 million | 3.5 | 4.3 | 4.7 | 2.7 | 1.9 |
| | Fewer than 500 000 | 14.0 | 19.4 | 22.1 | 3.2 | 2.2 |
| | Rural areas | 73.2 | 60.1 | 52.0 | 1.1 | 0.4 |
| | Total population | 100.0 | 100.0 | 100.0 | 1.9 | 1.3 |
| Least-developed countries | 10 million or more | 0.0 | 1.9 | 2.3 | – | 3.6 |
| | 5 million to 10 million | 0.0 | 0.8 | 3.5 | – | 12.2 |
| | 1 million to 5 million | 1.6 | 6.8 | 9.3 | 8.2 | 4.3 |
| | 500 000 to 1 million | 1.7 | 2.3 | 1.9 | 3.8 | 1.0 |
| | Fewer than 500 000 | 11.1 | 14.1 | 18.0 | 3.4 | 3.9 |
| | Rural areas | 85.6 | 74.0 | 64.9 | 1.9 | 1.4 |
| | Total population | 100.0 | 100.0 | 100.0 | 2.5 | 2.2 |

Source: United Nations (2001c).

by 2015 nearly twice as many people in the developed world are expected to live in small cities than in rural areas. In contrast, rural areas will likely remain the main areas of residence of the inhabitants of the less-developed regions, accounting for 52% of the total population in developing countries in 2015 and having more than double the population of the small cities in the developing world at that time.

Among major areas, cities with fewer than 500 000 inhabitants have also provided residence for the highest proportion of urban dwellers (Table 5.17). In Europe, Northern America, Oceania, and Latin America and the Caribbean, a higher percentage of the population lives in small cities than in rural areas. In 2000, the proportion of the population living in small cities was 47% in Europe, 36% in Latin America and the Caribbean, and close to 30% in Northern America and Oceania. In Asia and Africa those percentages were lower, at 17% and 22%, respectively. Over the next fifteen

**Table 5.17** Distribution of the total population of major areas by type of settlement and size of urban settlement, 1975, 2000, and 2015

| Major area | Type of settlement and number of inhabitants of urban settlement | Percentage distribution | | |
|---|---|---|---|---|
| | | 1975 | 2000 | 2015 |
| Africa | 10 million or more | 0.0 | 3.1 | 3.4 |
| | 5 million to 10 million | 1.5 | 0.6 | 2.3 |
| | 1 million to 5 million | 3.2 | 9.6 | 12.5 |
| | 500 000 to 1 million | 3.3 | 3.1 | 3.5 |
| | Fewer than 500 000 | 17.1 | 21.5 | 24.7 |
| | Rural areas | 74.8 | 62.1 | 53.5 |
| | Total population | 100.0 | 100.0 | 100.0 |
| Asia | 10 million or more | 1.3 | 4.1 | 5.5 |
| | 5 million to 10 million | 2.1 | 2.3 | 3.2 |
| | 1 million to 5 million | 5.9 | 9.0 | 11.7 |
| | 500 000 to 1 million | 3.2 | 4.4 | 5.0 |
| | Fewer than 500 000 | 12.1 | 16.9 | 19.3 |
| | Rural areas | 75.3 | 63.3 | 55.3 |
| | Total population | 100.0 | 100.0 | 100.0 |
| Europe | 10 million or more | 0.0 | 0.0 | 0.0 |
| | 5 million to 10 million | 5.4 | 5.2 | 5.3 |
| | 1 million to 5 million | 12.2 | 15.2 | 16.5 |
| | 500 000 to 1 million | 6.9 | 7.2 | 7.0 |
| | Fewer than 500 000 | 42.8 | 47.1 | 49.8 |
| | Rural areas | 32.7 | 25.2 | 21.4 |
| | Total population | 100.0 | 100.0 | 100.0 |
| Latin America and the Caribbean | 10 million or more | 6.6 | 11.4 | 10.4 |
| | 5 million to 10 million | 5.3 | 3.7 | 5.4 |
| | 1 million to 5 million | 9.9 | 17.1 | 21.1 |
| | 500 000 to 1 million | 5.2 | 7.2 | 6.7 |
| | Fewer than 500 000 | 34.2 | 35.9 | 36.3 |
| | Rural areas | 38.8 | 24.7 | 20.1 |
| | Total population | 100.0 | 100.0 | 100.0 |
| Northern America | 10 million or more | 6.5 | 9.6 | 9.2 |
| | 5 million to 10 million | 6.4 | 2.2 | 3.7 |
| | 1 million to 5 million | 21.3 | 27.2 | 27.9 |
| | 500 000 to 1 million | 7.0 | 8.3 | 7.2 |
| | Fewer than 500 000 | 32.6 | 29.9 | 32.9 |
| | Rural areas | 26.2 | 22.8 | 19.1 |
| | Total population | 100.0 | 100.0 | 100.0 |
| Oceania | 10 million or more | 0.0 | 0.0 | 0.0 |
| | 5 million to 10 million | 0.0 | 0.0 | 0.0 |
| | 1 million to 5 million | 25.8 | 39.2 | 36.6 |
| | 500 000 to 1 million | 15.4 | 0.0 | 4.3 |
| | Fewer than 500 000 | 30.6 | 31.0 | 30.2 |
| | Rural areas | 28.2 | 29.8 | 28.8 |
| | Total population | 100.0 | 100.0 | 100.0 |

Source: United Nations (2001c).

years the number of people living in small cities is expected to increase in all major areas except Oceania. The highest growth rates in small cities are projected for Africa (3% per year) and Asia (2% per year). Despite such rapid growth in the population of small cities, by 2015 the numbers of rural dwellers in both Africa and Asia are expected to be twice the number of residents of small cities. In other major areas, the population of small cities is expected to outnumber by wide margins the number of rural dwellers.

In Europe not only does the majority of the urban population (at least 63%) live in cities with fewer than 500 000 inhabitants but, in addition, cities with populations ranging from 1 million to 5 million inhabitants have attracted a growing share of the population to the detriment of larger cities. There are only five urban agglomerations in Europe with more than 5 million inhabitants, a number that has not changed since 1975. In comparison with Europe, Northern America has seen the share of the population in small cities decline while the concentration in medium-sized cities, particularly those with populations ranging from 1 million to 5 million inhabitants, and in mega-cities has risen. However, during 2000–2015, Northern America is expected to experience a slight increase in the proportion of the population living in cities with fewer than 500 000 inhabitants and declines in the proportions living in cities with 500 000 to 5 million inhabitants and in mega-cities.

In Latin America and the Caribbean there has been a tendency for the population to become more concentrated in medium-sized cities with populations ranging from 1 million to 5 million inhabitants and in mega-cities, and the trend towards a somewhat greater concentration of the population in the upper echelons of the urban hierarchy is expected to continue until 2015. In Asia the trend towards a greater concentration of the population in larger cities, particularly mega-cities, is more clear cut and is projected to continue, particularly as levels of urbanization rise. In Africa a similar trend is noticeable, especially if one considers jointly the proportion of the population living in urban agglomerations with 5 million to 10 million inhabitants and that living in mega-cities. The overall proportion in those agglomerations has increased from 4.4% in 1975 to 6.4% in 2000 and is projected to reach 8.7% in 2015.

For Oceania, the changes in the distribution of the population by size class are difficult to interpret because they are affected by the small number of cities in that major area and the discontinuities associated with the transfer of cities from one category to the next. In 1975 the two largest cities in Oceania had populations in the range of 1 million to 5 million inhabitants. By 2000 the number of cities in that category had increased to six and that number is expected to remain unchanged until 2015. Those six cities accounted in 2000 for 55.9% of the urban population of Oceania and are expected to have 51.5% of the corresponding population in 2015, indicating that the urban population of the region is highly concentrated in a few urban agglomerations.

To conclude, let us consider the mega-cities of the world. Those populous cities are not uniformly distributed among major areas, nor are they more likely to exist in the most highly urbanized regions (Table 5.18). Thus, only one of the five mega-cities that existed in 1975 was located in Northern America and there were none in Europe. At that time Asia and Latin America had two mega-cities each and Asia had the largest number of inhabitants living in mega-cities (31 million in two mega-cities). In 2000,

**Table 5.18** Population of cities with 10 million inhabitants or more, 1950, 1975, 2000, and 2015 (in millions)

| City | 1950 | City | 1975 | City | 2000 | City | 2015 |
|------|------|------|------|------|------|------|------|
| 1 New York | 12.3 | 1 Tokyo | 19.8 | 1 Tokyo | 26.4 | 1 Tokyo | 26.4 |
| | | 2 New York | 15.9 | 2 Mexico City | 18.1 | 2 Bombay | 26.1 |
| | | 3 Shanghai | 11.4 | 3 Bombay | 18.1 | 3 Lagos | 23.2 |
| | | 4 Mexico City | 11.2 | 4 Sao Paulo | 17.8 | 4 Dhaka | 21.1 |
| | | 5 Sao Paulo | 10.0 | 5 New York | 16.6 | 5 Sao Paulo | 20.4 |
| | | | | 6 Lagos | 13.4 | 6 Karachi | 19.2 |
| | | | | 7 Los Angeles | 13.1 | 7 Mexico City | 19.2 |
| | | | | 8 Calcutta | 12.9 | 8 New York | 17.4 |
| | | | | 9 Shanghai | 12.9 | 9 Jakarta | 17.3 |
| | | | | 10 Buenos Aires | 12.6 | 10 Calcutta | 17.3 |
| | | | | 11 Dhaka | 12.3 | 11 Delhi | 16.8 |
| | | | | 12 Karachi | 11.8 | 12 Metro Manila | 14.8 |
| | | | | 13 Delhi | 11.7 | 13 Shanghai | 14.6 |
| | | | | 14 Jakarta | 11.0 | 14 Los Angeles | 14.1 |
| | | | | 15 Osaka | 11.0 | 15 Buenos Aires | 14.1 |
| | | | | 16 Metro Manila | 10.9 | 16 Cairo | 13.8 |
| | | | | 17 Beijing | 10.8 | 17 Istanbul | 12.5 |
| | | | | 18 Rio de Janeiro | 10.6 | 18 Beijing | 12.3 |
| | | | | 19 Cairo | 10.6 | 19 Rio de Janeiro | 11.9 |
| | | | | | | 20 Osaka | 11.0 |
| | | | | | | 21 Tianjin | 10.7 |
| | | | | | | 22 Hyderabad | 10.5 |
| | | | | | | 23 Bangkok | 10.1 |

Source: United Nations (2001c).

Asia had more mega-cities than any other major area and the largest number of people living in mega-cities (150 million in 11 mega-cities). In addition, Latin America has four mega-cities, Northern America had two and Africa, with two mega-cities, had become the fourth major area having such populous cities. During 2000–2015 Asia is expected to continue having more mega-cities than any other major area and to have the largest population living in mega-cities. Yet the relative concentration of the population in mega-cities is and will continue to be considerably lower in Asia than in most of the other major areas. Thus, just 4.1% of the population of Asia is estimated to live in mega-cities in 2000, whereas 11.4% of that in Latin America and the Caribbean, and 9.6% of the population of Northern America does so.

Because mega-cities attract considerable attention from the media, policy-makers and the public at large, there seems to be a perception that they absorb a large share of urban growth and tend to grow very rapidly. In fact, the opposite is true. An analysis of past and future growth rates of the populations of mega-cities has indicated that as the city population rises its growth rate tends to decline (United Nations, 2001c). So, although some of today's mega-cities experienced very high rates of population growth when they were still medium-sized urban centers, their rates of growth moderate considerably as they approach the 10 million mark. Thus, in 1950, the only mega-city at the time, New York, also had the lowest rate of growth among all future mega-cities (1% per year during 1950–1975). During 1975–2000, four of the mega-cities or future mega-cities had rates of growth lower or equal to 1% – Beijing, New York, Osaka, and Shanghai – and all of them had populations of at least 8 million inhabitants. Furthermore, Tokyo, the largest urban agglomeration at the time, grew at just 1.2% per year during 1975–2000. Over the period 2000–2015, 11 of the 23 mega-cities of 2015 will have growth rates of at most 1% per year and two, Osaka and Tokyo, are expected to exhibit zero growth. Nevertheless, there are cities that maintain high growth rates even when their populations have already soared. Although a moderation of the rates of growth of all current mega-cities is expected during the period 2000–2015, cities such as Lagos, Dhaka, Karachi, and Jakarta are projected to grow at fairly rapid rates, ranging from 3% to 3.6% per year.

An analysis of the patterns of growth of all cities projected to reach a population of 5 million inhabitants or more by 2015 indicates that the population growth rates of those urban agglomerations have tended to be moderate or low, especially once their population surpasses the 2 million mark (United Nations, 2001c). The most populous urban agglomerations of the developed world have exhibited relatively low rates of growth since 1950 and are expected to grow very slowly if at all during 2000–2015. Among the urban agglomerations expected to reach the 5 million mark in the future, the highest rates of population growth have occurred in those agglomerations located in the less-developed regions of the world, especially over periods when they still had low numbers of inhabitants. But even among the large urban agglomerations of the developing world, rates of population growth above 5% sustained over lengthy periods have been exceptional.

# Conclusion

This review of past trends and future prospects of population growth, population aging, and urbanization has highlighted the crucial changes that world population dynamics have undergone over the course of the 20th century and the fact that the demographic transition, being a unique event in human history, still remains to play itself out to its full extent. Today, when most developing countries are already fairly advanced in the transition to low fertility and low mortality, the issue of whether the developing world will embark on the demographic transition has been largely put to rest. Nevertheless, some issues that had not been expected twenty or thirty years ago when the transition to low fertility in the developing world was beginning have now taken center stage and are leading to a reassessment of future prospects of population change.

The first of these developments is the persistence of low fertility in a large number of countries, especially in those that underwent the demographic transition early, since such persistence suggests that when couples master the means to control their fertility and live in societies where the risks of dying before old age are low, the number of children they will decide to have may be below the number needed to ensure the long-term replacement of the population. If this behavior becomes the norm rather than the exception in the countries that are today in the intermediate stages of the transition to low fertility, the prospects for a sustained and deep reduction of the world population over the coming century increase. However, this issue is only beginning to be addressed in a systematic way and the possibility of different outcomes cannot be ruled out, particularly given the heterogeneity that is still evident among the populations of the world. Furthermore, the persistence of high fertility in a significant number of countries and evidence suggesting a slowdown in the transition to low fertility in some of the most populous countries where fertility levels are still at an intermediate stage suggest that the universal adoption of low fertility norms is not so readily at hand.

The second development involves reversals of the transition to lower mortality, especially those stemming from a resurgence of infectious diseases as major causes of death and from the persistence of high rates of death caused by chronic and degenerative diseases such as those affecting the cardiovascular system. In addition, in a growing number of countries mortality due to violence and accidents has been increasing and although it is generally not sufficient to cause a sustained reversal of mortality trends, it may contribute to dampen further mortality reductions in many countries. These factors, among which the uncertainty about future levels of HIV prevalence is perhaps the most prominent, suggest that future assumptions about sustained mortality reductions in the majority of countries may turn out to be too optimistic. On the other hand, past experience has shown that projections of mortality decline have tended to err in the other direction, underestimating the reductions of mortality that have occurred in countries with advanced health systems where new medical interventions and behavioral change have contributed to reduce mortality in adult ages more rapidly than expected.

These considerations imply that the results of current projections can at best be taken as indicative of possible future developments. Nevertheless, as documented in this chapter, they already cover a wide range of outcomes and provide fairly solid basis for some key conclusions. The first is that the world population will continue to increase during the best part of the next fifty years and the potential for continued growth is large. The second is that population aging will continue and with it the rapid increase of the elderly population. The third is that the population of the future will be more urban and that growth of the rural population will be low or negative almost everywhere. The fourth is that the differences in demographic dynamics between the more-developed and the less-developed countries will persist for at least the next fifty years, and there will be considerable variation in the experiences of countries. A homogeneous world in which all populations have similarly low levels of fertility and mortality and are equally highly urbanized is still far away in the future.

# References

Biraben, J.N. (1979). Essai d'estimation du nombre des hommes. *Population* **1**, 13–26.

Champion, A. (1998). Population distribution in developed countries: has counter-urbanization stopped? *In* "Population Distribution and Migration". Proceedings of the United Nations Expert Group Meeting on Population Distribution and Migration,

Santa Cruz (Bolivia), 18–22 January 1993. United Nations publication, Sales No. E.98.XIII.12.

Clark, C. (1968). "Population Growth and Land Use". Saint Martin's Press, New York.

Korcelli, P. (1984). The turnaround in urbanization in developed countries. *In* "Population Distribution, Migration and Development". Proceedings of the Expert Group on Population Distribution, Migration and Development, Hammamet (Tunisia), 21–25 March 1983. United Nations publications, Sales No. E.84.XIII.3.

United Nations (1980). "Patterns of Urban and Rural Population Growth". United Nations publication, Sales No. E.79.XIII.9.

United Nations (2001a). "World Population Prospects: The 2000 Revision". Vol. I: Comprehensive Tables. United Nations publication, Sales No. E.01.XIII.8.

United Nations (2001b). "World Population Prospects: The 2000 Revision". Vol. II: Sex and Age Distribution of the World Population. United Nations publication, Sales No. E.01.XIII.9.

United Nations (2001c). "World Urbanization Prospects: The 1999 Revision". United Nations publication, Sales No. E.01.XIII.11.

Vallin, J. (1989). "La Population Mondiale". La Découverte, Paris.

# Biological Factors Affecting the Nutrition Transition

## PART II

6. The dynamics of the dietary transition in the developing world . . . . . . . .  111
7. Early nutrition conditions and later risk of disease . . . . . . . . . . . . . . . .  129
8. Obesity in the developing world . . . . . . . . . . . . . . . . . . . . . . . . . . . .  147
9. Diabetes . . . . . . . . . . . . . . . . . . . . . . . . . . . . . . . . . . . . . . . . . . .  165
10. Cardiovascular diseases . . . . . . . . . . . . . . . . . . . . . . . . . . . . . . . . .  191
11. The nutrition transition in China: a new stage of the Chinese diet . . . . .  205
12. Trends in under- and overnutrition in Brazil . . . . . . . . . . . . . . . . . . .  223
13. Policy implications . . . . . . . . . . . . . . . . . . . . . . . . . . . . . . . . . . . .  241

# The dynamics of the dietary transition in the developing world

*Barry M. Popkin*

## Introduction

Human history is characterized by a series of changes in the diet and nutritional status. This pace of change has quickened considerably over the last three centuries. In particular in the post-World War II period it appears to have changed at a much more rapid rate. Before that, major changes in diet and nutritional status occurred infrequently and one could argue that there were few changes in diet for the first several million years of existence of the human race. In this chapter, I consider dietary and overall nutritional change from a broad historical perspective. The concept of transitions or movement from one state or condition to another is used to capture the dynamic nature of diet, particularly large shifts in its overall structure. I begin with the premise that it is important to understand these broad changes in dietary patterns and the factors we consider as determinants or important correlates of the patterns of dietary change. The ultimate goal is to understand the various factors which cause or are associated with these dietary changes so that we can better understand how to promote dietary change systematically. I posit that the transitions which have occurred in nutrition are avoidable and that an understanding of the patterns and sources of change will serve as a basis for future interventions at the population level to lead to more healthful transitions.

The theory of the nutrition transition posits that these changes or stages relate to the complex interplay of changes in patterns of agricultural, health, and socioeconomic factors, among others. It is relatively easy to present a case that to understand the nutrition transition we require a broad-based examination of the patterns and determinants of dietary change. One needs to be concerned with food supply, which relates to agricultural systems and agricultural technology as well as to the factors which affect the demand and use of food. The latter include economic resources, demographic patterns, various cultural and knowledge factors associated with food choice, and also

The Nutrition Transition
ISBN: 0-12-153654-8

disease patterns, sociological considerations such as the role of women and family structure.

# Broad conceptualization of the nutrition transition

In Table 6.1 the conceptualization of the nutrition transition is laid out. This is a highly stylized synopsis of patterns of change, presenting the shifts in dietary intake and nutritional status and some of the possible correlates and/or causes of these trends. It is important to note the dearth of research which has tried to link dietary patterns across the centuries and millennia, particularly with some attention being paid to the pace of change and magnitude of structural shifts and the determinants of these changes. We have numerous examples of movements from one stage of the nutritional transition to another which occurred over various periods of time (e.g., the Japanese shift in diet after World War II produced a rapid change from the third to the fourth stage, in sharp contrast to much slower changes over the period of a century from the third to the fourth stage in North America and Western Europe). It is also important to note that such transitions occur highly unevenly over time and space and change varies greatly for different geographic and socioeconomic subpopulation groups.

The other factors presented in Table 6.1 represent some of the major relationships between the nutrition transition, and social, health, and technological change. Many of these factors have a role in determining the pattern and pace of the nutrition transition; others occur concurrently or follow this transition. The problem of causality represents a challenge that cannot be adequately addressed here. Does population growth lead to dietary change or vice versa? Examples of each abound. Is a stable food supply required to provide the resources for urban centers to grow or do the requirements of urban centers lead to increasing food production? Answers to such questions vary by stage of the nutritional transition and in some cases represent central elements in longstanding debates about the antecedents and consequences of economic and demographic change. In many cases, we can make clear statements about causality, in others, we can not. In many cases, the relationships discussed have not been considered because the questions have not been posed heretofore.

With the ability to control famines and to gain control over factors affecting the fluctuations in food supply which occur from season to season and over a series of years, it was possible for food to be available to fuel the labor force needed for the industrial revolution and the development of modern urban societies.

## Stage 1: Age of collecting food

For the first two–three million years of the existence of humans as we know them today, food was obtained by hunting and gathering and none was produced. Hunting only emerged as a significant component of the subsistence pattern in the last

**Table 6.1  The nutrition transition**

| Transition profile | Pattern 1: Collecting food | Pattern 2: Famine | Pattern 3: Receding famine | Pattern 4: Degenerative disease | Pattern 5: Behavioral change |
|---|---|---|---|---|---|
| **1. Nutrition profile** | | | | | |
| Diet | Plants, low-fat wild animals; varied diet | Cereals predominant; diet less varied | Fewer starchy staples; more fruits, vegetables, animal protein; low variety continues | More fat (especially from animal products), sugar and processed foods; less fiber | Less fat and processing; increased carbohydrates, fruits and vegetables |
| Nutritional status | Robust, lean, few nutritional deficiencies | Children, women suffer most from low fat intake; nutritional deficiency diseases emerge; stature declines | Continued MCH nutrition problems; many deficiencies disappear; weaning diseases emerge; stature grows | Obesity; problems for elderly (bone health, etc.); many disabling conditions | Reduced body fat levels and obesity; improved bone health |
| **2. Economy** | Hunter-gatherers | Agriculture, animal husbandry, home-making begin; shift to monocultures | Second agricultural revolution (crop rotation, fertilizer); Industrial revolution; women join labor force | Fewer jobs with heavy physical activity; service sector and mechanization; household technology revolution | Service sector mechanization, industrial robotization dominate; leisure exercise grows to offset sedentary jobs |
| Household production | Primitive; onset of fire | Labor-intensive, primitive technology begins (clay cooking vessels) | Primitive water systems; clay stoves; cooking technology advance | Household technology mechanizes and proliferates | Food preparation cost falls significantly with technological change |
| Income and assets | Subsistence; primitive stone tools | Subsistence; few tools | Increasing income disparity; agricultural tools; industrialization rises | Rapid growth in income and income disparities; technology proliferation | Income growth slows; home and leisure technologies increase |
| **3. Demographic profile** | | | | | |
| Mortality/fertility | Low fertility, high mortality, low life expectancy | Age of Malthus; high natural fertility, low life expectancy, high infant and maternal mortality | Slow mortality decline, later rapid; fertility static, then declines; small, cumulative population growth, later explodes | Life expectancy hits unique levels (60s–70s); huge fertility declines and fluctuations (e.g., postwar baby boom) | Life expectancy extends to 70s, 80s; disability-free period increases |
| Morbidity | Much infectious disease; no epidemics | Epidemics; endemic disease (plague, smallpox, polio, TB); deficiency disease begins; starving common | TB, smallpox, infection, parasitic disease, polio, weaning disease (diarrhea, retarded growth) expand, later decline | Chronic disease related to diet, pollution (heart disease, cancer); infectious disease declines | Increased health promotion (preventive and therapeutic); rapid decline in CHD, slower change in age-specific cancer profile |
| Age structure | Young population | Young; very few elderly | Chiefly young; shift to older population begins | Rapid fertility decline; elderly proportion increases rapidly | Increasing proportion of elderly >75 |
| Residency patterns | Rural, low density | Rural; a few small, crowded cities | Chiefly rural; move to cities increases; international migration begins; megacities develop | Urban population disperses; rural green space reduced | Lower density cities rejuvenate; urbanization of rural areas encircling cities increases |
| **4. Food processing** | Nonexistent | Food storage begins | Storage process (drying, salting); canning and processing technologies; increased food refining and milling | Numerous food transforming technologies | Technologies create foods and food constituent substitutes (e.g., macronutrient substitutes) |

Reprinted with permission from: Popkin, B.M. (1993) Nutritional patterns and transitions. *Popul. Dev. Rev.* **19**, 138–157.

million years (Gordon, 1987). The use or control of fire has been documented during this period in many locations. During this period in the age of collecting food, there was a balance of about 50–80% of food coming from plants and 20–50% from animals (coastal dwellers received more nutrition from fishing; inland residents received more from hunting; hunting progressed over time from small animals to larger mammals). Within this period, there were periods of increased consumption of animal food products and many subpopulations that were predominately meat-eaters.

- For the first several million years, humans were felt to be reasonably large in size and robust in skeletons and musculature (Truswell and Hansen, 1976; Schoeninger, 1982; Eaton *et al.*, 1988). These persons had short life spans but reasonable nutritional status, infectious diseases being the major source of morbidity and death.
- In general the diet was more varied in these traditional, preagricultural societies (Truswell, 1977). Seasonality and the need to combine hunting and gathering activities ensured this greater variety. The basic diet came from seeds of grasses, tree nuts, roots and tubers, fish and aquatic mammals, and herd ungulates (Harris, 1980). Fat content in the diet was low because of its high carbohydrate content and the low proportion of saturated fat in the meat consumed. Wild animal meat such as they consumed has five times the proportion of polyunsaturated fat as does the domestic animal meat consumed today (Eaton *et al.*, 1988). For example, the !Kung San who consume very high proportions of energy from meat, have a cholesterol level of 120 (Truswell and Hansen, 1978; Truswell, 1979). Although the hunter–gatherer societies studied in the past century live in far more precarious environments than their predecessors lived in a million years ago, it is unlikely that their diets differed significantly. Fiber intake, part of which came from indigestible roughage, was very high.
- Among the proportion of these persons who survived the infectious diseases and lived to be older, chronic diseases (e.g., coronary heart disease (CHD), hypertension, cancer, osteoporosis, dental caries, diabetes) were unknown problems (Cavalli-Sforza, 1981; Eaton *et al.*, 1988). These researchers are unanimous in their feeling that the absence of diet-related chronic diseases relates to living patterns rather than the short average live expectancy of these peoples. Obesity was not found; however, there is some debate as to whether the thin but robust persons who survived were malnourished or healthy (Harpending, 1976; Truswell and Hansen, 1978). More recent higher quality estimates of the hunter–gatherer diet lead to the following macronutrient composition: 19–35% of energy from protein; 22–40% of energy from carbohydrate; and the rest from fat (Cordain *et al.*, 2000). Thus most of these societies consumed more than 50% of their energy from animal foods.

## Stage 2: Age of famine

The age of famine began with the development of agriculture. Deemed the first agricultural revolution, this period saw society develop its first ability to produce food. Agriculture became dominant at different times in each region of the world (e.g., by about 7000 BC in Southeast Asia and 500 BC in Mexico (Tehuacan Valley agrarian-based economies were well-established) (Gordon, 1987)). The cause of this shift is unclear; however, population density increased considerably during the final stages of the age of collecting food and provides the most convincing explanation. It is important to note that the date of the early agricultural period varied from region to region and only in later periods (the two thousand or fewer years BC) does agriculture become more complex (e.g., Vargas, 1990). With this revolution, protein content in the diet declined modestly, complex carbohydrates increased from 50–70% of energy to 60–75%, and fat as a percentage of energy decreased from about 15–30% to 10–15% (Trowell, 1981). A disproportionate amount of food from plant sources occurred in some societies and in others, hunting/animal husbandry played a central role.

- In general the onset of animal husbandry and agriculture was associated with a significant decline in the proportion of meat in the diet and an increase in vegetable foods (up to 90% of the diet). There also appears to be an increasing specialization in activities other than agriculture which led to fewer persons being involved in farming. Associated with these changes was increased nutritional stress and a reduction in stature according to numerous studies of skeletal remains (e.g., Eaton and Konner, 1985; Vargas, 1990). It is estimated that stature declined by an average of 4 inches (10 cm) (Eaton *et al.*, 1988).
- There was a decrease in robustness as a result of changes in food procurement and activity levels. There was a shift to increasing dependence on dietary plant material. Changes in strontium:calcium ratios in bones somewhere between 10 000 and 15 000 years BC indicate a dietary shift in one region but similar data are unavailable for all regions of the world and patterns of dietary change and robustness appear to have varied greatly (Schoeninger, 1982).
- The shifts toward agriculture led to a less-varied diet with cereal grains predominant, an increase in alcohol consumption, and the onset of a variety of deficiency diseases, all directly related to the reduction in dietary variety (Yudkin, 1969). Social stratification began to appear during the later stages of this stage and resulted in "intragroup variation in diet along the lines of sex and social status" (Gordon, 1987).

## Stage 3: Age of receding famine

- The second agricultural revolution occurred in the 18th to 19th centuries when modern technology was first applied to agriculture, including the development of natural fertilizers and crop rotation systems. This development may partly relate to the excess food supply which allowed farmers to use rotted vegetables and animal manure for fertilizer. This technology was associated with an increase in animal protein. Later irrigation technology, transportation within and across national and regional borders, and other changes helped to reduce the effects of climatic fluctuations.
- The Industrial Revolution, in 19th-century Europe, found animal protein content of diet becoming increasingly adequate. During the second half and later in that

century, improved transportation, conquests of one people over another (e.g., the Spanish in the Americas), and other factors led to more complex diets with a greater mix of plant and animal products (e.g., the practice of animal husbandry increased). The result was an increase in stature.

- Changes in diet included reduced consumption of all starchy foods (bread and potatoes); increased consumption of sugar, vegetables, and fruits; and adaptation of dietary practices which eliminate major deficiency diseases (higher protein, fat consumption; changes in food processing; etc.). The introduction of techniques for milling grain led to a decline in fiber intake and to a short-term increase in selected deficiency diseases (e.g., pellagra and beriberi were caused by excessive milling of corn and rice, respectively).

- Additional features of this period were increases in social inequality, clustering of the poor in slums and ghettoes, and the evolution of a new set of dietary problems related to early weaning from the breast during the 17th to 19th centuries. Combined with poor sanitation and impure water supplies, a new set of infant nutrition problems occurred. This situation was followed rapidly in the late 19th and early 20th century by the development of formulations by medical practitioners for feeding infants, the development of tin cans, and the evolution of the commercial infant formula sector.

- Many lower-income countries have achieved remarkable economic or social progress during the past century and continue to move through the age of receding famine into the next stage. Keyfitz (1985) uses descriptive information to document some of the more subtle aspects of this shift for one village in Indonesia. One of the interesting shifts is a change from preoccupation with obtaining food which entered all aspects of life to one in which it takes much less time to earn a kilogram of rice and the focus of life has shifted. During this stage, the quality of the staple increases first, often reducing the consumption of inferior staples (e.g., cassava consumption is reduced and rice consumption increased as in Indonesia (Keyfitz, 1985)). Such changes in the quality of the diet during this stage of the nutrition transition fits our experience in many low-income countries.

## Stage 4: Age of degenerative diseases

This age began with rapid growth in animal husbandry, urbanization, and economic change, which combined to create the basis for a major shift toward a lower nutrient density diet which was excessively high in saturated fat and refined sugar.

- Hughes and Jones (1979) document long-term shifts from food balance studies in rural Wales. Table 6.2 shows the dietary changes which are related to this phase of the nutrition transition. This is an example of the diet high in fat, sugar, and processed foodstuffs, and low in fiber and natural foodstuffs, so often found in combination with an increasingly sedentary life. An increase in the consumption of sugar, processed foods, total fats, and cholesterol and decreased consumption of polyunsaturated fatty acids (PUFA) and dietary fiber are general trends.

- The proportion and type of animal fat in meat differs significantly from that consumed today and during the age of famine (now there is much more fat in

| Table 6.2  Dietary intake trends in rural Wales | | |
|---|---|---|
| Diet components | 1870 | 1977 |
| Fat as a percentage of energy | 25 | 40 |
| PUFA as percentage of total fat | 18.5 | 9.1 |
| PUFA : SFA ratio | 0.42 | 0.20 |
| Cholesterol (mg/day) | 130 | 517 |
| Sucrose (g/day) | 26 | 133 |
| Dietary fiber (g/day) | 65 | 21 |

Source: Hughes and Jones (1979).

subcutaneous tissue and facial planes, and as marbling within the muscle itself). Domesticated animals not only contain more fat but earlier undomesticated animal meat was much more likely to be polyunsaturated; also free-living animal meat has fewer calories and more protein. As an interesting aside, not only does this explain some of the effects of increased fat-related degenerative diseases such as coronary heart disease (CHD), but may also explain why our species does not provide more effective protection (e.g., different modes of utilization) against high-fat intake from animal products.

- The diet associated with modernization and industrialization is spreading to all developing countries at a time when the higher-income countries have drastically altered their diet and face problems of excess rather than deficit. The composition of the diets of most urban residents and in many rural regions in the low-income world is beginning to resemble Western diets and there are few exceptions to this pattern. This is a diet with over 20% of the calories from sugar and a very low fiber intake.
- Also many Mediterranean countries (Portugal, Italy) are rapidly changing their healthful, traditional diet (high in olive oil and carbohydrates in Italy and olive oil, cod, and legumes in Portugal) to a diet similar to that consumed in Western Europe and North America. This change has meant a significant increase in fat as a proportion of energy (e.g., Amorin-Cruz, 1987 as cited in Milio, 1990).

## Stage 5: Age of behavioral change to revise diet to reduce degenerative diseases and prolong health

The societal changes that brought us to the reduction in the importance of famine and infectious diseases and an increase in the importance of degenerative diseases, have begun to trigger a set of behavioral changes in diet felt to be associated with the desire to prevent degenerative diseases. Whether these changes will be sufficient to produce large-scale changes in the structure of diet and body composition remains to be seen. To some extent, the push is to change dietary behavior and return to a diet low in fat – particularly saturated fat – high in fiber, accompanied by extensive exercise. A number of researchers have shown that such behavioral changes are particularly important because they will extend the period of healthful living, that is time free of disability (Manton and Soldo, 1985; Rogers and Hackenberg, 1987).

- There has been a significant shift in public knowledge about the relationship between diet and disease, particularly related to cardiovascular disease, hypertension, osteoporosis, and to a lesser extent selected cancers. Related dietary changes have occurred mainly in certain higher-income countries and offer the promise of shaping the next stage of the nutrition transition. Increases in consumption of low-fat products, reductions in intake of higher fat products, careful attention to cholesterol intake, and less significant but emerging concern for fiber intake are evidence of a potentially new phase in the nutrition transition. For example, there have also been important changes in coronary heart disease patterns in several countries which have led to speculation that dietary change was responsible for them.
- To a very considerable extent, the changes in eating patterns associated with the recent reduction in fat intake in the United States (Popkin *et al.*, 2001), Norway (Milio, 1990), and other higher income countries and the shift toward increased lower fat food consumption has fueled a revolution in the food industry (Popkin *et al.*, 1989; Milio, 1990).

Some of the broad outlines of dietary change have been laid out here. As we head into the new millennium, it is important to present the more recent changes in the developing world against this backdrop. First, the two major defining characteristics are focused on – increased dietary diversity and a shift in the structure of the diet toward more added sugar and fats and a change of staples.

## Dietary diversity has improved

The diets of poor societies have been based on a very limited number of foods, and often consist of little more than starchy roots and coarse grains. Though low in fat and high in fiber, these foods offer little in the way of diversity or variety, essential components of eating pleasure. The nutrition transition typically involves a shift from a limited number of high-carbohydrate staples to a more diverse diet that becomes available to progressively more people. Improved diversity is not only important for improving the quality of life but probably has had a marked impact on improved reproductive outcomes and growth and development. As incomes grow, diets become more diverse, and more people incorporate meat and fish, milk, eggs, and cheese, as well as vegetables and fresh fruit into their habitual diets. Insofar as new foods are being introduced into the diet, they invariably include meat, eggs, and sweets that had been previously inaccessible to most low-income people. Some of these new foods are high in fats, simple sugars, or both. As a result, dietary diversity and the proportion of fats in the diet are sometimes directly linked.

Chapter 11 presents a more careful analysis of the Chinese nutrition transition. Here, a brief analysis of the Chinese diet, assessed by the 1989–97 China Health and Nutrition Survey (CHNS) surveys is presented. The 1989 diet of the poor was largely based on rice, millet, sorghum, cabbage, salted vegetables, soybean sauce, and salt, with some meat (pork). Higher income respondents replaced coarse grains and starchy

| Food groups consumed[a] | Urban | | Rural | | Low income tertile | | Mid income tertile | | High income tertile | | Total | |
|---|---|---|---|---|---|---|---|---|---|---|---|---|
| | 89 | 97 | 89 | 97 | 89 | 97 | 89 | 97 | 89 | 97 | 89 | 97 |
| Mean number | 9.9 | 11.6 | 8.3 | 9.1 | 7.6 | 8.6 | 9.0 | 9.8 | 10.1 | 11.0 | 8.8 | 9.9 |
| <8 | 23.5% | 7.3% | 41.6% | 26.6% | 52.8% | 34.1% | 31.5% | 17.9% | 20.6% | 11.3% | 35.6% | 20.3% |
| 8–10 | 23.3% | 15.8% | 29.3% | 33.3% | 29.0% | 33.9% | 29.1% | 30.2% | 23.4% | 20.5% | 27.3% | 27.6% |
| 10– | 53.2% | 76.9% | 29.1% | 40.1% | 18.2% | 32.0% | 39.4% | 51.8% | 56.0% | 68.2% | 37.1% | 52.1% |

**Table 6.3  Diversity in the Chinese diets, CHNS 1989 and 1997 among adults aged 20–45**

[a] Using the UNC-CH-INFH food groups that contain 39 food groups based first on the major food groupings and then on nutrient-based subgroups.

Source: Popkin *et al.* (in press).

tubers with more rice and wheat. As incomes rose, vegetables and pickled vegetables were replaced with more meat, poultry and eggs, more dairy products, and more fresh fruit. As more different foods were consumed, portion sizes (g/day/user) generally dropped for all foods, except meat, fresh fruit, and alcohol.

The analyses of dietary diversity in China are summarized in Table 6.3. The University of North Carolina at Chapel Hill Institute of Nutrition and Food Hygiene (UNC-CH-INFH) food grouping system was used. This food grouping system separates all foods into 39 useful descriptive and nutrient-based groups. Initially major food groups were based on food groupings used by the INFH. Then fat and beta-carotene compositions were used to develop more refined food groupings, and nutrient thresholds were used to separate major food groups into more distinct, nutrient-based food groups. The number consumed by each person was then summed and presented as mean intake and the proportion with high, medium, and low numbers of food groups consumed. What is noteworthy about this is that there is a marked increase in diversity of the Chinese diet across all socioeconomic status groupings. The urban effect is particularly noticeable. Over time, the proportion of Chinese of all income groups who consume less than eight food groups has declined whereas those who consume more than 10 increased considerably.

# The structure of the diet is shifting: more fat and more added sugar is found

Whereas high-fat diets and Western eating habits were once restricted to the rich industrialized nations, elsewhere evidence has been presented that the nutrition transition now occurs in nations with much lower levels of gross national product (GNP) than previously. Even low-income societies now have access to a high-fat and high-added-sugar diet. Food disappearance data from the Food and Agriculture Organization of the United Nations (FAOUN) is used to present first the average diet in the 1960s and then to show how this has shifted in the 1990s for low and high urban areas.

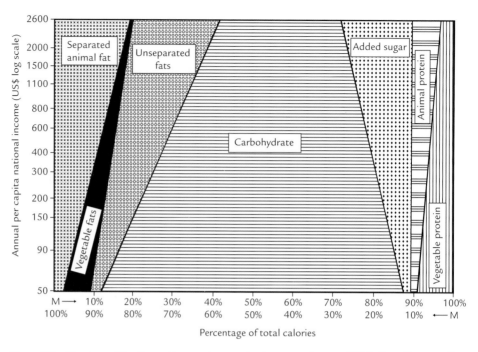

**Figure 6.1** Structure of the diet and income (country-level sources of energy, 1962) (from Drewnowski and Popkin, 1997).

Diets high in fats, especially meat and milk products, used to be tied to a high level of income, whether at national or individual level. A direct relationship between the GNP per capita and the global diet structure was documented three decades ago in a classic study (Perisse *et al.*, 1969; FAOUN, 1970). As shown in Fig. 6.1, analysis of food balance sheets from the Food and Agriculture Organization (FAO) of the United Nations for 85 countries in 1962 showed that high GNP levels were associated with greater percentages of energy derived from sugars and from vegetable and animal fats. Although the proportion of energy from protein remained constant, diets of rich nations were largely based on animal rather than vegetable proteins. The proportion of energy from complex carbohydrates diminished sharply as a function of growing incomes, a characteristic feature of the nutrition transition.

The estimated regression lines displayed in Fig. 6.2 show that the aggregate income–fat relationship had undergone a dramatic change from 1962 to 1990. Most significantly, by 1990 even the poor nations had access to a relatively high-fat diet. Whereas in 1962, a diet deriving 20% of energy (kcal) from fat was associated with a GNP of $1475, the same diet in 1990 was associated with a GNP of only $750 (both in 1992 dollars). This dramatic change arose from a major increase in the consumption of vegetable fats by poor and rich nations alike. The proportion of energy from vegetable fats accounted for up to 13% of total energy in 1990, compared to 10% in 1962. The availability of animal fats continued to be linked to income, though less strongly than before. Vegetable fats in 1990 accounted for a greater proportion of

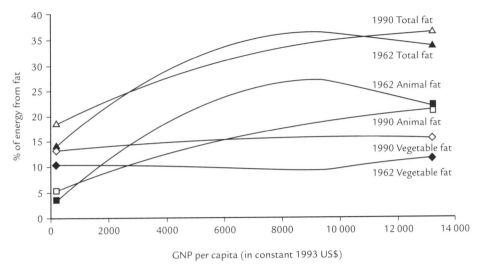

**Figure 6.2** Relationship between the percentage of energy from fat and GNP per capita, 1962 and 1990 (from Guo *et al.*, 2000). These are nonparametric regressions run with food balance data from FAOUN and GNP data from the World Bank.

dietary energy than animal fats for countries in the lowest 75% of the per capita income distribution. The absolute level of vegetable fat consumption increased, but there remained at most a weak association of GNP and vegetable fat intake in these aggregate data.

As a result of these diet adjustments, the lowest income countries now consume an additional 4–5% of energy from fat. Although meat consumption declined in high-income countries (by 6–9%), there was little overall reduction in fat intake. The results in Fig. 6.2 indicate that there has been a substantial shift in the relationship between GNP and the composition of diets over time. There was little information in the 1962 GNP–nutritional composition analysis, however, that would have predicted the form of the relationships in 1990.

There is evidence to show that the structure of the income–diet relationship has undergone a significant change. First, fat consumption is less dependent on GNP than ever before. Second, rapid urbanization has a major influence in accelerating the nutrition transition. The analyses were based on sequential FAO food balance sheets for the period 1962–90, now available in the FAOSTAT database. Data on food availability, expressed in percentage of daily energy from macronutrients were combined with the official estimates of GNP, as established by the World Bank. In both cases, GNP per capita was expressed in 1993 dollars to allow for an easier comparison of the results. Regression analyses were used to relate dietary data (the proportion of energy from vegetable and animal fats, carbohydrates, caloric sweeteners, and protein) for those countries for which full sets of data were available in 1962 and in 1990 to the logarithm of per capita GNP. This research used all countries for which both sets of data were available: 98 countries in 1962 and 133 in 1990. Using alternate samples that consisted of countries with full sets of data in both 1962 and 1990, the results were identical.

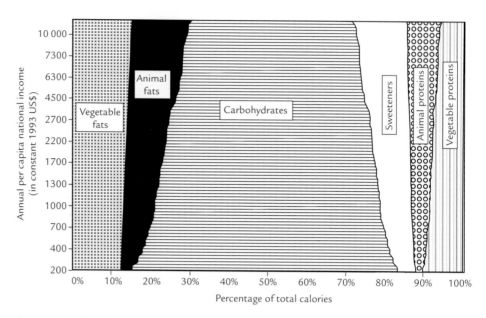

**Figure 6.3** Relationship between the proportion of energy from each food source and gross national product per capita with the proportion of the population residing in urban areas placed at 25%, 1990 (from Drewnowski and Popkin, 1997). Food balance data from the FAOUN; GNP data from the World Bank; regression work by UNC-CH.

The regression analysis also included an urbanization variable. Although GNP and the extent of urbanization were closely linked before World War II, this is clearly no longer the case and many lower income countries now experience very high rates of urbanization. In the regression analyses, the percentage of energy from each macro-nutrient was regressed on GNP per capita, the proportion of the population residing in urban areas that year, and an interaction term between GNP per capita and the proportion of urban residents. All variables in this regression were highly significant.

The data for 1990 (Figs 6.3 and 6.4) show that the income–fat relationship had undergone a dramatic change during the intervening three decades. Figure 6.2 showed the shift in fat intake. The relationship between incomes and energy from sweeteners also underwent a major change between 1962 and 1990. Figure 6.3 shows a very small proportion of energy from added sugar in lower-income countries. In contrast, lower-income urban societies in 1990 have more than 15% of their energy from added sugar and even less urban more rural societies that are low income have 5–7% of energy from added sugar.

# Urbanization contributes to dietary change

Persons living in urban areas consume significantly different diets from their rural counterparts. They have led the movement from stage 2 to 3 and 4 of the nutritional

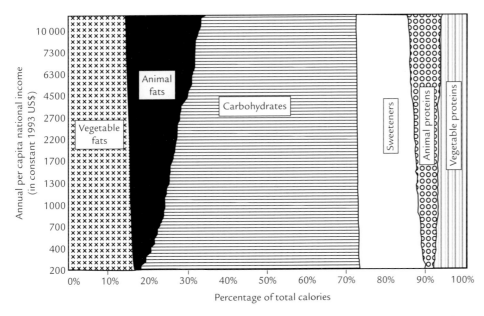

**Figure 6.4** Relationship between the proportion of energy from each food source and gross national product per capita with the proportion of the population residing in urban areas placed at 75%, 1990 (from Drewnowski and Popkin, 1997). Food balance data from the FAOUN; GNP data from the World Bank; regression work by UNC-CH.

transition. Among the distinct differences in eating patterns of urban and rural residents are the following:

- trend away from consumption of the inferior grains (e.g., corn or millet to rice);
- trend toward consumption of more milled and polished grains (e.g., rice, wheat);
- trend toward increased higher fat food prepared away from the home;
- trend toward more processed foods, higher sugar consumption;
- trend toward more animal protein and fats;
- the extent and duration of breast-feeding are shorter and supplementation occurs earlier.

These contrasts in eating patterns differentiate urban areas from rural ones to a greater extent in low-income countries than in higher-income ones. In higher-income countries, market penetration into rural areas is common and there are national integrated food distribution systems. Nevertheless, there are also important differences in eating patterns between urban and rural areas in higher-income countries. Foremost are distinct differences in consumption from away-from-home sources (Popkin *et al.*, 2001) and greater responsiveness to information and the influences of mass media (most likely because of the greater extent of media penetration into the denser urban markets). Even in higher-income countries urban and suburban food and labor markets differ greatly and, in combination with a variety of other factors related to residence, create distinct urban dietary and nutritional status patterns.

There are many reasons for the profound difference in dietary intake and the subsequent differences found in nutritional status. Key factors responsible for this difference include: the way improved transportation and marketing systems provide greater availability of foodstuffs during periods of seasonal shortage; more extensive penetration of marketing activities of the processed commercial food sector; more heterogeneous population with a wide range of dietary patterns; different occupational patterns, many of which are characterized by reduced compatibility of the jobs with home food preparation, child and elder care; different household structures related to a wide range of economic and social factors; and different disease and health service use patterns.

In relative terms, urban growth was modest before the industrial revolution. Since that time, rapid urban development occurred first in the higher-income countries and now lower-income countries are undergoing an even more rapid transformation into urbanized societies. As is shown in the review of demographic change, the last half of the 20th century has seen an unprecedented demographic revolution which appears to be continuing unabated into the 21st century. Urbanization brought on by migration and natural increase has become a dominant factor in all regions. Unlike urbanization in the world's higher-income countries, which is associated with major advances in science, technology, and social organization as well as absorption of large populations, urbanization in low-income countries has not been accompanied by the same level of economic and cultural progress (Popkin and Bisgrove, 1988).

An important dimension of urban growth is the pattern of migration found as part of it. Migration from rural areas either to other rural areas or to cities (and to a lesser extent from small to larger cities) and international migration has had profound effects on diet. The historical shifts in food staples are related to international migration in the Americas and even earlier (for instance in the Americas with corn and potatoes and in Ireland with potatoes). Similarly the studies of Samoans who moved to San Francisco, Polynesians and Maori who moved to New Zealand, Japanese who moved to the United States, and Yemenite Jews who moved to Israel all show a large change in diet with subsequent large increases in diet-related chronic diseases (Toor *et al.*, 1957; Marmot *et al.*, 1975; Worth *et al.*, 1975; Prior and Tasman-Jones, 1981). In addition, migration within countries is felt to have similar profound effects on the diets of the migrants and their communities of origin and destination. Most of the recent and future changes in population distribution will occur in lower-income countries where urban dietary patterns are quite different from those in rural areas and length of stay in urban areas is associated with a shift to adopt this new pattern of diet.

The results presented in Figs 6.3 and 6.4 summarize the profound ways that urbanization has affected the structure of diet.

# Income matters but there are other equally important factors

Based on complex longitudinal statistical methods summarized elsewhere, the effect of income on diet in China was examined (Guo *et al.*, 2000). In particular, the dynamic relationships were explored. The focus here is just on the income–food choice relationships, but the full model incorporated food prices and a large array of sociodemographic characteristics with time-varying variables, such as age, household size, educational level, and a vector of time-invariant variables, such as sex, place of residence and region. In the broader analysis, a study was made of how the effect of income on food choice changed in China for consumption of wheat and wheat flour, other grain products, rice, pork and edible oil, among others. Here the focus is on pork and edible oil consumption patterns.

To simplify the presentation for pork and edible oil, only the summary changes in income elasticities are presented in Figs 6.5 and 6.6. There was a positive income elasticity for the probability of consuming any pork in 1989. This income elasticity increased significantly over the 1989–93 period with the increase being somewhat larger among lower-income groups (Fig. 6.5a). The income elasticity for the quantity of pork consumed (conditional on positive consumption) became more positive among all income groups, but higher-income groups experienced the greatest increases in elasticities (Fig. 6.5b). These shifts are statistically significant for all per capita incomes above the first quartile. For edible oil, the income elasticity for the probability of consuming this product is quite small, and there has not been a significant change over time (Fig. 6.6a). The income elasticity for the amount of oil consumed (given positive consumption), surprisingly, was negative in 1989, but it was insignificantly different from zero over almost the entire income range. This income elasticity rose significantly by 1993, and it was positive at all income values and significantly different from zero for all but the top few percent of the income distribution.

During the 1989–93 time span higher-fat foods became much more responsive to income levels. Pork, edible oils, and eggs had significant increases in their income

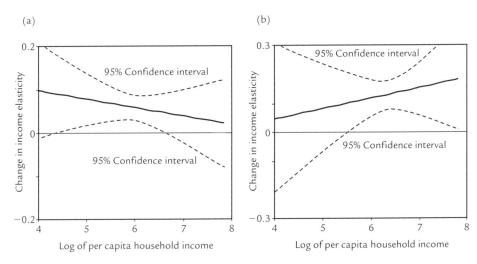

**Figure 6.5**  Changes in income elasticities pork consumption among adults aged 20–45 in China from 1989 to 1993. (a) Change in income elasticity for the probability of consuming any pork; (b) Change in income elasticity for the amount of pork consumers consume. From Guo *et al.* (2000).

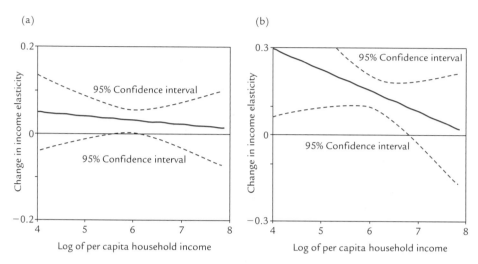

**Figure 6.6** Changes in income elasticities for edible oils consumption among adults aged 20–45 years in China from 1989 to 1993. (a) Change in income elasticity for the probability of consuming any edible oil; (b) Change in income elasticity for the amount of edible oils consumers consume. From Guo *et al.* (2000).

elasticities. The quantity of fat in the diets increased significantly and now appears to increase much more rapidly with increases in incomes.

## Instant access to modern mass media may explain partially these changes

One of the major shifts of this past few decades is in the area of communications. Predominantly through access to modern television, there has been a major shift in how persons in developing countries spend their leisure time. Television ownership has increased rapidly in the world. Elsewhere we have shown trends worldwide. It is most useful to look at the proportion of households that own television sets in a country. Again the CHNS data are used to reflect the types of changes one is setting. Figure 6.7 shows for households from low, middle and upper income tertiles the proportion that owned TVs during the 1989–97 period. Overall in China TV ownership increased from 64.7% of households in 1989 to 88.5% in 1997. It is noteworthy that in China, not only was TV viewing shifting, but also the types of programs and access to western influences were shifting. In the 1980s, cable systems in China did not provide outside programming but by 1997 many provinces provided access to China Star, a system from Hong Kong that relies heavily on US and British programming and provides modern TV advertising.

## Discussion

There is no doubt that dietary changes around the world are rapid and appear to be accelerating. There is limited evidence for this acceleration. The Chinese case study

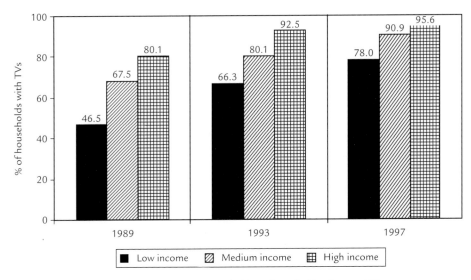

**Figure 6.7** TV ownership in China, 1989–97 (% of Chinese households who own TV).

provides evidence for one country. The food balance data that show a shift in the way lower-income countries have changed their consumption patterns between the 1960s and 1990s is another.

What is most important is that the dietary changes that appear to be occurring are related to an increased energy density of the diet and reduced intake of many of the more important nutrients and food constituents such as fiber. Although food diversity has increased and malnutrition is receding as a threat in many countries, these food shifts point toward the potential for a rapid increase in diet-related noncommunicable diseases in the developing world.

# References

Cavalli-Sforza, L.L. (1981). *In* "Food, Nutrition and Evolution: Food as an Environmental Factor in the Genesis of Human Variability" (D.N. Walcher, and N. Kretchmer, eds.), pp. 1–7. Masson, New York.

Cordain, L.J., Miller, B., Eaton, S.B., Mann, N., Holt, S.H.A., and Speth, J.D. (2000). *Am. J. Clin. Nutr.* **71**, 682–692.

Drewnowski, A., and Popkin, B.M. (1997). The nutrition transition: new trends in the global diet. *Nutr. Rev.* **55**, 31–43.

Eaton, S.B., and Konner, M. (1985). *N. Engl. J. Med.* **312**, 283–289.

Eaton, S.B., Shostak, M., and Konner, M. (1988). "The Paleolithic Prescription: A Program of Diet and Exercise and a Design for Living". Harper and Row, New York.

Food and Agriculture Organization of the United Nations (FAOUN) (1970). "Income Effect on the Structure of Diet. Provisional Indicative World Plan for Agricultural Development", Vol. 2, pp. 500–505. Rome, Italy.

Gordon, K.D. (1987). *In* "Nutritional Anthropology" (F.E. Johnson, ed.). Liss, New York.

Guo, X., Mroz, T.A., Popkin, B.M., and Zhai, F. (2000). *Econ. Dev. Cultural Change* **48**, 737–760.

Harpending, H. (1976). *In* "Kalahari Hunter-gatherers: Studies of the !Kung San and Their Neighbors" (R.B. Lee, and I. DeVore, eds.). Harvard University Press, Cambridge, MA.

Harris, D.R. (1980). *In* "Food, Nutrition and Evolution: Food as an Environmental Factor in the Genesis of Human Variability" (D.N. Walcher, and N. Kretchmer, eds.). Masson, Paris.

Hughes, R.E., and Jones, E. (1979). *BMJ* **1**, 1145.

Keyfitz, N. (1985). *Popul. Dev. Rev.* **11**, 695–719.

Manton, K.G., and Soldo, B.J. (1985). *Health Society* **63**, 206–285.

Marmot, M.G., Syme, S.L., Kagan, A., Hiroo, K., and Rhoads, G. (1975). *Am. J. Epidemiol.* **102**, 514–525.

Milio, N. (1990). "Nutrition Policy for Food-rich Countries: A Strategic Analysis". The Johns Hopkins University Press, Baltimore.

Perisse, J., Sizaret, F., and Francois, P. (1969). *FAO Nutr. Newsl.* **7**, 1–9.

Popkin, B.M., and Bisgrove, E.Z. (1988). *Food Nutr. Bull.* **10**, 3–23.

Popkin, B.M., Haines, P.S., and Reidy, K.C. (1989). *Am. J. Clin. Nutr.* **49**, 1307–1319.

Popkin, B.M., Siega-Riz, A.M., Haines, P.S., and Jahns, L. (2001). *Prev. Med.* **32**, 245–254.

Popkin, B.M., Lu, B., and Zhai, F. (2002). *Publ. Health Nutr.*

Prior, I., and Tasman-Jones, C. (1981). *In* "Western Diseases: Their Emergence and Prevention" (H.C. Trowell, and D.P. Burkett, eds.). Harvard University Press, Cambridge, MA.

Rogers, R.G., and Hackenberg, R. (1987). *Soc. Biol.* **34**, 234–243.

Schoeninger, M. (1982). *Am. J. Phys. Anthropol.* **58**, 37–52.

Toor, M., Katchalsky, A., Agmon, J., and Allalouf, D. (1957). *Lancet* **i**, 1270–1273.

Trowell, H.C. (1981). *In* "Western Diseases: Their Emergence and Prevention" (H.C. Trowell, and D.P. Burkitt, eds.). Harvard University Press, Cambridge, MA.

Truswell, A.S. (1977). "Health and Diseases in Tribal Societies", Ciba Foundation Symposium 149. Elsevier, Amsterdam.

Truswell, A.S. (1979). *In* "Human Nutrition and Dietetics" (S. Davidson, R. Passmore, J.F. Brock, and A.S. Truswell, eds.), 7th edn. Churchill-Livingstone, Edinburgh.

Truswell, A.S., and Hansen, J.D.L. (1976). *In* "Kalahari Hunter-gatherers: Studies of the !Kung San and Their Neighbors" (R.B. Lee, and I. DeVore, eds.). Harvard University Press, Cambridge, MA.

Vargas, L.A. (1990). *In* "Disease in Populations in Transition" (A.C. Swedlund, and G.J. Armelagos, eds.). Greenwood, Westport, CT.

Worth, R.M., Kato, H., Rhoads, G.G., Kagas, K., and Syme, S.L. (1975). *Am. J. Epidemiol.* **102**, 481–490.

Yudkin, J. (1969). *In* "The Domestication and Exploitation of Plants and Animals" (P.J. Ucko, and G.W. Dimbleby, eds.). Aldine, Chicago.

# Early nutrition conditions and later risk of disease

7

*Linda S. Adair*

## Introduction

Increased attention has been paid, in the past decade, to the hypothesis that chronic diseases in adulthood have origins in the fetal and early postnatal period. The fetal programming hypothesis holds that, in response to undernutrition during critical periods of growth and development, the structure and function of organs and tissues are "programmed", or permanently altered in ways that predispose individuals to chronic disease in later life, most notably diabetes and cardiovascular disease (CVD). The predisposition may take the form of increased susceptibility to chronic disease risk factors, such as atherogenic diets, excess energy intake and reduced physical activity. If this is the case, the programming hypothesis may be particularly relevant in the context of the nutrition transition in developing countries. Rates of fetal growth retardation remain relatively high in these developing countries, while at the same time, rapid socioeconomic changes are accompanied by an increase in sedentary activity and a transition to higher energy density diets. Thus, today's older children and adults in developing countries are more likely than those in earlier decades to have been small at birth, but subsequently exposed to more environmental and behavioral risk factors for chronic disease during their childhood and adult years.

Evidence to support the fetal programming hypothesis has accumulated at a rapid rate over the past decade. Hundreds of published papers have assessed the relationship of birth weight to blood pressure, type 2 diabetes, glucose and insulin dynamics, serum lipids, and cardiovascular disease, among others. The vast majority of studies have been conducted in the US and Western Europe, where more detailed hospital and research records allow scientists to identify indicators of poor maternal or fetal nutrition. Relatively few studies have been conducted in developing countries, but this is

The Nutrition Transition
ISBN: 0-12-153654-8

changing rapidly, with a substantial increase in papers published since 1995. This chapter will focus on the relationship of pre- and early postnatal nutrition to the development of chronic disease in developing countries. Research on populations undergoing changes in diet, activity, and other chronic disease risk factors may provide particularly valuable insights into the role of early nutrition in the rapid spread of chronic diseases.

Rates of obesity and noncommunicable disease are increasing throughout the developing world (see Chapters 9 and 10). For example, in India, the dramatic increases in coronary heart disease (CHD) and diabetes have been termed an epidemic. There has been a fourfold increase in prevalence of type 2 diabetes, from less than 3% in the 1970s to about 12% in the 1990s (Ramachandran et al., 1997), and a fivefold increase in CHD in the same time period (Gupta and Gupta, 1996). It is projected that CHD will be the leading cause of mortality in India by 2010. The World Health Organization (WHO) estimates that if current trends continue, 60% of deaths in Africa in 2030 will be caused by noncommunicable diseases, compared to 41% in 1990. Currently, close to 20 million Africans suffer from hypertension, and diabetes rates range as high as 20% in some urban populations of Africa.

At the same time, poor maternal nutrition, infections, and other prenatal stresses continue to produce poor birth outcomes. DeOnis et al. (1998) estimated the regional incidence of low birth weight related to growth restriction, rather than prematurity (intrauterine growth retarded low birth weight, IUGR-LBW, is defined as full term but weighing less than 2500 g at birth). They estimated that at least 13.7 million infants are born annually with IUGR-LBW. This number represents 11% of all newborns in developing countries. Rates of IUGR-LBW are highest in Asia, ranging to nearly 40% in Bangladesh. Rates in excess of 15% were estimated in Africa for Zaire, Angola, Guinea and The Gambia. Small size for gestational age (<10th percentile of birth weight for gestational age) is estimated to occur in nearly 30 million newborns per year, with 75% of those affected living in Asia. These children, who are likely to have suffered from inadequate intrauterine nutrition, may be at increased risk of developing CVD, diabetes, and other noncommunicable diseases as adults.

# Epidemiologic studies of fetal programming in developing countries

Much of the early programming literature focused on samples of European or North American adults that included individuals already diagnosed with chronic disease. Many of these studies were limited by a lack of detailed or accurate information on maternal nutrition during pregnancy, and birth outcomes other than birth weight. Birth outcome information was typically obtained from hospital records or existing research studies. Later, more sophisticated prospective studies, as well as retrospective studies with more detailed maternal and birth outcome data were conducted to take us "beyond birth weight." There is now an extensive literature on human epidemiologic studies testing the programming hypothesis, but the majority of studies are still conducted in developed countries.

In developing countries, a shortage of good population-based, maternal nutrition and birth outcome data that can be associated with long-term, chronic disease risk factors or outcomes in adults, limits the ability to test the programming hypothesis. A small number of retrospective studies have used hospital records, but in developing countries, historically, hospital births may over-represent higher socioeconomic status women or those with pregnancy complications. Examples include the studies of adults born in the Holdsworth Memorial Hospital in Mysore, India (Kumaran and Fall, 2001), a study of adults born in the Peking Union Medical College (Mi *et al.*, 2000) and a study of children born in the King Edward Memorial Hospital in Pune, India (Fall *et al.*, 1995; Yajnik *et al.*, 1995).

An increased appreciation of the potential contribution of early nutrition to the development of chronic disease risk, and of the importance of studying antecedents of disease, has resulted in more studies on children and young adults. Some studies are adding research on fetal programming to ongoing prospective studies of child growth. For example, the Birth to Ten (BTT) study follows a birth cohort of predominantly black South Africa children born in 1990 (Levitt *et al.*, 1999; Crowther *et al.*, 2000). The Cebu Longitudinal Health and Nutrition Survey (CLHNS) follows a cohort of Filipino youths born in 1983–84 (Adair *et al.*, 2001). The follow-up of the Guatemala study examines adults who, as children, received nutrition supplementation (Stein *et al.*, 2001). Recently, several new studies, such as the Pune Maternal Nutrition Study, were designed and implemented specifically to test the programming hypothesis (Fall *et al.*, 1999). Most of the studies relate to components of the insulin resistance syndrome and cardiovascular disease, although there are also several studies on programming of the immune system (Moore *et al.*, 1997, 1999; McDade *et al.*, 2001a,b).

# Cardiovascular disease, blood pressure, and lipids

## Studies among adults

Studies in Mysore, India were motivated by the observation of dramatic increases in CVD in Indian adults in the absence of high rates of typical CVD risk factors such as high blood pressure, obesity, high dietary saturated fat intakes and smoking (Kumaran and Fall, 2001). Researchers took advantage of hospital birth records, maintained since 1934, and recruited a sample of 517 individuals (ages 38–60) who could be matched to their birth records. CVD prevalence was higher among men and women who had underweight mothers, and who themselves were shorter, lighter, and had smaller head circumference at birth. Systolic blood pressure tended to be higher among those who were longer length at birth (Stein *et al.*, 1996). Kumaran *et al.* (2000) found no relationship of blood pressure, arterial compliance or left ventricular mass to small size at birth in a follow-up study of the same sample designed to examine the basis of elevated CVD risk in more detail. These results led to the authors' suggestion that CVD in Indian adults is more related to the insulin resistance syndrome.

A lack of association of small size at birth with blood pressure in adulthood was also found among Guatemalan young adults who had been participants in a nutrition supplementation trial in infancy and childhood. Stein *et al.* (2001) found no relationship of birth weight to blood pressure in young adult women, but a positive association of birth weight and weight at one year of age to blood pressure in men. Birth weight was positively correlated with adult body mass index (BMI) and blood pressure in a sample of 317 Australian Aboriginal adults (ages 20–38) with a low birth weight prevalence of 35% (Hoy *et al.*, 1999).

Results from a study of 137 young adult, urban, South Africans are more consistent with the inverse association of birth weight to blood pressure found in European and US populations. Levitt *et al.* (2000) compared adults who had been underweight (<10th percentile of birth weight for gestational age) or normal weight (25th–75th percentile). Those who were underweight for gestational age were shorter, had lower BMI, but had higher systolic and diastolic blood pressure. Similarly, in a cohort of 122 Hong Kong adults (30 years old), Cheung *et al.* (2000) found that systolic blood pressure was inversely related to birth weight and length, but positively related to increases in ponderal index during infancy. They also found diastolic blood pressure was inversely related to birth length only. Mi *et al.* (2000) studied 627 adults (41–47 years of age) who were born at the Peking Union Medical College. After adjusting for sex and BMI, each kilogram increase in birth weight was associated with a 2.9 mm decrease in systolic and a 1.7 mm decrease in diastolic blood pressure in men and women.

In the absence of birth outcome data, several studies used adult height as a proxy for fetal growth retardation. In a study of adult Nigerian civil servants, Olatunbosum and Bella (2000) found no relationship of current height with blood pressure. Sichieri *et al.* (2000) found a U-shaped relationship among Brazilian adults, with the lowest systolic blood pressure observed in the 3rd quartile of height. In both of these studies, it is assumed that short stature represents early growth retardation, but there are no data to identify the timing (pre- or postnatal) of growth retardation.

Many studies in Europe and the US have found that the relationship of birth weight to blood pressure is strongest among those who were small at birth, but relatively large at the time of measurement (Law and Schiell, 1996; Huxley *et al.*, 2000). This pattern is not so clearly evident in the studies cited above.

Several other risk factors for CVD have been studied. Stein *et al.* (1996) found no relationship between size at birth and serum lipids, plasma fibrinogen or factor VII in Indian adults. Kolacek *et al.* (1993) examined 192 young adult Croatians and found total cholesterol and low density lipoprotein cholesterol (LDL-C) were highest among males who were the leanest in the first 3 years of life, but the fattest as adults. However, there was no significant association of birth weight to lipids in adulthood. Adult males who were shorter as adults, but of lower socioeconomic status (SES) during childhood had the highest total cholesterol and LDL-C levels. In Chinese adults, Mi *et al.* (2000) found an inverse relationship of birth weight to serum triglycerides, total cholesterol and LDL-C.

Hoy *et al.* (1999) found that birth weight was inversely correlated with a marker of renal disease (urine albumin/creatinine ratio) in Australian Aboriginal adults, and low birth weight explained 27% of the population-based prevalence of overt albuminuria.

## Studies of precursors of disease among children and adolescents

Biological changes which foreshadow CVD are already present in childhood (see Misra, 2000 for a review). Several large studies in the US have documented disease risk profiles in children. Similarly, a pattern of elevated blood pressure and altered lipid profiles has been observed in young children in South Africa (Steyn *et al.*, 2000). Given the tendency for tracking of risk factors throughout life, it is important to identify determinants of cardiovascular disease risk factors, including elevated blood pressure and altered serum lipid profiles, early in childhood.

Based on large-scale systematic reviews of studies throughout the world, investigators concluded that a relationship of size at birth to blood pressure later in life is less consistently found or is weaker in children and adolescents than in adults (Law and Schiell, 1996; Leon and Koupilova, 1999; Huxley *et al.*, 2000). The literature from developing countries shows inconsistencies in all age groups.

There is typically a strong relationship of height and weight to blood pressure in children and adolescents. In fact, US reference data for blood pressure in children and adolescents are age-, sex- and height-specific. Thus, it is important to take current body size into account when assessing the relationship of birth size to later outcomes. However, this complicates the interpretation of results, since children's current size may also be related to their size at birth. Lucas *et al.* (1999) recommended that researchers examine crude effects of birth size, birth size after accounting for current size, and birth size interacted with current size as a means of understanding the relative importance of size at birth versus postnatal growth.

The relation of birth size to blood pressure in children and adolescents is typically stronger, or in some cases, observed only after accounting for current size. Results have been interpreted as indicating that size at birth potentiates the effects of current size or that it is the combined effect of small size at birth with rapid postnatal growth that is important. Size at birth, since it reflects a variety of prenatal physiological adaptations, may influence susceptibility or response to subsequent risk factors such as diet and sedentary lifestyle. Although continuing growth retardation into adulthood remains in many poor communities in developing countries, there are substantial subgroups of children who were growth restricted at birth, but who grew more rapidly in the postnatal period. In some cases, there is more compensation in weight than in linear growth, resulting in children who are relatively heavy but short in stature (Martorell *et al.*, 1987; Popkin *et al.*, 1996). This combination of being small at birth, but relatively heavy or fat in childhood is the pattern most often associated with elevated blood pressure, altered serum lipid profiles and altered glucose and insulin metabolism.

Law *et al.* (2001) conducted a multicountry study of blood pressure in young children from China, Chile, Guatemala, Nigeria, and Sweden. They found a strong association of systolic blood pressure with current weight in all samples, and after accounting for current size, an inverse relationship of systolic blood pressure to some aspect of size at birth except in Nigerian children was found. A relationship with birth *weight* was only found in Guatemalan and Chilean children, whereas the significant birth measures were head and chest circumference in China, and ponderal index in Sweden. This points to the importance of assessing other indicators of fetal growth. However, such indicators are often lacking because they are not routinely collected. The overall picture that emerges from this comparative study is that elevated systolic blood pressure in childhood relates most strongly to proportionate growth retardation that is most often the result of chronic undernutrition throughout gestation. Based on this study and earlier reviews, Law *et al.* (2001) suggested that a relation between size at birth and blood pressure in childhood is less consistent among Africans or those of African descent. However, this may reflect an imbalance in the number of studies conducted among blacks compared to other race/ethnic groups.

Among 1- to 9-year-old Gambian children, Margetts *et al.* (1991) found no associ- ation of birth weight to blood pressure. In contrast, Levitt *et al.* (1999) found a significant inverse relation between blood pressure and birth weight among 5-year-old children who were participants in the BTT Study, and Woelk *et al.* (1998) found a similar relationship among children in Harare, Zimbabwe. Several investigators have studied children of African descent living in Jamaica. Forrester *et al.* (1996) found an inverse association of birth weight to blood pressure in a sample of 1610 Jamaican school children. In Jamaican children (1–4 years of age), Thame *et al.* (2000) found an inverse relationship of systolic blood pressure to birth weight. Blood pressure was also found to be negatively related to placental volume at 17 weeks, and fetal abdomen circumference at 20 weeks. Maternal nutritional status during pregnancy was related to infant birth weight, but not to blood pressure.

Gaskin *et al.* (2000) compared 120 children (7–8 years old) who were stunted between 9 and 24 months of age to 220 nonstunted children. Although stunted chil- dren remained shorter and thinner at age 7–8 years and had higher systolic blood pressure, their birth weights did not significantly predict blood pressure. In the same study population assessed at ages 11–12 years, Walker *et al.* (2001) found that birth weight significantly predicted systolic blood pressure only after adjusting for current weight. The effects of current weight were stronger among children with a history of stunting, leading to the authors' conclusion that early postnatal growth retardation potentiates the relation of current weight to blood pressure.

Studies in other parts of the world are also inconsistent. Bergel *et al.* (2000) mea- sured systolic blood pressure in a sample of 518 children (ages 5–9) born in a clinic in Argentina. The mothers' hemoglobin during pregnancy was positively associated with blood pressure, but no other measure of maternal nutrition predicted the children's blood pressure. A weak inverse association of birth weight with systolic blood pres- sure was found only among children in the highest quartile of current BMI.

In a study of a large cohort of children born in 1983–84 in the Philippines longitu- dinal data from the prenatal period to the present allowed for detailed analysis of rela- tionships of maternal nutrition during pregnancy and birth outcomes to numerous aspects of current health status in about 2000 adolescents. In addition, fasting

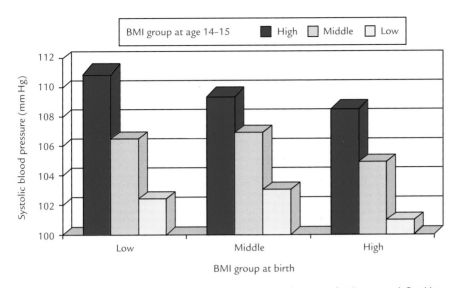

**Figure 7.1**   Mean systolic blood pressure of Cebu, Philippines adolescent males, in groups defined by thirds of BMI at birth and at age 14–15 years.

glucose, insulin, and serum lipids were measured on a subset of about 600 study participants. The subset was selected to over-represent those with IUGR. Among the full sample of adolescents, a significant inverse relationship of birth weight to adolescent systolic blood pressure was found only among males, and only after controlling for current body size (Adair *et al.*, 2001). The pattern typically seen, that is, of highest blood pressure among those relatively small at birth, but relatively large at the time of measurement is well illustrated in the Filipino sample of nearly 1000 males (ages 15–16) (Fig. 7.1). Our studies also controlled for other factors which may affect current blood pressure, including maturation status, physical activity, smoking, and diet. Overall, the strongest determinants of adolescent blood pressure were measures of current size, including height and BMI.

Overall, the magnitude of significant effects on blood pressure across all of the studies range from about 1.4 mm Hg per kg of birth weight in 1–4-year-old Jamaican children (Thame *et al.*, 2000) to 4.9 mm Hg per kg of birth weight in Chilean children (Law *et al.*, 2001). Although these mean changes may seem small, and of questionable biological significance, it is important to note that there may be greater impact when considering the occurrence of high blood pressure. For example, despite the relatively weak linear association of birth weight to adolescent male blood pressure in the Philippines study, we found a strong decline in the likelihood of having relatively high systolic and diastolic blood pressure with each kilogram increase in birth weight. Given the changes in blood pressure associated with age and height in adolescents, high blood pressure was defined as systolic and diastolic values falling in the top 10% of the age-, sex- and height-specific distribution of the sample of about 2000 participants. The predicted probability of high blood pressure decreases from about 23%, if birth weight is 2 kg, to about 6%, if birth weight is 4 kg (controlling for birth length, current age, height, BMI, maturation status, diet, and SES) (Fig. 7.2).

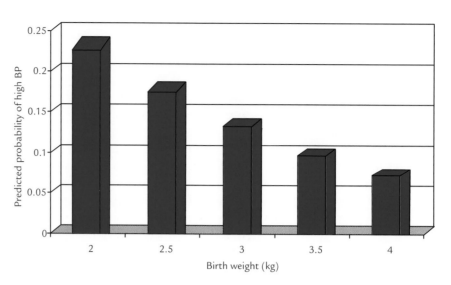

**Figure 7.2** Predicted probability of elevated blood pressure in Cebu, Philippines adolescent males, according to birth weight. Simulation based on birth weight coefficient from logistic regression model, outcome = high systolic and diastolic BP, controlling for birth length, current age, height, BMI, maturation status, energy and fat intake, socioeconomic status.

Very few studies in developing country studies have probed the "black box" represented by size at birth. It is widely assumed that prenatal nutrition is the most important programming stimulus (Harding, 2001). However, the few studies that include measures of maternal nutritional stress or nutritional status during pregnancy provide mixed support for the hypothesis that maternal nutrition is key to programming in humans.

In our study of Filipino adolescents (Adair *et al.*, 2001), we found a significant inverse relationship of mothers' triceps skinfold thickness during pregnancy to systolic blood pressure among male adolescents, and to diastolic blood pressure in males and females. Systolic blood pressure among males was significantly inversely related to mothers' percentage of energy from protein. Among females, systolic and diastolic blood pressure were inversely related to mothers' percentage of calories from fat. These relationships were not confounded by adolescents' diet, maturation status, physical activity, or socioeconomic status.

There are fewer studies related to other CVD risk factors in children. Relatively little information is available on the relationship of maternal nutrition during pregnancy or birth outcomes on serum lipids in children in any setting, much less in developing countries. Forrester *et al.* (1996) found no clear or strong relationships of size at birth to serum lipids in Jamaica. They did observe an inverse association of total cholesterol with crown–heel length in prepubertal children. In a study of adolescents in Hungary, Antal *et al.* (1998) found lower LDL-C and higher ApoA1 in boys who had been low birth weight. Among Indian children, Bavdekar *et al.* (1999) reported an inverse relationship of birth weight to LDL-C but no relationship with plasma triglycerides or high density lipoprotein cholesterol (HDL-C).

# Diabetes and its precursors

## Adults

Rates of type 2 diabetes are increasing dramatically in Asian, Latin American, and African populations. Of particular note is the suggestion that in Asian populations, abnormalities of glucose metabolism and type 2 diabetes occur at lower levels of BMI than is typically observed in Western populations (Ko et al., 1999; International Diabetes Institute, 2000). Compared to Caucasians, Asians have increased abdominal or central adiposity at similar levels of BMI (Deurenberg et al., 1998, 1999). Abdominal obesity is a well-known risk factor for insulin resistance and CVD. The observation of high rates of CVD in association with the insulin resistance syndrome (McKeigue et al., 1991, 1993) has led to a series of studies in India, designed to explain the unexpectedly high rates of diabetes in nonobese individuals. Yajnik (2001a) has described the clinical picture of diabetes in India: type 2 diabetics are relatively hyperinsulinemic and insulin resistant, with elevated triglycerides and elevated blood pressure. This pattern is associated with a high waist–hip ratio, even at lower levels of BMI.

The Mysore studies of Indian adults described above, with respect to blood pressure, also assessed glucose and insulin dynamics. In response to an oral glucose tolerance test (OGTT), 30-minute insulin values were significantly lower among participants with a higher birth weight and ponderal index. Type 2 diabetes, which occurred in 15% of the sample, was more prevalent in subjects who were short at birth with a relatively high ponderal index. Insulin resistance was predicted by birth weight in men, but not women (Fall et al., 1998).

Based on another study of Indian young adults, Raghupathy et al. (2001) presented preliminary data on the relation of maternal nutrition and fetal growth to CVD risk factors. They found the risk of diabetes or glucose intolerance was much higher, at the same level of BMI, in those who weighed less versus those who weighed more than 3 kg at birth. Mi et al. (2000) studied 41–47-year-old Chinese men and women born in Beijing. Fasting and 2-hour plasma glucose levels (after an oral glucose load), as well as fasting and 2-hour insulin levels were inversely related to birth weight after adjusting for sex and current BMI. In addition, 2-hour plasma glucose and insulin levels were inversely associated with maternal BMI at 38 weeks of pregnancy, with and without simultaneously adjusting for birth weight.

The importance of abdominal adiposity as a mediator of the relationship of birth weight to insulin sensitivity in Asians was questioned in a study of Korean young adults. Choi et al. (2000) found an inverse association of birth weight and insulin sensitivity, but no relationship of birth weight to measures of abdominal obesity in healthy young men.

Levitt et al. (2000) undertook a study to elucidate biological mechanisms that might explain the observed relationship of impaired glucose tolerance and elevated blood pressure to low birth weight, in nonobese young South African adults. They compared young adults whose birth weights were below the 10th to those between the 25th and 75th percentile of birth weight for gestational age. Those who were underweight for gestational age were shorter and had lower BMI as adults, but higher fasting glucose. Despite an absence of differences in mean glucose-stimulated insulin levels or homeostasis model insulin resistance (HOMA) between the groups, a higher proportion of those who had been underweight at birth had impaired glucose intolerance. Furthermore, they had higher plasma cortisol levels and a greater cortisol response to adrenocorticotropic hormone (ACTH) stimulation, leading the authors to suggest that the hypothalamic-pituitary-adrenal (HPA) axis is a target for early programming. It is notable that in this young adult population, as well as the populations studied in India, alterations in insulin sensitivity and glucose tolerance occur in the absence of obesity.

## Children

Crowther *et al.* (2000) assessed glucose and insulin dynamics in a sample of 152 children who were part of the South Africa BTT study. Seven-year-old children were categorized as above or below the sample median weight at birth and at age seven. Those who were small at both time periods had low pancreatic beta-cell activity. In contrast, those who were small at birth, but relatively large at age seven, had relatively high beta cell activity. The authors suggested that poor fetal and neonatal growth gives rise to low beta-cell numbers but increased efficiency of conversion of proinsulin into insulin. Despite this adaptation, they still had low insulin concentrations, and ultimately higher blood glucose concentrations and poorer glucose tolerance. Poor fetal growth followed by rapid postnatal growth resulted in beta cell dysfunction and insulin resistance. Both groups have elevated risk of type 2 diabetes later in life, particularly if they become obese.

A series of informative studies focus on urban children in India. In the first, reported by Yajnik *et al.* (1995) and Fall *et al.* (1995), subjects were 4-year-old children born in the King Edward Memorial Hospital. All were full term and weighed more than 2000 g at birth. After accounting for current weight and skinfold thickness, glucose and insulin levels in response to a glucose load were inversely associated with birth weight. Fasting insulin-like growth factor (IGF)-1 levels were also inversely associated with birth weight.

Bavdekar *et al.* (1999) tracked these children, as well as an additional sample at age eight, in order to evaluate the relative importance of pre- and postnatal growth. In a sample of 477 children (190 of whom had been in the earlier study), they found that higher birth weight was associated with being taller, heavier, and having thicker skinfolds at age eight. However, they found a significant clustering of insulin resistance syndrome variables with low birth weight. Birth weight tended to be inversely related to fasting insulin, and 30-minute plasma glucose and insulin levels, but not to fasting or 120-minute glucose. As expected, a higher fat mass was associated with insulin resistance. The highest level of insulin resistance was found among relatively tall children with short parents.

A new, prospective study of the long-term effects of maternal nutrition during pregnancy has been initiated in India by Yajnik and colleagues. The Pune Maternal Nutrition Study is prospectively tracking live births from six villages near Pune. In a sample of 770 live births, 28% of infants were low birth weight. The Indian babies, despite their small size and relative thinness compared to British babies, had similar subscapular skinfolds. Their low weight was attributable to relatively less lean tissue, a finding that has important implications for later insulin resistance. Furthermore, the fattest babies had mothers who were relatively short and fat.

In a review of the "insulin resistance epidemic" in India, Yajnik (2001a,b) highlighted the importance of these studies. Cardiovascular risk, including elevated blood pressure, altered serum lipids, and insulin resistance, is exaggerated among children who are born small but have more rapid postnatal growth. Yajnik has termed this the energy adaptation maladaptation syndrome (ENAMAS). He also notes that, as in the studies of Indian adults, altered disease risk profiles occur in children who are not obese, despite their more rapid postnatal growth.

# The role of overweight and obesity

The epidemiologic evidence summarized above points to the importance of being small at birth, and relatively large later, as a risk factor for CVD and diabetes. This raises an important question about the role of body size or fatness as a *mediator* of the relationship between early growth and later health outcomes. If intrauterine nutritional stress results in enhanced metabolic efficiency (or a thrifty phenotype), individuals with a history of poor prenatal nutrition may grow faster and/or have a greater propensity to store excess energy as fat when they subsequently encounter improved nutritional circumstances. Based on their work among poor Brazilian children, Hoffman *et al.* (2000) proposed that fat oxidation is impaired in stunted children. Furthermore, they suggested that stunted children may opportunistically overeat, which in turn, may contribute to their higher risk of overweight.

Whitaker and Dietz (1998), and more recently Martorell *et al.* (2001) reviewed the role of prenatal nutrition as a determinant of later adiposity. In general, there is more substantial literature linking the risk of high birth weight or macrosomia to later risk of obesity. For example, Hediger *et al.* (1998) found, in a large US national sample, that large size for gestational age at birth was associated with persistent fatness in childhood. In contrast, children who were small for gestational age had persistent deficits in muscularity, but not in fatness. Evidence accumulating from developing countries suggests a relationship of early growth restriction, manifested as lower birth weight or stunting in early childhood, to later adiposity in children than in adults. For example, Popkin *et al.* (1996) found a significant association of stunting with overweight among children in China, Brazil, Russia, and South Africa. In contrast, Martorell *et al.* (1998) found that IUGR was related to shorter stature but not to percentage body fat in 17-year-old Guatemalan adolescents. However, in a slightly larger sample of Guatemalan adults, researchers found a positive association of birth weight to percentage body fat (Schroeder *et al.*, 1999). After controlling for overall fatness, adults who had been severely stunted as children had a higher waist-to-hip ratio, suggestive of increased abdominal adiposity. Similarly, Bavdekar *et al.* (1999) found that poor intrauterine growth predicted higher central adiposity in 8-year-old Indian children.

Increased body fat, particularly central adiposity, is a well-established risk factor for type 2 diabetes and CVD. An important question in the context of the programming hypothesis is whether fatness carries the same risk irrespective of the nutritional history of the individual. Studies of the interaction of size at birth with current adiposity or BMI suggest that at the same level of adiposity, risk is worsened in those who were small at birth. This, in turn, suggests the importance of additional pathways that are independent of current fatness. There is an extensive literature, based largely on animal models, on the biological mechanisms that may explain the relationship of small size at birth to later risk of noncommunicable diseases (see Waterland and Garza, 1999 and Harding, 2001 for reviews).

One basic theme relates to the "thrifty phenotype", or the proposed alterations in metabolic efficiency that preserve fetal brain growth at the expense of other organs and tissues. Eriksson *et al*. (2000) hypothesize that restricted growth permanently reduces cell numbers in vital organs, resulting in impaired function. When compensatory growth occurs in childhood, there is excessive metabolic demand on limited cell mass, resulting in elevated disease risk. Studies in India (Yajnik, 2001a,b), point to the importance of long-term deficits in lean body mass, which affect metabolic rate as well as insulin resistance. Gale *et al*. (2001) found long-term associations between birth weight and adult bone and lean mass, but only weak associations with fat. Further research which focuses on specific aspects of body composition and fat patterning is needed, particularly given the observations that signs of disease are observed in the absence of obesity.

Other lines of research suggest that disease risk is associated with early programming of the HPA axis, resulting in heightened responsivity to stress (see Clark, 1998 for a review). Few studies have directly tested this hypothesis in developing countries. However, Levitt *et al*. (2000) found that plasma cortisol levels were higher, and response to ACTH stimulation was greater in adults who were underweight for gestational age at birth, suggesting that this a promising line of research.

## Discussion

The link between fetal and early infant development and later risk of chronic disease is well established by a wealth of experimental animal and human epidemiologic literature. There remain questions about the mechanisms, and about the relative importance of pre- versus postnatal factors in the origins of disease. Although not shown in all studies, a recurring finding in many settings is that disease risk is enhanced by the combination of fetal growth retardation and higher current body size, typically measured by BMI. This pattern of early undernutrition and later overnutrition in subgroups of populations in developing countries is a likely *consequence* of the nutrition transition.

The key elements of the nutrition transition occur in association with rapid socioeconomic change. They include: (1) changes in the overall structure and composition of the diet favoring higher fat and sugar content and thus higher energy density; and

(2) an increase in sedentary activity associated with adoption of more labor-saving devices, a shift in the physical demands of many economic activities, and an increase in leisure time (Popkin, 1998, 2001). Economic development is also associated with improved water supply and better preventive health care, which reduce the prevalence of childhood diarrheal diseases. These changes are likely to be associated with improved child growth, and at the extreme, with overweight and obesity. At the same time, however, there are historically high rates of low birth weight which are relevant for today's adult populations, and continuing high rates of poor prenatal growth affecting younger children. Biologically, poor fetal nutrition results in altered structure and physiological functioning. In response to an inadequate supply of oxygen and nutrients, adaptations which enhance survival and preserve brain growth may result in deficits in organs and tissues, including smaller kidneys with fewer nephrons, a reduced number or altered function of pancreatic beta cells, a smaller liver, and reduced skeletal muscle mass. Furthermore, there is evidence that poor maternal nutrition or high levels of stress cause reprogramming of the HPA axis such that stress responses are altered. Together, these adaptations reflect a "thrifty phenotype" (Hales and Barker, 1992). A child equipped with this altered physiology, who encounters an adequate or excessive energy and nutrient supply relative to needs, may have an increased tendency to store energy as fat, and to develop insulin resistance. In countries undergoing the nutrition transition, the likelihood of encountering such an environment is increased, in light of increased availability and altered composition of foods, and a trend toward more sedentary activity.

Yajnik (2001) suggests that exposure to the urban environment also heightens risk of chronic disease. Levels of tumor necrosis factor (TNF) alpha and interleukin 6 (proinflammatory cytokines) were found to be elevated among urban Indian populations, particularly slum dwellers, compared to rural residents (Yudkin *et al.*, 1999a). Yajnik *et al.* (1999b) hypothesize that aspects of urban stress trigger the release of adipose-tissue-derived cytokines, which are in turn associated with endothelial damage and CVD. This hypothesis is an important one to pursue in urban populations of developing countries.

When comparing the long-term effects of small size at birth in developed and developing countries, it is also important to keep in mind that the usual reasons for small size differ. For example, if low-birth-weight (LBW) infants in the US or Western Europe are compared with those in developing countries, two major differences are apparent. First, a much higher percentage of LBW in developed countries is attributable to prematurity, whereas in developing countries, the majority of LBW babies are full term but small for gestational age. Furthermore, babies in developing countries are more likely to be proportionately growth retarded, most likely as a result of chronic nutritional stress throughout gestation. The Pune studies show that relative to British babies, Indian babies are lighter and thinner, but subcutaneous fat is preserved. Their weight deficits are in skeletal muscle and organs, and it is precisely these changes that may have long-term importance for the insulin resistance syndrome. For example, less skeletal muscle means fewer insulin receptors, and lower metabolic rates. Many studies show that altered metabolic profiles develop at lower levels of BMI, particularly among Asian children, such that effects are seen in the absence of overweight or obesity. The role of fat patterning and distribution is an important area for further research in children and adolescents.

In addition to the predominant pattern of countries in transition (early growth restriction followed by compensatory growth), we are also seeing a new pattern emerge. Impaired glucose tolerance among young adult women who were growth retarded at birth may affect fetal growth in the next generation: women with impaired glucose tolerance or gestational diabetes during pregnancy may produce offspring who are relatively large (Yajnik, 2001a). These macrosomic infants may, in turn, show alterations in glucose metabolism later in their lives. In either scenario, the risk of adult diabetes and its associated sequlae is elevated. Thus, there is a high level of complexity in the relationship of maternal nutrition and fetal programming, leading Yajnik to suggest that "the effects of nutritional factors may vary depending on the position of the population in the epidemiological and nutrition transition" (Yajnik, 2001b: p. 58).

In summary, the literature on early origins of chronic disease risk in developing countries is rapidly expanding. Despite some inconsistencies in results across countries, the following generalizations are supported.

1. Fetal growth restriction and/or poor growth during infancy are significantly associated with precursors of chronic disease including elevated blood pressure, altered serum lipid profiles and altered glucose/insulin metabolism, and altered immune responses in children, adolescents and young adults. Among older adults, fetal growth restriction and/or poor growth during infancy are significantly associated with precursors of chronic disease and with chronic disease morbidity and mortality related to type 2 diabetes, CVD, hypertension, and kidney disease.

2. There is an important synergism between early growth restriction and later rapid growth. The highest risk of adverse risk factors (hyperlipidemia, elevated blood pressure, hyperinsulinemia) and chronic disease are found among those who were small at birth but grew relatively fast during childhood.

3. The pattern of early growth restriction (manifested as low birth weight or thinness at birth) followed by more rapid growth (resulting in relatively higher BMI or fatness) is likely to be typical of populations undergoing the nutrition transition. In those populations, historically high rates of LBW are now often coupled with dramatic increases in child and adult overweight.

4. Early growth restriction is likely to be a relatively stronger risk factor for adult chronic disease in countries undergoing the nutrition transition, compared to developed countries (where rates of IUGR are low, but exposure to postnatal lifestyle and dietary risk factors is high).

Given the importance of early nutrition as well as nutrition during the entire period of growth and development, these findings have several logical and important implications for health policy. First, we must optimize maternal nutrition, and reduce maternal infection and stress during pregnancy to optimize fetal growth and infant health at birth. Second, we must promote a nutritional environment for children and adults that meets, but does not exceed needs. The latter involves not only attention to the quality and quantity of the diet, but also to the promotion of healthy levels of physical activity to maintain energy balance.

# References

Adair, L.S., Kuzawa, C., and Borja, J.R. (2001). *Circulation* **104**, 1034–1039.

Antal, M., Afgalvi, R., Nagy, K., Szepvolgyi, J., Babto, E., Regoly-Merei, A., Biro, L., and Biro, G. (1998). *Z. Ernahrungswiss.* **37** Suppl 1,131–133.

Bavdekar, A., Yajnik, C., Fall, C.V.D., Bapat, S., Pandit, A.N., Deshpande, V., Bhave, S., Kellingray, S.D., and Joglekar, C. (1999). *Diabetes* **48**, 2422–2429.

Bergel, E., Haelterman, E., Belizan, J., Villar, J., and Carroli, G. (2000). *Am. J. Epidemiol.* **151**, 594–601.

Cheung, Y.B., Low, L., Osmond, C., Barker, D., and Karlberg, J. (2000). *Hypertension* **36**, 795–800.

Choi, C.S., Kim, C., Lee, W.J., Park, J.Y., Hong, S.K., Lee, M.G., Park, S.W., and Lee, K.U. (2000). *Diabetes Res. Clin. Pract.* **49**, 53–59.

Clark, P.M. (1998). *Eur. J. Pediatr.* **157** Suppl 1, S7–10.

Crowther, N.J., Trusler, J., Cameron, N., Toman, M., and Graph, I.P. (2000). *Diabetologia* **43**, 878–885.

deOnis, M., Blossner, M., and Villar, J. (1998). *Eur. J. Clin. Nutr.* **52** Suppl 1, 5–15.

Deurenberg, P., Yap, M., and Staveren, W.A. (1998). *Int. J. Obes.* **22**, 1164–1171.

Deurenberg, P., Deurenberg-Yap, M., Wang, J., *et al.* (1999). *Int. J. Obes.* **23**, 537–542.

Eriksson, J., Forsen, T., Tuomilehto, J., Osmond, C., and Barker, D. (2000). *Hypertension* **36**, 790–794.

Fall, C.H., Pandit, A.N., Law, C.M., *et al.* (1995). *Arch. Dis. Child.* **73**, 287–293.

Fall, C.H., Stenin, C.E., Kumaran, K., Cox, V., Osmond, C., Barker, D.J., and Hales, C.N. (1998). *Diabetic Med.* **15**, 220–227.

Fall, C.H.D., Yajnik, C.S., Rao, S., and Coyaji, K.J. (1999). *In* "Fetal Programming Influences on Development and Disease in Later Life" (P.M. Shaughn O'Brien, T. Wheeler, and D.J.P. Barker, eds.), pp. 231–245. Royal College of Obstetricians and Gynaecologists, London.

Forrester, T.E., Wilks, R.J., Bennett, F.I., Simeon, D., Osmond, C., Allen, M., Chung, A.P., and Scott, P. (1996). *BMJ* **312**, 156–160.

Gale, C.R., Martyn, C.N., Kellingray, S., Eastell, R., and Cooper, C. (2001). *J. Clin. Endocrinol. Metab.* **86**, 267–272.

Gaskin, P.S., Walker, S.P., Forrester, T.E., and Grantham-McGregor, S.M. (2000). *Eur. J. Clin. Nutr.* **54**, 563–567.

Gupta, R., and Gupta, V.P. (1996). *Indian Heart J.* **48**, 241–245.

Hales, C.N., and Barker, D.J. (1992). *Diabetologia* **35**, 595–601.

Harding, J. (2001). *Int. J. Epidemiol.* **30**, 15–23.

Hediger, M.L., Overpect, M.D., Kuczmarski, R.J., McGlynn, A., Maurer, K.R., and Davis, W.W. (1998). *Pediatrics* **102**, E60.

Hoffman, D.J., Sawaya, A.L., Verreschi, I., Tucker, K.L., and Roberts, S.B. (2000). *Am. J. Clin. Nutr.* **72**, 202–207.

Hoy, W.E., Rees, M., Kile, E., Mathews, J.S., and Wang, Z. (1999). *Kidney Int.* **56**, 1072–1077.

Huxley, R.R., Shiell, A.W., and Law, C.M. (2000). *J. Hypertens.* **18**, 815–831.

International Diabetes Institute (2000). "The Asia-Pacific Perspective: Redefining Obesity and its Treatment". Health Communications Australia Pty Limited, Australia.

Ko, G.T.C., Chan, J.C.N., Cockram, C.S., *et al.* (1999). *Int. J. Obes.* **23**, 1136–1142.

Kolacek, S., Kapetanovic, K., Zimolo, A., and Luzar, V. (1993). *Acta Paediatr.* **82**, 699–704.

Kumaran, K., and Fall, C.H. (2001). *Int. J. Diabetes Developing Countries* **21**, 34–41.

Kumaran, K., Fall, C.V.D., Martyn, C.N., Vijayakumar, M., Stein, C., and Rhier, R. (2000). *Int. J. Diabetes Developing Countries* **83**, 272–277.

Law, C.M., and Schiell, A.W. (1996). *J. Hypertens.* **14**, 935–941.

Law, C.M., Egger, P., Dada, O., Delgado, H., Kylberg, E., Lavin, P., Tang, G.H., von Hertzen, H., Schiell, A.W., and Barker, D.J. (2001). *Int. J. Epidemiol.* **30**, 52–57.

Leon, D., and Koupilova, I. (1999). *In* "Fetal Origins of Cardiovascular and Lung Disease" (D.J.P. Barker, ed.). Marcel Dekker, New York.

Levitt, N.S., Steyn, K., and de Wet, T. (1999). *J. Epidemiol. Community Health* **53**, 264–268.

Levitt, N.S., Lambert, E.V., Woods, D., Hales, C.N., Andrew, R., and Seckl, J.R. (2000). *J. Clin. Endocrinol. Metab.* **85**, 4611–4618.

Lucas, A., Fewtrell, M., and Cole, T. (1999). *BMJ* **319**, 245–249.

Margetts, B.M., Rowland, M.G.M., Foord, F.A., Cruddas, A.M., Cole, T.J., and Barker, D.J.B. (1991). *Int. J. Epidemiol.* **20**, 938–943.

Martorell, R., Mendoza, F.S., Castillo, R.O., Pawson, I.G., and Budge, C.C. (1987). *Am. J. Phys. Anthropol.* **73**, 475–487.

Martorell, R., Ramakrishnan, U., Schroeder, D.G., Melgar, P., and Neufeld, L. (1998). *Eur. J. Clin. Nutr.* **52** Suppl 1, S43–52.

Martorell, R., Stein, A.D., and Schroeder, D.G. (2001). *J. Nutr.* **181**, 874s–880s.

McDade, T., and Adair, L.S. (2001). *Soc. Sci. Med.* **53**, 55–70.

McDade, T., Beck, M., Kuzawa, C., and Adair, L.S. (2001a). *Am. J. Clin. Nutr.* **74**, 543–548.

McDade, T., Beck, M., Kuzawa, C., and Adair, L.S. (2001b). *J. Nutr.* **131**, 1225–1231.

McKeigue, P.M., Shah, B., and Marmot, M.G. (1991). *Lancet* **337**, 382–386.

McKeigue, P.M., Ferrie, J.E., and Pierpoint, T. (1993). *Circulation* **87**, 152–161.

Mi, J., Law, C., Zhang, K.-L., Osmond, C., Stein, C., and Barker, D. (2000). *Ann. Intern. Med.* **132**, 253–260.

Misra, A. (2000). *J. Cardiovasc. Risk* **7**, 215–229.

Moore, S.E., Cole, T.J., Poskitt, E.M., and Sonko, B.J. (1997). *Nature* **388**, 434.

Moore, S.E., Cole, T.J., Collinson, A.C., Poskitt, E.M., McGregor, I.A., and Prentice, A.M. (1999). *J. Epidemiol.* **28**, 1088–1095.

Olatunbosum, S.T., and Bella, A.F. (2000). *J. Natl. Med. Assoc.* **92**, 265–268.

Popkin, B.M. (1998). The nutrition transition and its health implications in lower income countries. *Public Health Nutr.* **1**, 5–21.

Popkin, B.M. (2001). *In* "Fetal Origins of Cardiovascular and Lung Disease" (D.J.P. Barker, ed.). Marcel Dekker, New York.

Popkin, B.M., Richard, M.K., and Montiero, C.A. (1996). *J. Nutr.* **126**, 3009–3016.

Raghupathy, P., Antonisamy, B., Richard, J., Jose, P.C., and Joseph, S. (2001). Vellore Study – Preliminary data. Proceedings of the First World Congress on the Fetal Origins of Adult Disease. Mumbai, India. Abstract.

Ramachandran, A., Snehalatha, C., Latha, E., Vijay, V., and Viswanathan, M. (1997). *Diabetologia* **40**, 232–237.

Schroeder, D.G., Martorell, R., and Flores, R. (1999). *Am. J. Epidemiol.* **149**, 177–185.

Sichieri, R., Siqueira, K.S., Pereira, R.A., and Ascherio, A. (2000). *Public Health Nutr.* **3**, 77–82.

Stein, C.E., Fall, C.V.D., and Kumaran, K. (1996). *Lancet* **348**, 1269–1273.

Stein, A.D., Conlisk, A.J., Schroeder, D.G., Barnhart, H.X., Grajeda, R., Torun, B., and Martorell, R. (2001). Paper presented at the First World Congress on the Fetal Origins of Adult Disease, Mumbai, India.

Steyn, K., de Wet, T., Richter, L., Cameron, N., Levitt, N.S., and Morrell, C. (2000). *S. Afr. Med. J.* **90**, 719–726.

Thame, M., Osmond, C., Wilks, R.J., Bennett, F.I., McFarlane-Anderson, N., and Forrester, T.E. (2000). *Hypertension* **35**, 662–667.

Walker, S.P., Gaskin, P., Powell, C.A., Bennett, F.I., Forrester, T.E., and Grantham-McGregor, S. (2001). *J. Epidemiol. Community Health* **55**, 394–398.

Waterland, R.A., and Garza, C. (1999). *Am. J. Clin. Nutr.* **69**, 179–187.

Whitaker, R.C., and Dietz, W.H. (1998). *J. Pediatr.* **132**, 768–776.

Woelk, G.B., Emanuel, I., Weiss, N.S., and Psaty, B.M. (1998). *Arch. Dis. Child. Fetal Neonatal Ed.* **79**, F119–F122.

World Health Organization (1980). *World Health Statistics Quarterly* **33**, 197–224.

Yajnik, C.S. (2001a). *Nutr. Rev.* **59**, 1–9.

Yajnik, C.S. (2001b). *Int. J. Epidemiol.* **30**, 57–59.

Yajnik, C.S., Fall, C.H., and Vaidya, U. (1995). *Diabet. Med.* **12**, 330–336.

Yudkin, J.S., Yajnik, C.S., and Mohammed, A.V. (1999a). *Diabetes Care* **22**, 363–364.

Yudkin, J.S., Stehouwer, C.D.A., and Emeis, J.J. (1999b). *Arterioscler. Throm. Vasc. Biol.* **19**, 972–978.

# Obesity in the developing world

## 8

*Reynaldo Martorell*

## Introduction

Popkin and Doak (1998) wrote an article titled "The obesity epidemic is a worldwide phenomenon" and the World Health Organization (WHO) issued a report with the title "Obesity – Preventing and Managing the Global Epidemic" (WHO, 1998). These titles imply that obesity has emerged as a significant public health problem in developed as well as in developing countries and that rates are increasing rapidly worldwide; so much so in fact, that it can be labeled an "epidemic".

The objective of this chapter is to examine whether these claims are true for developing countries. Emphasis is placed on evidence from nationally representative surveys and comparisons of obesity levels found in various countries are made to the United States, where obesity is perceived to be a major threat to public health. Attempts are made to document trends in obesity, difficult to do because of the paucity of data, as well as to describe the "social mapping" of obesity. By this is meant quantifying how obesity varies by socioeconomic status, which has relevance to planning because it identifies the groups most affected within countries. Much of the information presented is based on prior work by Martorell *et al.* (2000a,b), with updates from surveys subsequently released to the public. Because of the variety of criteria used in previous research, the chapter begins by reviewing the assessment of obesity in adults and children. After reviewing the information available about obesity rates for women, men, school children and preschool children, consideration is given briefly to policy and program implications.

## Assessment

Obesity is a disease of complex, multifactorial causes leading to an imbalance between energy intake and output, and to the accumulation of large amounts of fat. In normal

The Nutrition Transition
ISBN: 0-12-153654-8

individuals, regulation of energy balance is achieved over the long term despite large fluctuations in both energy intake and output within and between days (Goran, 2000). Only a very small imbalance is necessary to produce obesity in an individual or a population. For example, in children, only a 2% discrepancy in energy is necessary to produce obesity. This is equivalent to about 125 kJ/day in terms of food intake or 15 minutes of daily play traded for watching television (Goran, 2000). These differences are very small relative to the precision of measurement of intakes and expenditures and it would be difficult in any population becoming obese to establish with certainty how much of the imbalance might be due to dietary or physical activity changes.

In adults, obesity is measured most often as excessive weight for a given height using the Body Mass Index (BMI), which is weight (kg) over height squared ($m^2$). The WHO assessed the relationship between BMI and health risks and defined overweight as a BMI between 25.0 and 29.9 $kg/m^2$ and obesity as a BMI of 30.0 $kg/m^2$ or greater (WHO, 1995). These cut off points are widely accepted.

BMI is not a perfect indicator, particularly for clinical use. For example, athletes with robust skeletal frames and substantial muscularity may appear to be overweight when in fact they may not be. Other methods are available to measure fatness directly. These include fat fold measures of the trunk and extremities (e.g., subscapular and triceps fat folds) and percentage body fat estimated from determinations of body density, tritiated or deuterated water and other techniques (Bray, 1996; Pi-Sunyer, 1999). BMI is linearly related to percentage body fat, with correlations between 0.6 and 0.8 in USA adults, similar to results found in other populations (Gallager et al., 1996).

The appropriateness of BMI has been called into question for populations with significant levels of early childhood stunting. Because growth failure occurs with greater intensity in the first two years of life, when growth of the extremities is faster than of the trunk, BMI may overestimate fatness among adults who suffered malnutrition as children and who may therefore have high sitting height to stature proportions (i.e., shorter legs). Adaptation to high altitude may also lead to large chest dimensions to house larger cardiovascular and respiratory capacities and this may also alter the relationship between BMI and fatness. It is not known how important these biases might be. Blacks have relatively longer lengths than whites (Martorell et al., 1988) but the relationship between BMI and percentage body fat is identical in both groups (Gallagher et al., 1996).

BMI, although a very good measure of overall fatness in adults, does not provide information about patterns of fat deposition, which carry health risks independent of overall fatness (Bray, 1996). For this reason measures of upper body and abdominal fatness are recommended in addition to BMI for epidemiological studies of risk factors.

Measuring obesity in children is complicated by the process of growth and maturation which leads to changes in body proportions, bone mass and percentage body fat; although BMI correlates well with measures of adiposity in children, these relationships are weaker than among adults (Troiano and Flegal, 1998). Thus, definitions of overweight and obesity in children take age into account by comparing values found for study subjects to the age-sex-specific distribution of a reference population.

In the USA, the recommended practice for school children is to define risk of overweight as a BMI between the 85th and the 94th percentiles and overweight as at or above the 95th percentile of the NCHS/CDC BMI-for-age percentile curves (Barlow and Dietz, 1998). Revised versions of these curves are being used by some USA investigators (Crawford *et al.*, 2001). For clinical purposes, the designation of "obesity" in children is reserved only when confirmed by further evaluation. For epidemiological studies, the designations of overweight for values between the 85th and 94th percentiles and obesity for those at or above the 95th percentile seem appropriate.

An international reference based on six nationally representative countries has been proposed for use in assessing children 2–18 years of age (Cole *et al.*, 2000). Cut off points at different ages are proposed that at 18 years pass through the "adult" cut off points of 25 and 30 kg/m$^2$. Averaging across the six data sets, the cut off point for overweight corresponds roughly to the 90th percentile of BMI for age and that for obesity more or less to the 97th percentile. Even though the cut off points correspond to those used in adults, which is the salient advantage of this approach, the authors caution that the health consequences for children above these cut off points may differ from those of adults. The approach proposed by Cole *et al.* (2000) may become widely adopted.

The practice for children less than 5 years of age is based on the use of weight for length (under two years) or weight for height (2–5 years) curves that originate from the USA but that have come to be known as the WHO/NCHS curves (Hamill *et al.*, 1979). Weight for length (or height) provides equivalent information as BMI for age in this age range. WHO defines obesity as any value greater than two standard deviations above the age- and sex-specific mean in the WHO/NCHS reference population (WHO, 1995) and Martorell *et al.* (2000b) also defined overweight as greater than 1 standard deviation. Others define overweight as any value greater than the 95th percentile of the reference curves (Ogden *et al.*, 1997) or as any value greater than two standard deviations above the reference mean (de Onis and Blössner, 2000). The various uses of the words "obesity" and "overweight" require careful attention to the criteria used across studies.

New reference data for preschool children based on multicountry studies of growth and development and on subjects that have been breastfed according to WHO recommendation are being developed by WHO and will be available in a few years (Garza and de Onis, 1999). These reference curves will replace the WHO/NCHS curves for international use.

# The consequences of obesity

The consequences of obesity for adults are well known. It contributes to the development of many diseases including diabetes, hypertension, stroke, cardiovascular disease, and some cancers (Solomon and Manson, 1997). Obesity also increases mortality from all causes, as well as from cardiovascular disease, cancer and other diseases (Seidell, 1997; Bender *et al.*, 1998; Stevens *et al.*, 1998). Increased mortality risk begins well below the established criterion of obesity, a BMI less than 30 kg/m$^2$, perhaps from as low as 22–25 kg/m$^2$ (Stevens *et al.*, 1998; Calle *et al.*, 1999).

Childhood obesity is viewed as a problem because it is an important predictor of adult obesity (Serdula *et al.*, 1993; Whitaker *et al.*, 1997). About a third of obese preschool children become obese adults and half of obese school-age children become obese adults (Serdula *et al.*, 1993). On the other hand, most obese adults were not obese as children (Strauss, 1999). The influence of childhood obesity on adult status rises with age. Serdula *et al.* (1993) report that the risk of adult obesity was 2.0–2.6 times greater in obese than in nonobese preschool children but 3.9–6.5 times greater for the same comparison at older ages. Whitaker *et al.* (1997) found that childhood obesity was not a significant predictor of adult obesity at 1–2 years of age, but that it did become a significant predictor at 3–5 years, and even a stronger one at older ages. Also, parental obesity magnifies the probability that an obese child will become an obese adult (Whitaker *et al.*, 1997).

There are also important consequences of obesity on child health per se (Dietz, 1998; Must and Strauss, 1999). The risk of hyperlipidemia, hypertension and abnormal glucose tolerance is increased somewhat among obese children, and in the United States, childhood obesity has important psychosocial consequences. Obese children frequently become targets of systematic discrimination and by adolescence, many suffer from low self-esteem (Dietz, 1998).

Obesity is recognized as an important public health problem in industrialized countries, but until recently, not in developing countries. WHO (1998) has called attention to the fact that obesity is increasing worldwide at an alarming rate in both developed and developing countries. WHO issued this conclusion despite the limited availability of nationally representative data and the lack of information about trends. This note of alarm led a team at Emory University (Reynaldo Martorell, Morgen Hughes) and at the Centers for Disease Control and Prevention (CDC) (Laura Kettel Khan and Laurence Grummer-Strawn) to analyze data from national nutrition surveys in the last 15 years to ascertain levels and trends in obesity in developing countries (Martorell *et al.*, 2000a,b). These surveys, mostly Demographic Health Surveys (DHS), were designed to assess health and malnutrition among women and young children. For this reason, they provide only limited information about patterns of obesity in developing countries. They include only height and weight information. Most surveys were from very poor countries and information from many of the advanced countries from Latin America and Asia is lacking. Most surveys excluded school children, adolescents, women past reproductive age and men.

## Levels of obesity in women

The percentages of women aged 15–49 years who were overweight ($25.0$–$29.9 \, kg/m^2$) or obese ($>30 \, kg/m^2$) are given in Table 8.1 for 35 developing countries (13 countries had two surveys) and the United States. The surveys included are all those previously analyzed and reported by Martorell *et al.* (2000a) as well as results from recently released surveys from DHS (Burkina Faso, 1998/99; Cameroon, 1998; Colombia, 2000; Ghana, 1998; Guatemala, 1998/99; Kenya, 1998; Nigeria, 1999; Tanzania, 1999;

**Table 8.1** Overweight and obesity levels in women aged 15–49 years in developing countries

| Country | Year | Sample size | % Overweight (25–29.9 kg/m²) | % Obese (30 kg/m²) |
|---|---|---|---|---|
| **Sub-Saharan Africa** | | | | |
| Benin | 1996 | 2266 | 6.9 | 2.1 |
| Burkina Faso | 1992/93 | 3161 | 5.9 | 1.0 |
| Burkina Faso[a] | 1998/99 | 3202 | 4.5 | 0.9 |
| Cameroon[a] | 1998 | 1537 | 17.8 | 3.5 |
| Central African Rep. | 1994/95 | 2025 | 5.5 | 1.1 |
| Comoros | 1996 | 773 | 15.9 | 4.4 |
| Côte d'Ivoire | 1994 | 3108 | 11.0 | 3.0 |
| Ghana | 1993 | 1773 | 9.3 | 3.4 |
| Ghana[a] | 1998 | 2068 | 11.0 | 5.0 |
| Kenya | 1993 | 3294 | 11.4 | 2.4 |
| Kenya[a] | 1998 | 3240 | 12.3 | 2.6 |
| Malawi | 1992 | 2323 | 8.1 | 1.1 |
| Mali | 1996 | 4237 | 7.2 | 1.2 |
| Namibia | 1992 | 2205 | 22.5 | 13.8 |
| Niger | 1992 | 3292 | 6.2 | 1.2 |
| Nigeria[a] | 1999 | 2094 | 15.6 | 7.3 |
| Senegal | 1992/93 | 2895 | 12.0 | 3.7 |
| Tanzania | 1991/92 | 4597 | 9.3 | 1.9 |
| Tanzania | 1996 | 3721 | 10.8 | 2.6 |
| Uganda | 1995 | 3199 | 7.3 | 1.2 |
| Zambia | 1992 | 3239 | 11.8 | 2.4 |
| Zambia | 1996/97 | 3838 | 10.5 | 2.3 |
| Zimbabwe | 1994 | 1968 | 17.4 | 5.7 |
| Zimbabwe[a] | 1999 | 5121 | 19.4 | 7.4 |
| **Middle East and North Africa** | | | | |
| Egypt | 1992 | 4855 | 33.9 | 23.5 |
| Egypt | 1995/96 | 6769 | 31.7 | 20.1 |
| Morocco | 1992 | 2850 | 22.3 | 10.5 |
| **South Asia** | | | | |
| Bangladesh | 1995/96 | 3997 | 2.2 | 0.6 |
| Nepal | 1996 | 3399 | 1.5 | 0.1 |
| **Latin America and the Caribbean** | | | | |
| Bolivia | 1994 | 2347 | 26.2 | 7.6 |
| Brazil | 1989 | 10 189 | 25.0 | 9.2 |
| Brazil | 1996 | 3158 | 25.0 | 9.7 |
| Colombia | 1995 | 3319 | 31.4 | 9.2 |
| Colombia[a] | 2000 | 3236 | 30.5 | 10.6 |
| Costa Rica[a,c] | 1996 | 865 | 33.2 | 12.7 |
| Dominican Rep. | 1991 | 2163 | 18.6 | 7.3 |
| Dominican Rep. | 1996 | 7356 | 26.0 | 12.1 |
| Guatemala | 1995 | 4978 | 26.2 | 8.0 |
| Guatemala[a] | 1998/99 | 2373 | 31.9 | 12.1 |
| Haiti | 1994/95 | 1896 | 8.9 | 2.6 |
| Honduras | 1996 | 885 | 23.8 | 7.8 |
| Mexico | 1987 | 3681 | 23.1 | 10.4 |
| Mexico[a,b] | 1998 | 13 887 | 35.2 | 24.4 |
| Peru | 1992 | 5200 | 31.1 | 8.8 |
| Peru | 1996 | 10 747 | 35.5 | 9.4 |
| **Central Eastern Europe/Commonwealth of Independent States (CEE/CIS)** | | | | |
| Kazakstan | 1995 | 3538 | 21.8 | 16.7 |
| Turkey | 1993 | 2401 | 31.7 | 18.6 |
| Uzbekistan | 1996 | 4077 | 16.3 | 5.4 |
| United States | 1988–94 | 5219 | 20.7 | 20.7 |

[a] Data not analyzed by Martorell *et al.* (2000a).
[b] Women 18–49 years.
[c] Women 20–44 years.

Zimbabwe, 1999). Also in Table 8.1 point estimates for Costa Rica for 1996 (Ministerio de Salud, 1996) and for Mexico for 1998 (Rivera *et al.*, in press) are included but these refer to women aged 18–49 and 20–44 years respectively.

Regional summaries were then obtained by weighting the latest point estimates for the countries listed in Table 8.1 by population estimates of women 15–49 years for 1996 and these are given in Fig. 8.1. Regional designations are those used by UNICEF. Levels of overweight (25.0–29.9 BMI) and obesity (≥30 BMI) were extremely low in South Asia, represented by Bangladesh and Nepal, relatively rare in sub-Saharan Africa, but nearly as common in other regions as found in the United States. Although many countries from sub-Saharan Africa and Latin America were included in generating the estimates in Fig. 8.1, many countries were not and representation for other regions was much poorer or absent.

The region of East Asia and the Pacific is not represented in Fig. 8.1 but some data exist for this region. A representative survey of eight provinces of China in 1991 found a prevalence of obesity of 4.3% among women aged 20–45 years (Popkin *et al.*, 1995). Pacific island nations are known to have extremely high levels of obesity. In Western Samoa, for example, the prevalence of obesity among women aged 25–74 years was 66% in 1991 (Hodge *et al.*, 1994). Other data from the Middle East and North Africa confirm that this region has among the highest levels of obesity in the world. A national sample drawn from primary health care clinics in Kuwait found a prevalence of obesity of 40.2% among women older than 18 years in 1993 (Al-Isa, 1997). Prevalences for women aged 20–60 years and estimated from national surveys were reported to be 18.3% for Morocco in 1998 and 22.7% for Tunisia in 1997 (Mokhtar *et al.*, 2001). On the other hand, in southern Iran, only 8% of women and 2.5% of men were obese in 1993/94 (Pishdad, 1996).

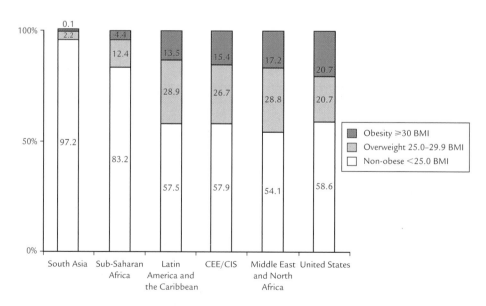

**Figure 8.1** Percentage distribution of obesity in women aged 15–49 years in different regions of developing countries and in the United States.

# The social mapping of obesity

Knowing how obesity is distributed across socioeconomic groups is important for policy makers because it informs them of the groups that need to be targeted by programs. A review of the literature found that whereas obesity among women increases with greater wealth in developing countries, it decreases in developed countries (Sobal and Stunkard, 1989). From these findings, WHO (1995) hypothesized that in very poor countries, few people and only those of high socioeconomic status would be heavy. In mid-income developing countries, more people would be obese and both high and low socioeconomic groups would be affected. Finally, in an affluent society, thinness would become culturally desirable, the rich would become thinner and obesity would become a marker of poverty.

Martorell *et al.* (2000a) have tested elements of this hypothesis by examining how the relationship between socioeconomic status and obesity varies according to level of national economic development, as defined by gross national product (GNP) per capita. They defined high socioeconomic status in these data sets in two ways: residence in urban areas and at least one year of secondary schooling. In Table 8.2, data are provided for each of the largest countries of the regions included in Fig. 8.1: Bangladesh (South Asia), Tanzania (sub-Saharan Africa), Egypt (Middle East and North Africa), Brazil (Latin America and the Caribbean), Turkey (Central and Eastern Europe). Bangladesh and Tanzania are very poor countries and have low levels of obesity. Further, obesity levels are much greater among urban and better-educated women. Using multivariate analysis, obesity was estimated to be between 4 and 7 times more probable in such women. Egypt is a country with very high levels of obesity for its level of income; although the relationship between socioeconomic status and obesity was not as strong as in Bangladesh and Tanzania, values were still over twice as likely among Egyptian women of higher socioeconomic status. Brazil and Turkey represent countries well along the nutrition transition defined by Popkin (1994). In these countries, the

**Table 8.2** Obesity prevalence in women aged 15–49 years by residence (urban/rural) and education[a] in selected countries (data from Martorell *et al.*, 2000a)

| Country | 1992 GNP per capita (US$) | % Obese total | % Obese | | % Obese | | Odds ratios[b] | |
|---|---|---|---|---|---|---|---|---|
| | | | Urban | Rural | High education | Low education | Residence (urban/rural) | Education (high/low) |
| Bangladesh (1995/96) | 220 | 0.6 | 2.7 | 0.4 | 1.9 | 0.3 | 7.50[c] | 7.07[c] |
| Tanzania (1996) | 110 | 2.6 | 6.0 | 1.7 | 8.4 | 2.3 | 4.27[c] | 4.22[c] |
| Egypt (1995/96) | 640 | 20.1 | 30.0 | 13.0 | 26.1 | 17.0 | 2.72[c] | 2.09[c] |
| Brazil (1996) | 2770 | 9.7 | 9.9 | 8.9 | 8.8 | 11.0 | 1.15 | 0.81 |
| Turkey (1993) | 1980 | 18.6 | 19.5 | 17.1 | 10.5 | 20.5 | 1.24 | 0.46[c] |

[a] Education: low, none to completed primary school; high, at least 1 year of secondary schooling.
[b] Estimated from multivariate logistic regressions that included obesity (0 = No, 1 = Yes) as the dependent variable and area of residence (0 = rural, 1 = urban) or educational level (0 = low, 1 = high) as the independent variable and age squared as a covariate.
[c] $P < 0.001$.

relationship with socioeconomic status became weaker or even reversed to a point where there was less obesity among those of higher socioeconomic status. For example, in Turkey, women with higher education had half the levels of obesity found in women with lower levels of education.

The relationship between GNP per capita and the within-country distribution of obesity by socioeconomic level is examined in Fig. 8.2 for the group of countries analyzed by Martorell *et al.* (2000a). As in Table 8.2, the odds ratios measure the concentration of obesity in urban and higher educated women. Three groups of countries are defined, those with odds ratios lower than 2, those between 2 and 4.99 and those greater than 5. There is a significant relationship with GNP. Countries with attenuated

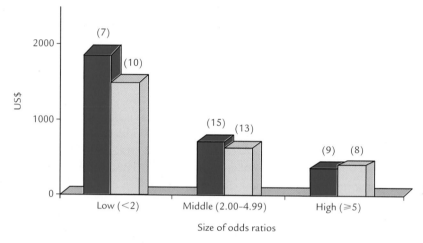

**Figure 8.2** Strength of the relationship between obesity and social class, as indexed by odds ratio sizes, and gross national product in 1992 (not including the USA). ■ Residence odds ratios, $F = 19.4$, $P < 0.0001$; ■ Education odds ratios, $F = 8.5$, $P < 0.001$; ( ) Number of countries.

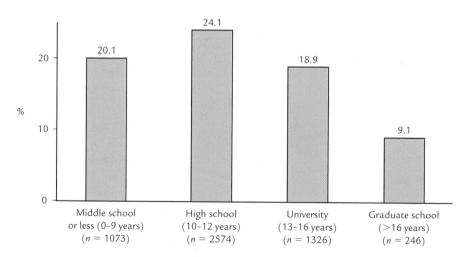

**Figure 8.3** Obesity ($>30\,\mathrm{kg/m^2}$) by years of schooling in the United States among women aged 15–49 years included in NHANES III (1988–1994).

relationships between socioeconomic status and obesity (i.e. odds ratios less than 2) have higher national incomes than countries with a strong positive relationship between these variables (i.e. odds ratios $\geqslant 5$).

The level of obesity among women in the United States is similar in urban and rural areas (Martorell *et al.*, 2000a). Level of education, on the other hand, is related to obesity as shown in Fig. 8.3. However, it is only highly educated women that have strikingly lower prevalences than the rest: 9% among women with graduate training versus over 20% among women with no university training.

The social mapping of obesity has clear implications for how obesity might be perceived as a national public health problem. If obesity is rare and found only among the elite, then it will be difficult to assign a high priority to programs to prevent it. On the other hand, in countries in transition, levels will be high and well distributed across socioeconomic levels, making it easier to assign a high level of priority to the problem of obesity.

# Trends in obesity

Obesity has increased dramatically in the United States among adults (Flegal *et al.*, 1998). Serial data are available from four national surveys: NHES I (1960/62), NHANES I (1971/74), NHANES II (1976/80) and NHANES III (1988/94). Rates of obesity among men aged 20–74 years were 10.4, 11.8, 12.3, and 20.0% and among women 15.0, 16.2, 16.5, and 24.9%, respectively. Most of the change is between the last two surveys, that is, between 1976/80 and 1988/94. Serial data from Europe also show that obesity is increasing in some countries (Björntorp, 1997; Seidell, 1997; Popkin and Doak, 1998). Is there also an epidemic of obesity in developing countries? This is a difficult question to answer with precision given the low number of countries with repeat nationally representative surveys. Martorell *et al.* (2000a) analyzed existing trend data (see Table 8.1) and reviewed the published literature. They found that obesity appears to be increasing in Latin America, the Middle East and North Africa and among Pacific Islanders but not in sub-Saharan Africa. Trends should be examined, as done in this volume for China and Brazil, by urban/rural residence and by socioeconomic status, in order to better inform policies and programs.

Since the analysis by Martorell *et al.* (2000a), several national surveys have become available for countries with prior data (see Table 8.1). The prevalence of obesity remained low and similar in Burkina Faso (1.0 in 1992/93 to 0.9% in 1998/99) and Kenya (2.4 in 1993 to 2.6% in 1998) but increased in two other sub-Saharan countries (Ghana, 3.4 in 1993 to 5.0% in 1998; Zimbabwe, 5.7 in 1994 to 7.4% in 1999).

New data from Mexico reveal dramatic increases in obesity (Fig. 8.4). In just 10 years, the prevalence of obesity among women 18 to 49 years increased from 9.4% to 24.4% and that of overweight and obesity from 33.4 to 59.6% (Rivera *et al.*, in press). All regions of Mexico (north, central, Mexico City and south) show these pronounced trends. Obesity also increased alarmingly among Mexican American women aged 15–49 years, specifically from 19.5 in 1982–84 to 28.7% in 1988–94. Women in Mexico

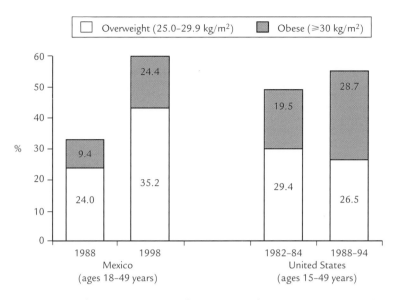

**Figure 8.4**  Increases in obesity among women of Mexican origin living in Mexico (Rivera *et al.*, in press) and the United States (Martorell *et al.*, 1998).

are now as fat as women of Mexican origin living in the United States. Women of Mexican origin are among the heaviest in the American continent. New DHS data for Colombia for 2000 show a prevalence of obesity of 10.5% among women aged 15–49 years, up from 9.2% in 1995. Similarly, new DHS data for Guatemala for 1998/99 show that 12.1% of women aged 15–49 years were obese, a rate greater than the 8.0% found in 1995.

Rapid increases, particularly among women, have been reported recently for North Africa (Mokhtar *et al.*, 2001). In Tunisia, rates of obesity increased among women aged 20–60 years old from 8.7 in 1980 to 22.7% in 1997 and in Morocco, rates increased among women 18 years or older from 5.0 in 1984/85 to 18% in 1998 (these values were not included in Table 8.1 or used to generate the regional estimates given in Fig. 8.1 because of the different age range used, 20–60 versus 15–49 years). The increases in obesity in Morocco and Tunisia are similar in magnitude to those that occurred in Mexico.

The new data support the previous conclusion by Martorell *et al.* (2000a). There continue to be insufficient data about trends in obesity from nationally representative data but it would appear that rates are increasing dramatically in many countries in Latin America, in North Africa and the Middle East and in Pacific Island nations but not in sub-Saharan Africa.

## Levels of obesity in men

Few surveys include men but those that do almost always find higher levels of obesity in women compared to men (Hodge *et al.*, 1994, 1995, 1996; Pishdad, 1996; Al-Isa, 1997). As an example, data are presented in Fig. 8.5 for Morocco and Tunisia

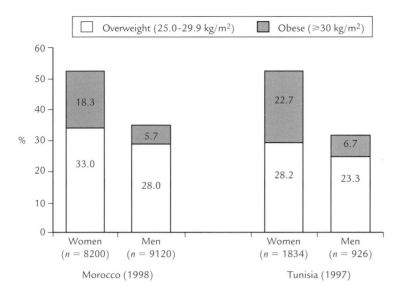

**Figure 8.5** Obesity among women and men in Morocco ($\geq$18 years) and Tunisia (20–60 years). (Data from Mokhtar *et al.*, 2001.)

(Mokhtar *et al.*, 2001). In Morocco, 51.3% of women were overweight or obese compared to 33.7% in men; the corresponding values for Tunisia were 50.9% in women and 30.0% in men. From Fig. 8.5, it is clear that the significant difference between women and men is in the extent of obesity, which was more than 3 times more common in women compared to men.

# Obesity in preschool children

As noted earlier, nationally representative data are available from many nutrition surveys for children less than 5 years of age. Two analyses of such data have been published (Martorell *et al.*, 2000b; de Onis and Blössner, 2000). Data from 50 countries for children aged 12–60 months were used by Martorell *et al.* (2000b). Infants (<12 months) were excluded because their greater levels of overweight compared to older children, particularly if breastfed, may represent normal growth (Dewey, 1998; Victora *et al.*, 1998). Obesity was defined as greater than two standard deviations above the mean, using the NCHS reference population (Hamill *et al.*, 1979). By definition, the prevalence of obesity in the reference population is 2.3%. Values for obesity by region are given in Fig. 8.6. Each point represents a country and the dashed line represents the value in the reference population, 2.3% (Uzbekistan had an extreme value of 12.5%, which may be erroneous, and is therefore not shown). With the exception of Pakistan, where 2.6% of children were obese, obesity was rare in South Asia (including representation from India) and in Thailand. Sub-Saharan Africa also had low levels of obesity, with only one country having high values, Malawi with 5.2%. Seven of 13 countries in Latin America and the Caribbean, one of two in the CEE/CIS region,

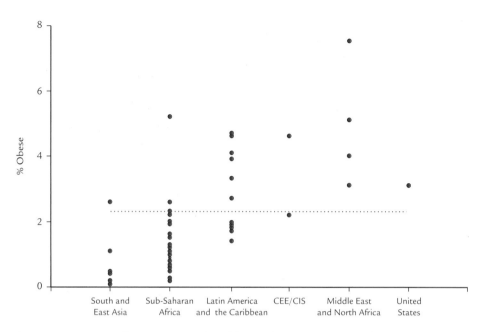

**Figure 8.6** Percentage obese ($\geq 2$ Wt/HtZ) in children aged 12–60 months in developing country regions and in the United States. (Data from Martorell *et al.*, 2000b.)

and all four Middle Eastern and North African countries exceeded 2.3%. In the United States, 3.1% of children were obese. Obesity was more common in urban areas, in children of mothers with higher education, and in girls. At country level, child obesity was positively related to GNP, negatively related to per-capita income and stunting. As in the case of women, the assessment of trends was severely constrained by lack of data.

The analyses by de Onis and Blössner (2000) involved a larger number of national surveys (160 surveys from 94 countries). They used the same criterion as Martorell *et al.* (2000b) but called weight for length/height values greater than two standard deviations above the WHO/NCHS reference mean "overweight" rather than "obesity". An important difference in sample selection is that de Onis and Blössner (2000) included children younger than 12 months whereas Martorell *et al.* (2000b) did not. Thus, obesity prevalences for surveys common to both analyses and which included children less than 12 months of age will be greater when reported by de Onis and Blössner (2000).

The conclusions of de Onis and Blössner (2000) were similar to those of Martorell *et al.* (2000b): rates of obesity among preschool children were lowest in sub-Saharan Africa and Asia and highest in the Middle East, North Africa, and Latin America. Of 11 countries from the Middle East and North Africa, only Oman had a prevalence lower than 2.3%, the value above two standard deviations in the reference population. The value reported for Oman was 0.9%, which seems oddly low. Several countries exceeded a rate of 4.6%, which is twice the prevalence of the reference population: Egypt, 8.6%, Algeria, 9.2%; Morocco, 6.8%; Qatar, 6.8%; Jordan, 5.7%; Kuwait, 5.7% and Bahrain, 4.7%. Similarly, of 23 countries from Latin America and the Caribbean included, only Honduras, one of the poorest countries in the region, had prevalences lower than 2.3%, with a value of 1.4%. Several countries equaled or exceeded rates of 4.6%: Argentina, 7.3%; Chile, 7.0%, Bolivia, 6.5%; Peru, 6.4%; Uruguay, 6.2%; Costa Rica, 6.2%; Jamaica, 6.6% and Brazil, 4.9%. De Onis and Blössner (2000) analyzed a total of 38 countries with trend data but they were unable to make firm conclusions. Although 18 of the 38 countries had values that appear to be rising, there was no particular regional pattern; a variety of countries in Latin America, the Middle East and North Africa as well as sub-Saharan Africa had increasing prevalences. Eight countries had values that appeared to be falling and 14 values that appeared not to have changed. Thus, the overall impression is one of increases being more common than decreases but without a particularly defined pattern. On the other hand, there are well entrenched regional differences in preschool obesity levels, with North Africa and the Middle East and Latin America and the Caribbean having high levels of obesity.

Documenting trends in preschool children is also difficult in the United States. Rates of overweight (greater than the 95th percentile of weight for height or length) did not increase for children younger than three years of age between 1971/74 and 1988/94; however, overweight increased in girls 4 and 5 years old from 5.8 to 10.8% over the same period. In boys 4 and 5 years old, the increases were only from 4.4 to 5.0% (Ogden *et al.*, 1997).

# Obesity in school children

Most of the available information for school age children is not from nationally representative samples. This does not allow for quantification of the problem or for estimation of trends. However, the information available suggests that although the problem of obesity begins in preschool children, it is among school children where the problem becomes more manifest.

Obesity rates in the United States have tripled over the last two decades among children 6–19 years old (Crawford *et al.*, 2001) and have more than doubled in Japan among children aged 6–14 years (Kotani *et al.*, 1997). Rapid changes may also be occurring in developing countries but this is difficult to demonstrate.

There are many studies of school children in developing countries and many of these express concern about the high rates of obesity found. Most studies from the Middle East, for example, suggest that school children in this region are considerably fatter than the US reference population (Al-Nuaim *et al.*, 1996; Al-Isa and Moussa, 2000; Musaiger and Gregory, 2000; Musaiger *et al.*, 2000; Hasan *et al.*, 2001; Moktar *et al.*, 2001).

One study from Kuwait was representative of the country's elementary school population, 6–10 years of age, and provided data for 1985 (*n* = 4942) and 1995 (*n* = 8425) (Al-Isa and Moussa, 2000). The percentage of boys whose weight for height equaled or exceeded the 95th percentile of the NCHS/CDC reference population was 12.1% in 1985 and 21.1% in 1995. The values for girls were 13.8% and 22.7% for 1985 and 1995, respectively. For a rough comparison, the percentage of children exceeding the 95th percentile of the 2000 CDC BMI for age charts was 13% in preliminary data for 1999 for US children 6–11 years from NHANES IV

(Crawford *et al.*, 2001). In a separate study (Al-Isa, 1997), higher levels of obesity were found in adults from Kuwait during 1980–81 and 1993–94 than reported for the USA for roughly the same years. Obesity in men increased from 16.9 to 32.3% and in women from 32.2 to 40.6% across these years in Kuwait; corresponding rates in the USA were 12.3 and 20.0% for men and 16.5% and 24.9% for women, respectively for 1976/80 and 1988/94 (Flegal *et al.*, 1998).

Lower levels of fatness than for Kuwait were found among Brazilian adolescents 10–19 years of age in a nationally representative survey ($n = 13\,715$) conducted in 1989 (Neutzling *et al.*, 2000). The Brazilian researchers used a lower cut off point, the 85th percentile of the BMI for age reference curves from the USA, but found only 4.8% of boys and 10.6% of girls above the criterion. Recent data from other Latin American populations suggest high levels of fatness among adolescents. A representative survey of 10–13-year-old school children from the urban area of San José, Costa Rica ($n = 683$) found that 31% of children were overweight (85th to 94th percentile); it is not clear whether this figure also includes obese children (at or above the 95th percentile) (Monge *et al.*, 2000). A study of school children aged 9–16 years from a low to middle income town in the Mexico City area, found that 24% of children were obese in 1997, defined as higher than the 85th percentile of both the BMI and triceps skinfold USA reference curves (Hernandez *et al.*, 1999).

## Discussion

Any conclusion about obesity in developing countries needs to be viewed with caution because nationally representative data are lacking for many countries. Few countries have repeated surveys and information about trends is limited. There are also methodological concerns. The reference population used to assess obesity in children is derived from measurements of US children, who may have higher than desired levels of fatness and the interpretation of weight for height indices in populations with significant levels of stunting has been called in question. On the other hand, there is consensus that a BMI over $30\,kg/m^2$ in adults (the definition of obesity) represents a serious clinical concern. Risk appears at much lower levels of BMI and a value of 25 or greater (i.e., the definition of overweight) implies increased health and mortality risk.

Is obesity a problem in developing countries? It depends. Obesity remains rare in sub-Saharan Africa and in South Asia. In more developed countries of Latin America, the Middle East and North Africa, and the CEE/CIS region, obesity is as common as in the United States.

What accounts for the increases in obesity in many developing countries? Developing countries are undergoing fundamental changes as a result of the economic, epidemiological, demographic and nutritional transitions (Popkin, 1994; Martorell and Stein, 2001). Ultimately, these societal changes impact on dietary changes and on physical activity. The major shifts in diet include increases in the consumption of vegetable oils, displacement of course grains by refined ones, more meat and eggs, more processed foods and more eating away from home (Popkin and Doak, 1998). Among adults, there is a vast shift towards more capital-intensive and knowledge-based employment that relies far less on physical activity (Popkin and Doak, 1998). There is also a shift from active to sedentary recreation. Television viewing is thought to be a driving force behind the rise in childhood obesity in the United States (Dietz and Gortmaker, 1985; Robinson, 1999) and is likely to be also important in developing countries. Reduced energy expenditures from displacement of physical activity and increased dietary energy intakes due to snacking during viewing or as a result of food advertisement altering consumption patterns have been suggested as mechanisms (Robinson, 1999). School children from San José, Costa Rica watch about 2.5 hours of television per day, more than the 2.2 hours they spend in physical activity (Monge *et al.*, 2000). School children from low and middle income schools from the Mexico City area spend 2.4 hours per day watching television, and 1.7 hours watching videos or playing video games, more than the 1.7 hours of daily moderate and vigorous exercise they report (Hernandez *et al.*, 1999). The impact of these patterns of recreation cannot be known without information on what was replaced and what the dietary response to these changes in physical activity have been. Data of this nature are not generally available. Only small imbalances between energy intake and expenditure would be required to produce the obesity levels that have emerged over the last two decades.

Increased adult obesity may also be among the factors responsible for increased childhood obesity. Maternal obesity and gestational diabetes lead to large birthweights, which increase the risk of increased fatness later in life among affected children and adults (Parsons *et al.*, 1999; Martorell *et al.*, 2001). The decline in breastfeeding in many parts of the world may also be a cause of increasing levels of childhood obesity, but its relative importance in developing countries is unknown (Dietz, 2001). Also unclear is whether undernutrition *in utero* and infancy is an important factor behind the obesity epidemic (Martorell *et al.*, 2001).

Some of the countries with high levels of obesity still report significant rates of childhood stunting and of nutritional deficiencies (ACC/SCN, 2000; de Onis and Blössner, 2000). The existence of a dual nutrition agenda presents a difficult challenge because resources are limited. In addition, many countries are poorly prepared to face the changing epidemiology. For many, there is limited information about how important obesity and related chronic diseases are in the population and hence little recognition of these entities as public health problems. There is also limited experience and expertise about chronic diseases as the focus of nutrition policy in many countries continues to be only undernutrition.

Many measures need to be taken by developing countries to prevent obesity and related chronic diseases. For example, information systems need to collect data about chronic diseases in order to generate the data needed for advocacy and for policy and program definition. These efforts must include school children, elderly women and men, and not just women of reproductive age and young children. Professionals will need to be trained to design, monitor, and evaluate programs aimed at the prevention of chronic diseases. Nutrition and healthy lifestyles should be topics covered well in the school curriculum and physical activity should be promoted in schools and in the general population. Urban planners should support this aim by building recreational facilities, such as parks and playgrounds. Public education should be aggressive and effective, as much as commercial advertisement is, in order to promote healthy diet and lifestyles food and agricultural policies should stimulate the consumption of healthy diets. Nutrition labeling should be required for all industrially prepared foods to assist consumers in food selection and the role of industry in developing healthier products and in promoting public health and nutrition should be recognized and encouraged. In much of the developing world, the prevention of obesity and related chronic diseases should be a priority of governments, as well as of international, bilateral and national organizations. At the same time, efforts must continue to eliminate nutritional deficiencies.

# References

ACC/SCN (United Nations Administrative Committee on Coordination, Sub-Committee on Nutrition) and IFPRI (International Food Policy Research Institute) (2000). Fourth Report on The World Nutrition Situation. WHO, Geneva.

Al-Isa, A. (1997). *Eur. J. Clin. Nutr.* **51**, 743–749.

Al-Isa, A.N., and Moussa, M.A.A. (2000). *Int. J. Food Sci. Nutr.* **51**, 221–228.

Al-Nuaim, A.R., Bamgboye, E.A., and Al-Herbish, A. (1996). *Int. J. Obes.* **20**, 1000–1005.

Barlow, S.E., and Dietz, W.H. (1998). *Pediatrics* **102**, e29.

Bender, R., Trautner, C., Spraul, M., and Berger, M. (1998). *Am. J. Epidemiol.* **147**, 42–48.

Björntorp, P. (1997). *Lancet* **350**, 423–426.

Bray, G.A. (1996). *In* "Present Knowledge in Nutrition", 7th edn (E.E. Ziegler, and L.J. Filer, Jr, eds.), pp. 19–32. ILSI Press, Washington, DC.

Calle, E.E., Thun, M.J., Petrelli, J.M., Rodriguez, C., and Heath, Jr, C.W. (1999). *N. Engl. J. Med.* **341**, 1097–1105.

Cole, T.J., Bellizzi, M.C., Flegal, K.M., and Dietz, W.H. (2000). *BMJ* **320**, 1240–1243.

Crawford, P.B., Story, M., Wang, M.C., Ritchie, L.D., and Sabry, Z.I. (2001). *Pediatr. Clin. North Am.* **48**, 855–878.

de Onis, M., and Blössner, M. (2000). *Am. J. Clin. Nutr.* **72**, 1032–1039.

Dewey, K.G. (1998). *J. Human Lact.* **14**, 89–91.

Dietz, W.H. (1998). *Pediatrics* **101**, 518–525.

Dietz, W.H. (2001). *JAMA* **285**, 2506–2507.

Dietz, W.H., and Gortmaker, S.L. (1985). *Pediatrics* **75**, 807–812.

Flegal, K.M., Carroll, M.D., Kuczmarski, R.J., and Johnson, C.L. (1998). *Int. J. Obes.* **22**, 39–47.

Gallagher, D., Visser, M. Sepúlveda, D., Pierson, R.N., Harris T., and Heymsfield, S.B. (1996). *Am. J. Epidemiol.* **143**, 228–239.

Garza, C. and de Onis, M. (1999). *In* "Human Growth in Context" (F.E. Johnston, B. Zemel, and P.B. Eveleth, eds.), pp. 85–94. Smith-Gordon, London.

Goran, M.I. (2000). *Am. J. Clin. Nutr.* **73**, 158–171.

Hamil, P.V.V., Drizd, T.A., Johnson, C.L., Reed, R.B., Roche, A.F., and Moore, W.M. (1979). *Am. J. Clin. Nutr.* **32**, 607–629.

Hasan, M.A., Batieha, A., Jadou, H., Khawaldeh, A.K., and Ajlouni, K. (2001). *Eur. J. Clin. Nutr.* **55**, 380–386.

Hernández, B., Gortmaker, S.L., Colditz, G.A., Peterson, K.E., Laird, N.M., and Parra-Cabrera, S. (1999). *Int. J. Obes.* **23**, 845–854.

Hodge, A.M., Dowse, G.K., Toelupe, P., Collins V.R., Imo, T., and Zimmet, P.Z. (1994). *Int. J. Obes. Metab. Dis.* **18**, 419–428.

Hodge, A.M., Dowse, G.K., Zimmet, P.Z., and Collins, V.R. (1995). *Obes. Res.* **3**, 77S–87S.

Hodge, A.M., Dowse, G.K., Gareeboo, H., Tuomilehto, J., and Alberti, K.G.M.M. (1996). *Int. J. Obes.* **20**, 137–146.

Kotani, K., Nishida, M., Yamashita, S., Funahashi, T., Fujioka, S., Tokunaga, K., Ishikawa, K., Tarui, S., and Matsuzawa, Y. (1997). *Int. J. Obes. Rel. Metab. Dis.* **21**, 912–921.

Martorell, R., and Stein, A.D. (2001). *In* "Present Knowledge in Nutrition", 8th edn (B.A. Bowman, and R.M. Russell, eds.), pp. 665–685. ILSI Press, Washington, DC.

Martorell, R., Malina, R.M., Castillo, R.O., Mendoza, F.S., and Pawson, I.G. (1988). *Hum. Biol.* **60**, 205–222.

Martorell, R., Kettel Khan, L., Hughes, M.L., and Grummer-Strawn, L.M. (1998). *J. Nutr.* **128**, 1464–1473.

Martorell, R., Kettel Khan, L., Hughes, M.L., and Grummer-Strawn, L.M. (2000a). *Eur. J. Clin. Nutr.* **54**, 247–252.

Martorell, R., Kettel Khan, L., Hughes, M.L., and Grummer-Strawn, L.M. (2000b). *Int. J. Obes.* **24**, 959–967.

Martorell, R., Stein, A.D., and Schroeder, D.G. (2001). *J. Nutr.* **131**, 874S–880S.

Ministerio de Salud (1996). "Encuesta Nacional de Nutrición". Fascículo Antropometría, San José, Costa Rica.

Mokhtar, N., Elati, J., Chabir, R., Bour, A., Elkari, K., Schlossman, N.P., Caballero, B., and Aguenaou, H. (2001). *J. Nutr.* **131**, 887S–892S.

Monge, R., Holst, I., Faiges, F., and Rivero, A. (2000). *FNB* **21**, 293–300.

Musaiger, A.O., and Gregory, W. B. (2000). *Int. J. Obes.* **24**, 1093–1096.

Musaiger, A.O., Al-Ansari, M., and Al-Mannai, M. (2000). *Ann. Hum. Biol.* **27**, 507–515.

Must, A., and Strauss, R.S. (1999). *Int. J. Obes.* **23**, S2–S11.

Neutzling, M.B., Taddei, J.A.A.C., Rodrigues, E.M., and Sigulem, D.M. (2000). *Int. J. Obes.* **24**, 869–874.

Ogden, C.L., Troiano, R.P., Briefel, R.R., Kuczmarski, R.J., Flegal, K.M., and Johnson, C.L. (1997). *Pediatrics* **99**, 1–7.

Parsons, T.J., Power, C., Logan, S., and Summerbell, C.D. (1999). *Int. J. Obes.* **23**, S1–S107.

Pishdad, G.R. (1996). *Int. J. Obes.* **20**, 963–965.

Pi-Sunyer, F.X. (1999). *In* "Modern Nutrition in Health and Disease", 9th edn (M.E. Shils, J.A. Olson, M. Shike, and A.C. Ross, eds.), pp. 1395–1418. Williams & Wilkins, Baltimore.

Popkin, B.M. (1994). *Nutr. Rev.* **52**, 285–298.

Popkin, B.M., and Doak, C.M. (1998). *Nutr. Rev.* **56**, 106–114.

Popkin, B.M., Paeratakul, S., Ge, K., and Fengying, Z. (1995). *Am. J. Public Health* **85**, 690–694.

Rivera, J.A., Barquera, S., Campirano, F., Campos, I., Safdie, M., and Tovar, V. (in press). *Pub. Nutr.*

Robinson, T.N. (1999). *JAMA* **282**, 1561–1567.

Seidell, J.C. (1997). *Horm. Metab. Res.* **29**, 155–158.

Serdula, M.K., Ivery, D., Coates, R.J., Freedman, D.S., Williamson, D.F., and Byers, T. (1993). *Prev. Med.* **22**, 167–177.

Sobal, J., and Stunkard, A.J. (1989). *Psychol. Bull.* **105**, 260–275.

Solomon, C.G., and Manson, J.E. (1997). *Am. J. Clin. Nutr.* **66**, 1044S–1050S.

Stevens, J., Cai, J., Pamuk, E.R., Williamson, D.F., Thun, M.J., and Wood, J.L. (1998). *N. Engl. J. Med.* **338**, 1–7.

Strauss, R. (1999). *Curr. Probl. Pediatr.* **29**, 5–29.

Troiano, R.P., and Flegal, K.M. (1998). *Pediatrics* **101**, 497–504.

Victora, C.G., Morris, S.S., Barros, F.C., de Onis, M., and Yip, R. (1998). *J. Nutr.* **128**, 1134–1138.

Whitaker, R.C., Wright, J.A., Pepe, M.S., Seidel, K.D., and Dietz, W.H. (1997). *N. Engl. J. Med.* **337**, 869–873.

World Health Organization (1995). Report of a WHO Expert Committee, WHO Technical Report Series 854. WHO, Geneva.

World Health Organization (1998). Report of a WHO Consultation on Obesity, 3–5 June. WHO, Geneva.

# Diabetes

9

*Kerin O'Dea and Leonard S. Piers*

## Prevalence of diabetes in the developing world, current and historical trends

The emergence of type 2 diabetes is a feature of the growing wave of chronic diseases and can be viewed as a symptom of the changing social norms and lifestyle resulting from urbanization and economic development. The high and rising prevalence of diabetes, its impact on mortality and morbidity, its disproportionate effect on disadvantaged individuals, communities and nations, and its high human and economic costs clearly position diabetes as a significant global public health problem (Vinicor, 1994; IDF, 1997; King *et al.*, 1998; Fagot-Campagna *et al.*, 2000, 2001).

The burden of diabetes worldwide is great and continues to grow (King *et al.*, 1998). Overall, 90–95% of diabetes is type 2, and this form of the disease (traditionally considered rare in young people) is now increasingly affecting children and adolescents (Rosenbloom *et al.*, 1999). Type 2 diabetes is being reported in children and adolescents from the United States, Canada, Japan, Hong Kong, Singapore, Bangladesh, Libya, the United Kingdom, Australia, and New Zealand (Fagot-Campagna *et al.*, 2000, 2001). It is type 2 diabetes that is so strongly associated with urbanization and its accompanying changes in diet and lifestyle, and this chapter will therefore focus exclusively on this form of diabetes.

Prevalence varies widely by ethnic group and country. Adult rates range from <2% in rural Bantu people in Tanzania to nearly 50% in US Pima Indians and South Pacific Nauruans (Amos *et al.*, 1997). Rates are also relatively high in migrant and "transplanted populations", such as Asians in Europe (McKeigue *et al.*, 1991) and African Americans (Harris *et al.*, 1998). The projected increase in rates, however, is universal. Although it is estimated that 30–50% of diabetes cases remain undiagnosed, there were approximately 30 million people worldwide diagnosed with diabetes in 1985 (IDF, 1997). By 1995 this had increased to 135 million (4.0% of the world population), and conservative projections indicate there may be 300 million people with diabetes (5.4% of the world population) by 2025 (King *et al.*, 1998). Between 1995 and 2025, the number of people with diabetes is projected to increase from 51 million to 72 million (a 42% increase) in industrialized countries, and from 84 million to 228 million (a 170% increase) in industrializing countries. The countries currently with the largest number of people with diabetes are India, China, and the United States of America and this will still be the case in 2025. The majority of people with diabetes in industrialized countries will be aged 65 years and older. However, the majority of people with diabetes in industrializing countries will be relatively younger, between 45 and 65 years old. Thus, it appears that the diabetes epidemic disproportionately affects not only industrializing countries, but also people in their economically productive years in these countries (Narayan *et al.*, 2000).

Many indigenous populations are at high risk for type 2 diabetes when they make the transition to western lifestyle. The extremely high prevalence of diabetes in association with severe obesity in Pima Indians and Nauruans has already been noted. Other populations, such as Australian Aborigines and Torres Strait Islanders, are also at high risk for early onset type 2 diabetes and its complications (Rowley *et al.*, 1997). Although obesity is the strongest predictor of diabetes risk in Aboriginal populations, risk is already increased at the upper end of the "healthy weight" range for Europeans, i.e. body mass index (BMI) above $22 \, \text{kg/m}^2$ (Daniel *et al.*, 1999).

In industrialized countries, the disease and its complications appear to disproportionately affect individuals from economically disadvantaged and racial/ethnic minority communities (CDC, 1998a). In relation to end-stage renal disease among indigenous Australians not only is there a very strong link to social disadvantage (Cass *et al.*, 2001), 47% of those on dialysis have diabetes. This compares with 14% of nonindigenous patients on dialysis (Kerr, 2000). Based on data from several countries, the World Health Organization (WHO) estimated that in 2000, 30–45% of people with diabetes worldwide had retinopathy, 10–20% had nephropathy, 20–35% had neuropathy and 10–25% had cardiovascular disease (CVD) (IDF, 1997). Hence, the burden of diabetes complications is large worldwide.

# Race, ethnicity, genetic dimensions

Explanations of mechanisms underlying ethnic variability in disease usually focus on differences between groups in the prevalence of individual factors such as genetics, family history and lifestyle. However, there are at least two important gaps in our understanding of this relation. First, we need to better understand what "ethnicity" actually is and how to measure it. Ethnicity transcends racial designation or genotypic groupings and represents instead the aggregate of cultural practices, lifestyle patterns, social influences, religious pursuits and racial characteristics that shape the distinctive identity of a community. Within a single ethnic designation there can be as much or more variability in disease and in the determinants of disease than between ethnic groups. Asian and Pacific Islanders, for example, comprise 30–50 ethnic subgroups with tremendous diversity in language, culture and health status (O'Loughlin, 1999).

Categorizing such groups under a single label can mask the rich diversity that we should be striving to describe and understand. Ethnic labels may provide guidance in targeting interventions or research efforts, but they do little to help us understand the underlying causal mechanisms. Moreover, labels such as white, Caucasian, black, European and minority have little scientific, biologic or anthropologic value (Bhopal and Donaldson, 1998). Such terminology often carries social meanings that are best avoided, as well as the assumption that one population represents the standard or norm. Careful descriptions of the ancestry, geographic origin, birthplace, language, religion and migration history of populations studied are needed to make the basis for classification into ethnic groups clear (Bhopal and Donaldson, 1998).

Another major problem is that many studies investigating the relation between ethnicity and disease do not take potentially confounding factors into account. It is well established that ethnic minority groups tend to be disproportionately poor, making socioeconomic status a probable confounder of the relation. Therefore, research that does not take socioeconomic status into consideration can lead to incorrect conclusions, such that susceptibility attributed to ethnicity may really relate to poverty (O'Loughlin, 1999). Further, socioeconomic status is difficult to measure comprehensively because it comprises many factors; these include, among others, educational attainment, income, employment, access to goods, services and labor markets, access to healthy foods, safe and inexpensive places to exercise, smoke-free environments, and educational, economic, political and cultural discrimination. Therefore, even when socioeconomic status is taken into account, confounding can still be a problem if measurement of socioeconomic status is incomplete (O'Loughlin, 1999).

Hence, ethnicity is difficult to define, but most definitions reflect self-identification with cultural traditions that provide both a meaningful social identity and boundaries between groups (Barot, 1996). This section has considered evidence that uses various definitions of ethnicity. However, in the main these definitions are those that people apply to themselves. Thus ethnicity as used here includes cultural identity, place of origin and skin color, and so includes white and nonwhite groups.

Research comparing health attributes between racial or ethnic groups has a long history. Notably higher rates of morbidity, mortality or both have been observed with respect to stroke among Afro-Caribbeans in the UK (Chaturvedi and Fuller, 1996), diabetes and coronary artery disease among south Asians in the United Kingdom (Chaturvedi and Fuller, 1996; Yudkin, 1996; Cappuccio, 1997; Mather *et al.*, 1998) and Canada (Sheth *et al.*, 1999), diabetes, stroke and hypertensive disease among Hispanic people in New York City (Fang *et al.*, 1997). However, explanations for between-country differences in health will require an appreciation of the complex interactions of history, culture, politics, economics, and the status of women and ethnic minorities (Lynch *et al.*, 2001).

# Risk factors: environmental, genetic

It is generally assumed that type 2 diabetes arises from an interaction between genetic and lifestyle factors. Much of the evidence for a genetic base for type 2 diabetes comes from studies in twins, with higher rates of concordance in monozygotic (MZ) than in dizygotic (DZ) twin pairs (Kaprio *et al.*, 1992). If conducted and analyzed properly, studies of the similarities and differences within both MZ and DZ twin pairs can be used to make guarded inference about the roles of genetic and nongenetic factors on the etiology of disease. Twin studies can never prove the existence of a genetic susceptibility, however, and at best can indicate the extent of genetic determination consistent with a specific model, under certain important assumptions (Hopper, 1999).

A widely cited study from the UK reported rates of concordance for type 2 diabetes in MZ twin pairs at 1, 5, 10, and 15 years follow-up that were 17%, 33%, 57%, and 76%, respectively. The concordance rate for any abnormality of glucose metabolism (either type 2 diabetes or impaired glucose tolerance) at 15 years follow-up was 96% (Medici *et al.*, 1999). However, lower rates of concordance in a study conducted within the Danish Twin Registry (Poulsen *et al.*, 1999) suggest that there may have been unintended selection bias in the relatively small sample in that original landmark study (Hopper, 1999). The population-based Danish study suggests that whereas MZ pairs are concordant for diabetes, and more so than DZ pairs, the difference is not large and consistent with chance (Poulsen *et al.*, 1999). However, twins share more than genes *in utero*. Nongenetic intergenerational mechanisms related to the metabolic milieu include amniotic fluid growth factors and a range of hormones, plus other maternal exposures.

## Lifestyle interventions

Type 2 diabetes has long been linked with behavioral and environmental factors such as overweight, physical inactivity, and dietary habits. Obesity is by far the strongest predictor of diabetes risk in all populations examined to date and almost certainly underlies the increase of type 2 diabetes in most societies, for example "whites" in the US (Flegal *et al.*, 1998). This change probably underlies the "insulin resistance syndrome", which for many people is likely to increase both the incidence of diabetes and, through its multiple risk factor associations, cardiovascular risk (Haffner and Miettinen, 1997). Epidemiological data support the roles of obesity (Haffner *et al.*, 1986), fat intake (Marshall *et al.*, 1994), and low physical activity (Helmrich *et al.*, 1991) as risk factors for diabetes and have led to a wave of trials to prevent type 2 diabetes by lifestyle or drug interventions (Hammersley *et al.*, 1997; NIDDK, 2001). These trials have been preceded by positive results in a large community-based intervention in Da-Qing, China (Pan *et al.*, 1997) and the beneficial metabolic effects seen in a small group of urbanized Australian Aborigines who returned temporarily to a traditional lifestyle about 20 years ago (O'Dea, 1984). In a study on the relationships between lifestyle and cardiovascular risk factors among the Brazilian Amondava, one of the world's most isolated populations Pavan *et al.* (1999) also concluded that a traditional lifestyle (no contact with "civilization", diet based on complex carbohydrates and vegetables, high energy expenditure) may protect against the development of hypertension, hypercholesterolemia, and diabetes.

In a randomized trial of 522 middle-aged, overweight people with impaired glucose tolerance Tuomilehto *et al.* (2001) showed that lifestyle changes can reduce the risk of progression to diabetes by a striking 58% over four years. Each person in the intervention group received individualized counseling aimed at reducing weight, reducing intake of total fat and saturated fat and increasing intake of dietary fiber and increasing physical activity. The net weight loss at the end of two years, 3.5 kg in the intervention group and 0.8 kg in the control group, was modest. However, the cumulative incidence of diabetes after four years was 11% in the intervention group and 23% in the control group. The reduction in the incidence of diabetes was directly associated with the changes in lifestyle. One case of diabetes was preventable for every five subjects with impaired glucose tolerance treated for five years, or for every 22 subjects treated for one year. Two earlier studies from Sweden (Eriksson and Lindgarde, 1991) and China (Pan *et al.*, 1997) showed that lifestyle interventions may delay progression from impaired glucose tolerance to diabetes. However, the Swedish study was not randomized and the Chinese study was randomized by clinic, rather than by individual. Thus, the Finnish study offers us the best evidence so far that lifestyle modification can indeed prevent diabetes.

## The putative "thrifty genotype"

The alarmingly high prevalence of diabetes among Pima Indians and Nauruans provides further important clues to causation. It has been postulated that until recently such people were hunter–gatherers or agriculturalists and may have acquired an insulin-sensitive metabolism favoring fat storage at times of plenty but would not necessarily require a similar degree of insulin sensitivity in muscle tissue, where glucose entry to cells might be largely stimulated by high activity levels (Orchard, 1994). With westernization, a plentiful supply of energy-dense food has been accompanied by a reduction in physical activity. Both factors may therefore cause the previously favorable metabolic profile seen in "survivors" to become a handicap: the "thrifty genotype rendered detrimental by 'progress'" (Neel, 1962). Reaven (1998) has recently further developed this "muscle resistance-thrifty genotype" hypothesis by suggesting that muscle insulin resistance will favor survival by preserving muscle protein, thus enhancing the ability to hunt and gather.

On the basis of our research on the impact of lifestyle change on diabetes and associated conditions in Australian Aborigines, we have proposed an alternative hypothesis of "selective insulin resistance" to explain how the "thrifty genotype" could have operated to favor survival under conditions of the hunter–gatherer lifestyle, but promote the development of obesity and type 2 diabetes when populations became urbanized (O'Dea, 1992). Under conditions of the hunter–gatherer lifestyle, a metabolism that could efficiently convert excess energy intake into depot fat would confer survival advantage. The feasts for hunter–gatherers were usually provided by large animals (terrestrial or marine). In general wild animals have low carcass fat contents, in stark contrast to domesticated meat animals such as beef cattle and sheep (Crawford, 1968; Naughton *et al.*, 1986; O'Dea *et al.*, 1990). Thus the feasts may have often been high in protein and relatively low in carbohydrate and fat. An efficient system for converting excess dietary protein into glucose and fat as readily available forms of energy could be achieved by a high capacity for hepatic gluconeogenesis, *which was not sensitive to insulin suppression*, coupled with a high capacity for hepatic lipogenesis *which was sensitive to stimulation by insulin*. Thus, an efficient system for fat accumulation to take advantage of the "feasts" could be achieved under conditions of hyperinsulinemia in which there was resistance to the hypoglycemic actions of insulin but normal sensitivity to those actions of insulin involved in fat deposition. We have made observations consistent with this possibility utilizing glucose turnover studies in Aborigines at high risk of type 2 diabetes (Proietto *et al.*, 1992). A key question of course is whether the selective insulin resistance is genetic or acquired.

The "thrifty genotype" hypothesis is now being down played (Bjorntorp, 2001) – even by its original proposer (Neel, 1999). Over the past 35 years, it has become increasingly clear that essential hypertension and obesity share many of the epidemiological features of type 2 diabetes. Both are diseases of urbanization, with a very gradual onset. Both are familial, with the disease the result of a complex interplay of genetic and environmental factors. It has also become clear that genetically type 2 diabetes is an etiologically heterogeneous entity. A good illustration is the recognition of a distinctive maturity-onset-type diabetes of youth (MODY) in which the impairment of glucose metabolism has an early onset, progresses slowly, and appears to be inherited as a simple dominant trait (Spielman and Nussbaum, 1992; Fajans *et al.*, 1994). In the 25 years since its recognition, MODY has by now been divided into some five subtypes, each associated with a specific aspect of glucose metabolism, and the locus for each subtype generally characterized by numerous different mutations at the molecular level (Spielman and Nussbaum, 1992; Fajans *et al.*, 1994). There are also a number of other rare genetic syndromes that seem to carry an increased risk of type 2 diabetes. It does not appear that these rare, monogenically inherited subtypes will collectively comprise more than about 10% of what is commonly diagnosed as type 2 diabetes (Neel, 1999).

## Obesity

Many investigators studying metabolic diseases have simply used body mass index (BMI) as a measure of relative body size or obesity and attempted to match groups for this variable, without considering that BMI does not account for the fact that people with similar BMI may have widely varying amounts and distribution of their adipose tissue. When the relationship between insulin sensitivity and BMI in a group of 93 healthy subjects <45 years old was examined by Kahn *et al.* (1993), it was found that these two variables are not simply linearly related. Even individuals who would be considered to be lean (BMI <25 kg/m$^2$) had a broad range of insulin sensitivity with some of these apparently lean subjects having insulin sensitivity values that were as low as those observed in individuals who would be considered to be obese and insulin resistant. The reason(s) for this lack of a simple relationship between body size and insulin sensitivity, especially in relatively lean subjects, is complex because it is well recognized that insulin sensitivity can be influenced by factors such as dietary nutrients (Mann, 2000), body fat distribution (Bjorntorp, 1993; Fujimoto *et al.*, 1994; Abate *et al.*,. 1995; Goodpaster *et al.*, 1999), genetics (Barroso *et al.*, 1999), acute exercise (Prigeon *et al.*, 1995), physical fitness (Kahn *et al.*, 1990), and medications (Kahn *et al.*, 1989).

## Body fat distribution

It is becoming abundantly clear that the pattern of body fat distribution is a major determinant of the residual variation of insulin sensitivity. Accumulation of body fat centrally is associated with insulin resistance, whereas distribution of body fat in a peripheral pattern is less metabolically important from the standpoint of impairing insulin action (Kahn *et al.*, 2001). However, although it is clear that central adiposity is of greater importance metabolically (Despres *et al.*, 1990; Bjorntorp, 1993), there is still debate about which of the central depots is more important. Although many groups have proposed the role of the intra-abdominal depot (Bjorntorp, 1993; Fujimoto *et al.*, 1994), others have argued that it is central subcutaneous fat accumulation that is the critical determinant of reduced insulin sensitivity (Abate *et al.*, 1995, 1996). Also, the association between abdominal obesity and hyperglycemia is stronger in the presence of a parental history of diabetes (van Dam *et al.*, 2001).

If intra-abdominal fat depot is an important contributor to insulin sensitivity, then interventions that reduce adipose tissue mass within the peritoneal cavity should be associated with improvements in insulin sensitivity. This is illustrated by the results of a 3-month weight loss program in 21 older men that was associated with an average 4.5 kg (10%) weight loss, of which 80% was fat. This decrease in fat mass was associated with a 24% reduction in intra-abdominal fat area, a 58% improvement in insulin sensitivity and the development of a less atherogenic lipid profile (Purnell *et al.*, 2000). Similar findings of the effect of weight loss on body fat distribution and insulin sensitivity were also reported by Goodpaster *et al.* (1999).

Although the issue of which of the central depots is the most important is still being debated and how these fat depots may predict this reduction in whole body insulin sensitivity is also unclear, it is apparent that marked variability in these parameters occurs even in healthy subjects and may contribute to differences in disease risk among these individuals.

## Public health implications of the obesity pandemic

The increase in obesity worldwide will have an important impact on the global incidence of cardiovascular disease, type 2 diabetes, cancer, osteoarthritis, work disability, and sleep apnea. Obesity has a more pronounced impact on morbidity than on mortality. Disability due to obesity-related type 2 diabetes will increase particularly in industrializing countries, as insulin supply is usually insufficient in these countries. As a result, in these countries, an increase in disabling macrovascular (atherosclerosis) and microvascular (nephropathy, neuropathy, and retinopathy) disease is expected. Increases in the prevalence of obesity will potentially lead to an increase in the number of years that subjects suffer from obesity-related morbidity and disability. A 1% increase in the prevalence of obesity in such countries as India and China leads to 20 million additional cases of obesity. Thus the focus should be on prevention programs to stem the obesity epidemic more efficiently than weight-loss programs, which have a poor record of sustainability over the long term (Visscher and Seidell, 2001).

## The role of physical inactivity

The goal of treatment in type 2 diabetes is to achieve and maintain near-normal blood glucose levels and optimal lipid levels, in order to prevent or delay the microvascular, macrovascular, and neural complications (Eastman *et al.*, 1993). Exercise is frequently recommended in the management of type 2 diabetes and can improve glucose uptake by increasing insulin sensitivity and lowering body adiposity. Either alone or when combined with diet and drug therapy, physical activity can result in improvements in glycemic control in type 2 diabetes. Exercise also modifies lipid abnormalities and hypertension. In addition, exercise can also help to prevent the onset of type 2 diabetes, in particular in those at higher risk, and has an important role in reducing the significant worldwide burden of this type of diabetes. Recent studies, described below, have improved our understanding of the acute and long-term physiological benefits of physical activity, although the precise duration, intensity, and type of exercise have yet to be fully elucidated.

From observational studies (Helmrich *et al.*, 1991; Manson *et al.*, 1991, 1992; Hu *et al.*, 1999, 2001a,b; Wei *et al.*, 1999) to clinical trials (Yamanouchi *et al.*, 1992, 1995; Uusitupa *et al.*, 2000; Tuomilehto *et al.*, 2001) in a variety of populations and age groups, evidence is mounting in support of the hypothesis that physical activity plays a significant role in the amelioration and/or prevention of type 2 diabetes. Based on the current findings, it is likely that physical activity can reduce the risk of development of type 2 diabetes and the protective benefit is especially pronounced in persons at the highest risk for the disease (Helmrich *et al.*, 1991). What is less clear is how much physical activity is necessary, and for how long (intensity, frequency). Obviously, we are more likely to see the anticipated physiological changes if the dose is maximized. Yet, although maximal is better from a physiological point of view, it is also recognized that a sedentary individual will most likely not sustain a high intensity activity exercise regimen. In contrast, evidence is mounting regarding long-term compliance to moderate levels of activity (Hu *et al.*, 1999), which appear to be easier to adopt in one's lifestyle and are less likely to result in injury (Kriska, 2000). More importantly, there appear to be beneficial changes in insulin sensitivity and glucose tolerance in the sedentary individual who incorporates moderate levels of activity, such as walking or low intensity bicycling, into their lifestyle (Helmrich *et al.*, 1991; Usui *et al.*, 1998). Regular physical exercise at least once a week, and even vigorous activity once a week at weekends, has been shown to be associated with a decreased risk of type 2 diabetes (Okada *et al.*, 2000). However, the onset of beneficial metabolic changes appear to occur much more slowly and less dramatically than what occurs with a high intensity regimen. Although the mechanism is still unclear, exercise seems to be effective in promoting long-term weight loss and has consistently been one of the strongest predictors of long-term weight control (Long, 1985). Exercise is, therefore, a valuable adjunct measure along with dietary changes in the long-term management of weight. Furthermore, individuals who exercise may adhere better to nutritional advice. Physical activity may improve mood and self-esteem and as a result contribute to better control of food intake (Schneider *et al.*, 1984).

It has also been shown that low cardiorespiratory fitness was associated with increased risk for impaired fasting glucose and type 2 diabetes and a sedentary lifestyle may contribute to the progression from normal fasting glucose to impaired fasting glucose and diabetes (Wei *et al.*, 1999). However, it is uncertain whether there is a dose–response effect of exercise on improved glucose control in type 2 diabetes. There does appear to be a limited amount of evidence suggesting that increasing levels of physical activity contribute to better diabetes control (Yamanouchi *et al.*, 1995). Clearly, additional studies are needed to determine the influence of physical fitness on the treatment and prevention of type 2 diabetes (Kelley and Goodpaster, 2001).

Dvorak *et al.* (1999) hypothesized that metabolically obese, normal-weight (MONW) women – a hypothesized subgroup of the general population – would display higher levels of total and visceral fat and lower levels of physical activity than normal women. They studied a cohort of 71 healthy nonobese women (21–35 years old), MONW women were identified based on cut off points for insulin sensitivity (impaired = glucose disposal $<8$ mg/min/kg of fat-free mass (FFM), $n = 13$ vs. normal = glucose disposal $>8$ mg/min/kg of FFM, $n = 58$). Body composition was measured by dual energy X-ray absorptiometry and body fat distribution by computed tomography, cardiorespiratory fitness from $V_{O_2max}$ on a treadmill, physical activity energy expenditure using doubly labeled water and indirect calorimetry, glucose tolerance with an oral glucose tolerance test, serum lipid profile, and dietary intake. They observed a higher body fat percentage and higher abdominal (both subcutaneous and visceral) adiposity in the MONW group versus the normal group. The MONW group showed a lower physical activity energy expenditure, but no difference in cardiorespiratory fitness was noted between groups. Hence, despite a normal body weight and lack of difference in cardiorespiratory fitness compared to controls, young apparently healthy MONW women had lower physical activity energy expenditure, which may have produced a cluster of high risk phenotypic characteristics that predispose to type 2 diabetes and cardiovascular disease (Dvorak *et al.*, 1999).

Even if activity is known to be beneficial, at the population level we are faced with the challenge of reaching sedentary individuals who would most likely benefit from an increase in physical activity. The protective nature of a physically active lifestyle in preventing type 2 diabetes does not have a lasting impact once a return to a sedentary way of life is made. Therefore, from a public health viewpoint, long-term commitments to increased activity are required. In the large prospective Da-Qing study (Pan *et al.*, 1997), both dietary and physical activity interventions reduced the incidence of type 2 diabetes considerably in a Chinese population. Whether this is also achievable in other ethnic populations at high risk for developing type 2 diabetes, and whether additional pharmacological measures are useful, is currently under investigation.

In conclusion, the question is no longer "can increased physical activity benefit the individual with type 2 diabetes?" The answer is yes. Future research needs to refine questions regarding type, dose, and magnitude of effects of physical activity (and its subcategory exercise) on glycemic control, insulin sensitivity, and on risk factors for cardiovascular disease within the context of program acceptability and feasibility (Tudor-Locke *et al.*, 2000). The issue of sustainability of increased levels of physical activity at both the individual and population level is the major challenge, as urban life becomes increasingly "obesigenic" (Egger and Swinburn, 1997).

## Insulin resistance and blood pressure

The relationship between physical activity and type 2 diabetes appears to be mediated by serum true insulin level and components of the insulin resistance syndrome

(Wannamethee *et al.*, 2000). Insulin resistance is associated with dyslipoproteinemia characterized by increased serum triglycerides, reduced high-density lipoprotein (HDL) cholesterol, and an increase in the small, dense particle subfraction of low-density lipoprotein (LDL). Physical activity and weight reduction are known to improve insulin resistance and dyslipoproteinemia (Halle *et al.*, 1999). A multiethnic epidemiological study examined whether physical activity was related to insulin concentrations in two populations at high risk for diabetes that greatly differ by location, ethnic group, and BMI (Kriska *et al.*, 2001). Physical activity was negatively associated with insulin concentrations both in the Pima Indians, who tend to be overweight, and in Mauritians, who are leaner. These findings suggest a beneficial role of activity on insulin sensitivity that is separate from any influence of activity on body composition. In fact, walking, which can be safely performed and easily incorporated into daily life, can be recommended as an adjunct therapy to diet treatment in obese type 2 diabetic patients, not only for body weight reduction, but also for improvement of insulin sensitivity (Yamanouchi *et al.*, 1995).

Risk for type 2 diabetes is elevated in older persons and those with high blood pressure, high body mass index, and triglyceride levels and a parental history of diabetes (Wei *et al.*, 1999). Hyperinsulinemia is linked to blood pressure elevation in some, but not all, populations. However, it is generally accepted as an independent risk factor for atherosclerosis. Furthermore, insulin *per se* does not elevate blood pressure, but rather reduces total peripheral vascular resistance in experimental studies. Blood pressure might be elevated by other mechanisms secondary to hyperinsulinemia, such as enhanced renal sodium retention, elevated intracellular free calcium, and increased activity of the sympathetic nervous system. Indeed, subjects whose blood pressure is salt-sensitive exhibit hyperinsulinemia after glucose loading, and normotensive subjects with glucose-induced hyperinsulinemia will develop hypertension within 5 years more often than normoinsulinemic subjects. In primary hypertension, the incidence of insulin resistance and hyperinsulinemia is much higher than in normotensive controls. However, not all reported studies show a relationship between hyperinsulinemia and blood pressure elevation, and in some experimental studies no blood pressure elevation could be induced by prolonged hyperinsulinemia. Therefore, it is still unclear whether hyperinsulinemia induces hypertension or is only casually associated with it (Bonner, 1994).

## Interventions

The Diabetes Prevention Program (DPP), a major clinical trial comparing diet and exercise to treatment with metformin in 3234 people with impaired glucose tolerance (IGT), ended a year early, because participants randomly assigned to intensive lifestyle intervention reduced their risk of getting type 2 diabetes by 58%. On average, this group maintained their physical activity at 30 minutes per day, usually with walking or other moderate intensity exercise, and lost 5–7% of their body weight. Participants randomized to treatment with metformin also reduced their risk of getting type 2 diabetes, but only by 31% (NIDDK, 2001).

As already noted, smaller studies in China (Pan *et al.*, 1997) and Finland (Tuomilehto *et al.*, 2001) have shown that diet and exercise can delay type 2 diabetes in at-risk people, but the DPP, conducted at 27 centers across the US, is the first major trial to show that diet and exercise can effectively delay diabetes in a diverse American population of overweight people with IGT. In the study of Finnish adults at high risk for type 2 diabetes showed that losing up to 5 kg, boosting exercise, and switching to a reduced fat, higher fiber diet reduced the risk of developing diabetes by 58% (Tuomilehto *et al.*, 2001). Researchers followed 522 Finns, for 2–6 years, who were all overweight and showed IGT. Half received intensive instruction from a dietitian in sessions at least once every 3 months and from fitness professionals at a health club to which participants got free memberships. Those participants developed diabetes less often than did people in the other half of the group, who received advice about the importance of a healthy diet and regular exercise but not periodic instruction.

Body weight and the prevalence of obesity are rising so rapidly in many countries that the World Health Organization has recognized that there is a "global epidemic of obesity" (WHO, 1997). The prevalence of type 2 diabetes is rising in parallel. While both obesity and type 2 diabetes have a combined genetic and environmental background, the epidemic must be due to major changes in the environment. There is a great, and still insufficiently understood, variation in prevalence of obesity and in the rate of change of the prevalence. The prevailing contention is that the epidemic is due to the changes in the society leading to overnutrition and a sedentary life. In Denmark, a steep rise has taken place in the prevalence of obesity among schoolboys and young men in two phases linked to the birth cohorts of the 1940s and of the mid-1960s and later (Sorensen, 2000). This rise is consistent with environmental influences operating early in life.

## Intrauterine factors

The maternal factors of diabetes, obesity, and pregnancy weight gain alter the intrauterine environment and thereby increase the risk of later obesity in the offspring. Of these maternal factors, evidence is strongest for the role of maternal diabetes. No single mechanism explains how these maternal factors could change the intrauterine environment to increase obesity risk. However, all potential mechanisms involve an altered transfer of metabolic substrates between mother and fetus, which may influence the developing structure or function of the organs involved in energy metabolism (Whitaker and Dietz, 1998).

Intrauterine exposure to diabetes *per se* conveys a high risk for the development of diabetes and obesity in offspring in excess of risk attributable to genetic factors alone (Dabelea *et al.*, 2000a). Pettitt and Knowler (1998) studied the long-term effect of the diabetic pregnancy on Pima Indian offspring to determine how the prevalence of diabetes during pregnancy was influenced by early life events, such as birth weight and type of infant feeding, that are known to influence the prevalence of diabetes in nonpregnant Pima adults. They found that diabetes during pregnancy was a major risk factor for early onset obesity and type 2 diabetes in the offspring during adolescence and early adulthood. Diabetes in the next generation was less common among children breast-fed for at least 2 months (6.9% and 30.1% among offspring of nondiabetic and diabetic women, respectively) than among bottle-fed children (11.9% and 43.6%, respectively). The apparent protective effect of breast-feeding may be related to attenuating the increased appetite in the babies of diabetic mothers secondary to their hyperinsulinemia at birth. It is possible that the increasing fat content of breast milk during each feed produces greater satiety and helps curb their overconsumption.

The prevalence of diabetes during pregnancy was influenced by other conditions, such as birth weight, which is known to influence the prevalence of diabetes in this population in general. The highest rates of diabetes during pregnancy at 25–34 years of age (25%) were found among women with a birth weight below 2.5 kg. The infant of the woman with diabetes during pregnancy was at risk of becoming obese and of developing type 2 diabetes at a young age. Hence, the effects of the diabetic pregnancy can be thought of as a vicious cycle, with consequences for the offspring extending well beyond the neonatal period. The young woman whose mother had diabetes during pregnancy is at risk of perpetuating the cycle by developing diabetes by her child-bearing years (Dabelea et al., 2000b). The prevalence of diabetes in women of child-bearing age is influenced by factors occurring early in life (i.e., birth weight and type of infant feeding). Whether or not the long-term adverse outcomes, including diabetic pregnancies in the next generation, can be lessened or prevented by meticulous control of diabetes during pregnancy, careful attention to intrauterine growth, or more general infant breast-feeding remains unknown (Pettitt and Knowler, 1998), although it has strong biological plausibility.

The standard risk factors – dyslipidemia, hypertension and smoking – do not fully explain the raised cardiovascular risk in diabetes. The observations of an association between short stature and microalbuminuria suggested that intrauterine or early infant nutrition may represent a common antecedent, these having also been shown to predict both components of the insulin resistance syndrome and cardiovascular disease in adult life (Yudkin, 1995). However, in a study on 169 subjects exposed to malnutrition in utero during the siege of Leningrad (now St Petersburg) in 1941–44, intrauterine malnutrition was not associated with glucose intolerance, dyslipidemia, hypertension, or cardiovascular disease in adulthood (Stanner et al., 1997).

In India there is a rapidly escalating epidemic of the insulin resistance syndrome and its major sequelae (diabetes and coronary heart disease). Contribution of genes and environment is under debate. Small size at birth coupled with subsequent obesity increases risk for insulin resistance syndrome in later life. The tendency of Indians to have higher body fat and central adiposity compared with other races may be programmed in utero. The adipose tissue releases not only fatty acids but also a number of proinflammatory cytokines, which increase insulin resistance and cause endothelial dysfunction. Crowding, infections, and environmental pollution in Indian cities may increase cardiovascular risk by stimulating cytokine production. Prevention of diabetes and coronary heart disease in India will need to be addressed through a comprehensive life course approach. It is clear that such an approach should encompass not only on the conventional adult risk factors (diet, exercise, lifestyle generally), but also on early life influences and other factors associated with poverty such as high burden of infectious diseases (Yajnik, 2001).

It has been shown that aspects of maternal diet exert an influence on fetal growth, especially the dietary intake of carbohydrate, protein and some micronutrients. However, these relationships are less strong than might have been predicted, especially when compared with the associations that can be drawn with maternal shape, size and metabolic capacity. Maternal height, weight and body composition relate to the metabolic capacity of the mother and her ability to provide an environment in which the delivery of nutrients to the fetus is optimal. Current evidence suggests that the size of the mother determines her ability to support protein synthesis, and that maternal protein synthesis, especially visceral protein synthesis, is very closely related to fetal growth and development. The extent to which the effect of an adverse environment *in utero* can be reversed by improved conditions postnatally is not clear (Jackson, 2000).

# Is there a role for diet? How might the transition that we find in the developed world in diet affect the diabetes trends independent of its effect on obesity?

The demographic and economic transition that many developing countries are undergoing is producing important changes in diet and lifestyle that greatly impact on disease risks. Among the risk behaviors associated with socioeconomic transition and urbanization are excessive dietary fat intake, sedentary lifestyle, smoking, and environmental contamination. Combined with a reduced infant mortality and increased life expectancy, those risk factors lead to an increasing prevalence of chronic disease like type 2 diabetes and coronary heart disease (Caballero and Rubinstein, 1997).

The average prevalence of obesity (BMI $\geqslant 30\,kg/m^2$) among European centers participating in the WHO-MONICA study between 1983 and 1986 was about 15% in men and 22% in women. Prevalence figures ranged in men from 7% in Gothenburg to 22% in Lithuania and in women from 9% to 45% in the same places. Some monitoring projects or repeated surveys suggest that the prevalence of obesity has been increasing during the past 15 years in some European countries. Data from The Netherlands suggest that average weight increase of the order of about 1 kg can be responsible for quite dramatic increases in the prevalence of obesity. This suggests that only small changes in the daily caloric balance may be sufficient to increase the number of obese subjects in populations (Seidell, 1997).

Prospective studies in the US have highlighted the potential role of saturated fat in increasing the risk of type 2 diabetes. For example, to further investigate the role of dietary fat and carbohydrate as potential risk factors for the onset of type 2 diabetes, current diet was assessed among a geographically based group of 1317 subjects without a prior diagnosis of diabetes who were seen in the period from 1984 to 1988 in two counties in southern Colorado. In this study, 24-hour diet recalls were reported prior to an oral glucose tolerance test. Persons with previously undiagnosed diabetes

($n = 70$) and impaired glucose tolerance ($n = 171$) were each compared with confirmed normal controls ($n = 1076$). The adjusted odds ratios relating a 40 g/day increase in fat intake to type 2 diabetes and impaired glucose tolerance were 1.51 (95% confidence interval (CI) 0.85–2.67) and 1.62 (95% CI 1.09–2.41), respectively. Restricting cases to diabetic persons with fasting glucose greater than 140 mg/dl and persons with impaired glucose tolerance confirmed on follow-up, the odds ratios increased to 3.03 (95% CI 1.07–8.62) and 2.67 (95% CI 1.33–5.36), respectively. The findings of this study support the hypothesis that high-fat, low-carbohydrate diets are associated with the onset of type 2 diabetes in humans (Marshall *et al.*, 1991). In a later study Marshall *et al.* (1994) concluded that fat consumption significantly predicts type 2 diabetes risk in subjects with IGT after controlling for obesity and markers of glucose metabolism.

High intake of *trans* and saturated fatty acids has been shown to increase the risk of coronary heart disease. Christiansen *et al.* (1997) studied the effects of diets enriched in various fatty acids on postprandial insulinemia and fasting serum levels of lipids and lipoproteins in obese patients with type 2 diabetes. They concluded that in the presence of unchanged glycemia, both dietary *trans* fatty acids and saturated fatty acids induce an increase in postprandial insulinemia in obese patients with type 2 diabetes.

However, most of these conclusions were reached based on data obtained from self-reported dietary intakes. Schaefer *et al.* (2000) conducted a study to investigate the efficacy of food-frequency questionnaires and diet records in subjects fed natural-food diets of known composition. They compared the validity of a semi-quantitative food-frequency questionnaire in assessing intakes of macronutrients (absolute amounts and percentages of energy) by 19 subjects fed natural-food diets of known composition. They also tested 3-day diet records in small subsets ($n = 5$ or 6). In their study each subject consumed three different diets for ≥6 weeks and self-reported his or her food intake by using a food-frequency questionnaire and a diet record. The diets varied in their chemically analyzed contents of fat (15–35% energy), saturated fat (5–14%), monounsaturated fat (5–14.5%), polyunsaturated fat (2.5–10.5%), carbohydrate (49–68%), and cholesterol (108–348 mg/day). The food-frequency questionnaire significantly underestimated fat, saturated fat, monounsaturated fat, and protein intakes and significantly overestimated carbohydrate intake with the high-fat diet. The percentage of energy from fat was significantly underestimated for the high-fat diet and significantly overestimated for the very-low-fat diet. Estimates from the food-frequency questionnaire differed significantly from actual intakes for fat (absolute and percentage), saturated fat (absolute and percentage), monounsaturated fat (absolute and percentage), and protein (percentage) in the high-fat diet and for polyunsaturated fat (absolute and percentage), saturated fat (percentage), fiber (absolute), and cholesterol (daily absolute; in mg/day) in the lower-fat diet. Estimates from the diet records agreed better with actual intakes than did estimates from the food-frequency questionnaire except for monounsaturated fat (absolute and percentage) in the high-fat diet and polyunsaturated fat (percentage) in the lower-fat diet and the very-low-fat diet. Their data indicated that the food-frequency questionnaire did not provide reliable estimates of absolute amounts of dietary fats or cholesterol (Schaefer *et al.*, 2000). Similarly, Livingstone *et al.* (1990) evaluated the seven day weighed dietary record, which is currently accepted as the most accurate technique for assessing habitual dietary intake in studies investigating the links between diet and health. Energy intake, as measured by the seven day weighed dietary record, was compared to total energy expenditure estimated concurrently by the doubly labeled water technique in 31 free-living adults (16 men and 15 women). Average recorded energy intakes were significantly lower than measured expenditure in the group overall (9.66 MJ/day vs. 12.15 MJ/day). Among those in the upper third of energy intakes the mean ratio of intake to expenditure was close to 1.0, indicating accurate records. In the middle and lower thirds the ratios for men were only 0.74 and 0.70, respectively and for women 0.89 and 0.61. These results show a serious bias in reporting habitual energy intake. Thus the conclusions of all studies using self-reported dietary intake data should be carefully evaluated.

To determine the relations of diet with risk of clinical type 2 diabetes, Colditz *et al.* (1992) analyzed data from a prospective cohort of 84 360 US women. During 6 years of follow-up 702 definite incident cases were identified. Because BMI is a powerful risk factor for diabetes, they examined the relations of fat (including type), fiber, sucrose, and other components of self-reported dietary intake to risk of diabetes, among women with BMI $<29$ kg/m$^2$. After controlling for BMI, previous weight change, and alcohol intake, they observed no associations between self-reported intakes of energy, protein, sucrose, carbohydrate, or fiber and risk of diabetes. Compared with women in the lowest quintile of energy-adjusted intake, and relative risks (and tests for trend) for those in the highest quintile were 0.61 ($P$ trend $= 0.03$) for vegetable fat, 0.62 ($P$ trend $= 0.008$) for potassium, 0.70 ($P$ trend $= 0.005$) for calcium, and 0.68 ($P$ trend $= 0.02$) for magnesium. These data are consistent with a protective effect of a diet rich in plant food. These inverse associations were attenuated among obese women (BMI $\geq 29$ kg/m$^2$). Furthermore, in a more recent study there are data that support a protective role for grains (particularly whole grains), cereal fiber, and dietary magnesium in the development of diabetes in older women (Meyer *et al.*, 2000).

## Increase in energy density – link with obesity

The association between type 2 diabetes and adiposity is arguably of even greater importance than the previously well described association with cardiovascular risk factors including hypertension, dyslipidemia and hypertension. Although the causes of obesity are the result of complex interactions between genetic predisposition and environmental trigger factors, the current epidemic has to be attributed to the "obesogenic environment" (Egger and Swinburn, 1997) as the human genome has not changed in this period. In addressing the environmental facilitators of obesity, we need to consider both food intake and energy expenditure.

Much of the discourse on the role of diet in the development of obesity highlights the role of fat, due to its high energy density (kJ/g of food or beverage) and its propensity, if consumed in excess, to be deposited as adipose tissue. However, there is now evidence that fat gain is similar with overfeeding of carbohydrate or fat (McDevitt *et al.*, 2000). Spontaneous energy intake is strongly influenced by energy density. Covert manipulation of energy density results in sustained changes in energy intake (Stubbs *et al.*, 1998). The increased use of low-fat products, many of which are energy dense due to their high sugar content, and sugar-containing beverages, now contribute significantly to total energy intake. Independent of fat content, low energy dense diets generate greater satiety than energy dense diets, suggesting that an important regulatory signal may be the weight or volume of food consumed. Epidemiological studies confirm that energy intake increases with energy density and thus weight loss may be best achieved on a low energy dense diet (Poppitt and Prentice, 1996).

## Sweetened drinks – link with childhood obesity

Evidence is accumulating that the form in which the sucrose is consumed is also important. A recent prospective study from Ludwig *et al.* (2001) demonstrated a clear cut, graded relation between the consumption of sugar-sweetened drinks and development of obesity in children. The prevalence of obesity among children in the United States doubled between 1980 and 1994 so that 11% are now above the 95th reference percentile of BMI for age and sex. The observation that this increase paralleled the increase in sugar-sweetened soft drinks prompted Ludwig *et al.* (2001) to enroll 548 ethnically diverse school children (average age 11.7 ± 0.8 years) in four Massachusetts communities in a prospective study for 19 months. The difference in measures of obesity was related to differences in consumption of sugar-sweetened drinks and other possible determinants of obesity including physical inactivity and fat intake. For each additional serving of sugar-sweetened drinks both BMI (mean 0.24 kg/m$^2$) and frequency of obesity (odds ratio 1.6) increased after adjustment for anthropometric, demographic, dietary and lifestyle variables. Differences in diet soda intake were not related to obesity incidence.

Of course an observational study does not prove causality, but it is of interest that another recently published study in an entirely different group of older individuals produced similar results. Elmslie *et al.* (2001) compared a group of bipolar (manic depressive) patients and matched controls; the patient group had higher rates of overweight and obesity than the controls. The bipolar patients reported a higher energy intake, the increased energy being derived almost entirely from sucrose in sweetened drinks. Energy from drinks (regardless of whether it is from sugar, fat, or alcohol) adds to total energy intake, and does not displace energy from other forms (Poppitt *et al.*, 1996). Furthermore, compensation at subsequent meals for energy consumed in the form of liquid appears to be less complete than for energy consumed in solid form (Mattes, 1996).

Although these new data suggest a potentially untoward effect, in terms of promoting obesity, of sugar-containing beverages it may also be relevant to recall data published some thirty years ago (Mann *et al.*, 1970). Free-living middle-aged men were asked to replace as far as possible sucrose with foods rich in starch in order to maintain energy balance. Despite regular advice and encouragement from a dietitian they were unable to maintain energy balance and lost weight presumably because of the greater satiety-promoting qualities of the starchy foods. Although not providing direct evidence for sugar as an etiological factor these observations do suggest that recommending a reduction in sugar (in both beverages and food) may be a potentially useful public health measure in countries where obesity and its co-morbidities have reached epidemic proportions.

## Type of dietary fat

Although a low-fat diet is recommended for diabetic and nondiabetic patients (ADA, 1994), findings from epidemiological studies on the association of total dietary fat with type 2 diabetes or insulin sensitivity have been inconsistent (Feskens and Kromhout, 1989; Lundgren *et al.*, 1989; Marshall *et al.*, 1991). However, more recent epidemiologic and metabolic studies suggest that dietary fat subtypes may be relevant to diabetes pathophysiology. The impact of various dietary fatty acids on the risk of type 2 diabetes was examined in the Iowa Women's Health Study (Meyer *et al.*, 2001), which studied 35 988 women, aged 55–69 years, free of diabetes, and followed them for 11 years, resulting in 1890 new cases of type 2 diabetes. Intake of fat and fatty acids was assessed from a validated food-frequency questionnaire. After adjustments for main risk factors, including BMI, waist-to-hip ratio, physical activity, dietary fiber, magnesium, and other dietary fat subtypes, substituting polyunsaturated fatty acid (PUFA) intake for saturated fatty acid (SFA) was inversely associated with diabetes risk, with a 16% reduction in the highest quintile. The consumption of vegetable fat was associated with a 22% reduction in new cases of diabetes in the highest quintile. Interestingly, in another study on patients with type 2 diabetes, relative to high-monounsaturated-fat diets, high-carbohydrate diets also caused persistent deterioration of glycemic control and accentuation of hyperinsulinemia, as well as increased plasma triglyceride and very-low-density lipoprotein cholesterol levels, which is undesirable (Garg *et al.*, 1994). People with diabetes in Spain have near-optimal serum lipid levels and maintain reasonably good blood glucose control and BMI, indicating that diabetes management that includes the usual Spanish diet, which is low in carbohydrates and high in fat, especially monounsaturated fat (mostly olive oil), might be a useful model (DNCT, 1997). Furthermore, diets enriched with polyunsaturated fatty acids augment insulin secretion significantly more than a diet comprising primarily saturated fatty acids (Lardinois *et al.*, 1987). Borkman *et al.* (1993) observed significant inverse relations between fasting serum insulin and the content of n-3 and n-6 fatty acids within skeletal-muscle phospholipids. This implies that the *type* of polyunsaturated fat (the n-6/n-3 ratio) may also be critical.

Although the mechanism for this increased insulin sensitivity in response to unsaturated fats is unknown, there are several mechanisms that have been proposed. Saturated fatty acids have been shown to decrease insulin binding to receptors and to impair glucose transport (Pelikanova *et al.*, 1989). Specific dietary fatty acids may modify the phospholipid composition of cell membranes, which in turn may alter the function of the insulin receptor (Boden, 1996). Dietary PUFAs (n-6 and n-3) have been shown to reduce triglyceride accumulation in skeletal muscle and possibly in β-cells, by upregulating the expression of genes encoding proteins involved in fatty acid oxidation while simultaneously downregulating genes encoding proteins of lipid synthesis (Clarke, 2001). Fatty acids are also known to affect gene expression directly as they act as natural ligands for genes, such as peroxisome proliferator-activated receptors (PPAR)

(Kliewer *et al.*, 1997). Other potential pathways relating PUFA and vegetable fat to diabetes risk involve low-grade inflammation. Proinflammatory cytokines, such as tumor necrosis factor-$\alpha$, may induce insulin resistance by influencing the function of the insulin receptor (Hotamisligil *et al.*, 1996). Interestingly the production of these inflammatory cytokines is affected by the ratio of n-6/n-3 PUFA in the diet (Leaf, 1999).

# Implications for health care and quality of life

Diabetes is a lifelong condition that seriously affects a person's quality of life. Individuals with the disease have to make major lifestyle changes and learn to live with monitoring blood glucose, using multiple drugs and injections, and dealing with complications of the disease and their treatment. Diabetes is a complex and multifactorial disease that is associated with considerable mortality, morbidity, and loss of quality of life. The complications of type 2 diabetes are both microvascular and macrovascular in nature and include the following: retinopathy, peripheral and autonomic neuropathy, nephropathy, peripheral vascular disease, atherosclerotic cardiovascular and cerebrovascular disease, hypertension, and susceptibility to infections and periodontal disease.

The onset of type 2 diabetes is insidious and is usually recognized only 5–12 years after hyperglycemia develops. During this period of undiagnosed diabetes, hyperglycemia, in combination with lifestyle factors (physical inactivity, alcohol use, smoking), and other metabolic (dyslipidemia, obesity, insulin resistance) and hemodynamic (hypertension) abnormalities frequently associated with type 2 diabetes, promote the initiation and progression of micro- and macrovascular complications. Furthermore, when blood glucose levels are increased only slightly and no symptoms are apparent, the physician may be reluctant to diagnose type 2 diabetes or start treatment. A delay in diagnosing the disease results in a high prevalence of chronic complications at the time of actual diagnosis. Indeed, when type 2 diabetes is diagnosed, cardiovascular disease and neuropathy are found in approximately 10% of cases, and retinopathy and nephropathy in 15–20% (Muggeo, 1998).

Much of the direct costs of diabetes result from its complications, and hospitalization costs are particularly high (IDF, 1997). On average people with diabetes are three times more likely to be hospitalized than nondiabetic individuals. The risk for hospitalization is slightly diversified, venous complications being the least risky (1.7 times) and heart-related complications the most risky (3.1 times). The risk of premature death is higher for persons with diabetes compared to those without diabetes, and the life expectancy is 10–15 years shorter. US data show that diabetes is the leading cause of blindness and accounts for 40% of the new cases of end-stage renal disease. The risk for leg amputation is 15–40 times higher and the risk for heart disease and stroke is two to four times higher for people with diabetes compared with people without diabetes. Recent studies show that the health care expenditures are as much as five times higher for individuals with diabetes compared to individuals without diabetes. In Sweden in 1994, three times more resources were spent on treating complications compared to what was spent on control of the disease. Studies show that intensive treatments cost more than traditional treatment, but also cut costs substantially for the treatment of late complications (Bjork, 2001).

Nephropathy has been considered a rare complication of type 2 diabetes in patients from European or North American populations, in which the highest incidence of this disease is recorded in individuals aged over 70 years. Other ethnic groups such as Pima Indians in the USA, Pacific Islanders, and Australian Aborigines have markedly different incidence patterns of type 2 diabetes, with a high incidence in the 20–50-year age group. These patients live long enough to develop nephropathy, and they do so at a similar or higher rate to type 1 diabetes patients. Since the prevalence of type 2 diabetes is increasing worldwide, particularly in the developing world, diabetic nephropathy will be a growing problem in patients with this disease. The prevention of end-stage renal failure is possible in most patients, but the treatment of end-stage renal disease is very expensive (Borch-Johnsen, 1995).

The United Kingdom Prospective Diabetes Study (UKPDS), conclusively demonstrated that improved blood glucose control in these patients reduces the risk of developing retinopathy and nephropathy and possibly reduces neuropathy (UKPDS, 1998a,b; Stratton et al., 2000). The overall microvascular complications rate was decreased by 25% in patients receiving intensive therapy versus conventional therapy. Epidemiological analysis of the UKPDS data showed a continuous relationship between the risk of microvascular complications and glycemia, such that for every percentage point decrease in hemoglobin (Hb)$A_{1c}$ (e.g., 9 to 8%), there was a 37% reduction in the risk of microvascular complications (Stratton et al., 2000).

The proportion of family income spent on diabetes care is higher in disadvantaged socioeconomic groups in both industrialized and industrializing countries. Diabetes is expensive for people with the disease and their families and also for nations. For example, in households with a diabetic patient, a substantial portion of the family income, 5–25% in India, and 5–10% in the United States, is devoted to diabetes care (IDF, 1997). At the national level, diabetes exerts a substantial toll on the direct health care costs in all countries. A person with diabetes costs the health care sector ~2.5 times more than a person without the disease (Selby et al., 1997). The estimated total annual direct health care cost of diabetes in 1998 in industrialized countries varied from US$ 0.54 billion in Denmark to US$ 60 billion in the United States (IDF, 1997). Within the ambit of economic aspects of the population in a developing country, the direct cost of diabetes health care is very high for many people. One study estimated the annual direct cost of diabetes in India at US$ 2.2 billion (Shobhana et al., 2000). These large variations in the estimated national costs of diabetes reflect a number of factors. There may be variations in (a) the methods used for measuring and estimating costs, (b) differences in clinical practice patterns, (c) differences in the purchasing power for the same amount of resources, and (d) the effect of competing priorities on the level of resources allocated for treating diabetes (Narayan et al., 2000).

O'Brien et al. (1998) estimated the direct medical costs of complications resulting from type 2 diabetes in the US. They calculated event costs (associated with resource use that is specific to the acute episode and any subsequent care occurring in the first year) and state costs (the annual costs of continued management), expressed in 1996

US dollars. They concluded that more severe or debilitating events associated with diabetes, such as acute myocardial infarction ($27 630 event cost; $2185 state cost), generate a greater financial burden than do early-stage complications, such as micro-albuminuria ($62 event cost; $14 state cost). However, complications that are initially relatively low in cost (e.g., microalbuminuria) can progress to more costly advanced stages (e.g., end-stage renal disease, $53 659 state cost). In the CODE-2 Study (Costs of Diabetes in Europe-Type 2) performed in eight European countries, the total expenses for type 2 diabetics in Germany were evaluated and analyzed for the first time. In the German arm of the study, the annual costs caused by type 2 diabetes patients in Germany in 1998 amounted to 31.4 billion DM. Of these costs, 61% were covered by statutory and private health insurance. The annual expenses of the Statutory Health Insurance (SHI) for these patients amounted to 18.5 billion DM, 50% being spent for inpatient treatment, 13% for ambulatory care, and 27% for medication. Diabetes medication (insulin, oral antidiabetic drugs) accounted for only 7% of total SHI costs. Only 26% of all diabetic patients had $HbA_{1c}$ values <6.5%, the therapeutic target of the European Diabetes policy group. Around 50% of the type 2 diabetic patients exhibited severe macro- and/or microvascular complications. The costs per patient compared to the average expenses for SHI insured patients increased with complication state from the 1.3-fold (no complications) up to the 4.1-fold (macro- and microvascular complications). Diabetes-related complications and concomitant diseases are the predominant reasons for these high costs (Liebl *et al.*, 2001).

In conclusion, there is strong evidence that improved glycemic control is effective at lessening the risks of retinopathy, neuropathy, and nephropathy in type 2 diabetes. The evidence about the effect on coronary heart disease is limited and equivocal. The hypoglycemic risk from improved glycemic control is significantly less in type 2 diabetes than in type 1, and weight gain seems to be modest. Although glycemic goals should be individualized based on several clinical factors, most patients with type 2 diabetes would probably benefit from glucose lowering to a $HbA_{1c}$ level between 7% and 8% (Gaster and Hirsch, 1998).

In addition to these direct costs, diabetes takes a toll on society through several indirect costs, such as lost productivity due to worker sickness, absences, disability, premature retirement, and premature mortality. These indirect costs may be as high, if not higher, than direct costs, and estimates vary from US$ 330 million per year in Mexico to US$ 54 billion per year in the United States (IDF, 1997).

## Population health implications

Both obesity and type 2 diabetes are common consequences of urbanization (increased sedentary lifestyles and increased energy density of diets). Both are potentially preventable through lifestyle modification on a population level, but this requires coherent and multifaceted strategies. The development and successful and sustainable implementation of such strategies is a major public health challenge globally. There is an urgent need to develop global and national plans for the prevention and manage-ment of obesity and type 2 diabetes mellitus (Seidell, 2000). Early diagnosis and treatment through opportunistic screening of type 2 diabetes may reduce the lifetime incidence of major microvascular complications and result in gains in both life-years and QALYs. Although current recommendations in industrialized countries like Australia and the US are that screening should begin at age 45 years, it is becoming apparent that screening can be more cost-effective at younger ages (CDC, 1998b). This is particularly the case in developing countries and in other populations at high risk (minority groups in affluent western countries).

# References

Abate, N., Garg, A., Peshock, R.M., Stray-Gundersen, J., and Grundy, S.M. (1995). *J. Clin. Invest.* **96**, 88–98.

Abate, N., Garg, A., Peshock, R.M., Stray-Gundersen, J., Adams-Huet, B., and Grundy, S.M. (1996). *Diabetes* **45**, 1684–1693.

ADA (1994). *Diabetes Care* **17**, 519–522.

Amos, A.F., McCarty, D.J., and Zimmet, P. (1997). *Diabet. Med.* **14** Suppl 5, S1–S85.

Barot, R. (1996). "The Racism Problematic: Contemporary Sociological Debates on Race and Ethnicity". Edwin Mellen Press, Lewiston, NY.

Barroso, I., Gurnell, M., Crowley, V.E., Agostini, M., Schwabe, J.W., Soos, M.A., Maslen, G.L., Williams, T.D., Lewis, H., Schafer, A.J., Chatterjee, V.K., and O'Rahilly, S. (1999). *Nature* **402**, 880–883.

Bhopal, R., and Donaldson, L. (1998). *Am. J. Public Health* **88**, 1303–1307.

Bjork, S. (2001). *Diabetes Res. Clin. Pract.* **54** Suppl 1, 13–18.

Bjorntorp, P. (1993). *Adv. Exp. Med. Biol.* **334**, 279–285.

Bjorntorp, P. (2001). *Lancet* **358**, 1006–1008.

Boden, G. (1996). *Diabetes Care* **19**, 394–395.

Bonner, G. (1994). *J. Cardiovasc. Pharmacol.* **24** Suppl 2, S39–S49.

Borch-Johnsen, K. (1995). *Pharmacoeconomics* **8** Suppl 1, 40–45.

Borkman, M., Storlien, L.H., Pan, D.A., Jenkins, A.B., Chisholm, D.J., and Campbell, L.V. (1993). *N. Engl. J. Med.* **328**, 238–244.

Caballero, B., and Rubinstein, S. (1997). *Arch. Latinoam. Nutr.* **47**, 3–8.

Cappuccio, F. P. (1997). *J. Hum. Hypertens.* **11**, 571–576.

Cass, A., Cunningham, J., Wang, Z., and Hoy, W. (2001). *Aust. NZ J. Public Health* **25**, 322–326.

CDC (1998a). "National Diabetes Fact Sheet". Center for Disease Control and Prevention, Atlanta.

CDC (1998b). *JAMA* **280**, 1757–1763.

Chaturvedi, N., and Fuller, J. H. (1996). *J. Epidemiol. Community Health* **50**, 137–139.

Christiansen, E., Schnider, S., Palmvig, B., Tauber-Lassen, E., and Pedersen, O. (1997). *Diabetes Care* **20**, 881–887.

Clarke, S.D. (2001). *J. Nutr.* **131**, 1129–1132.

Colditz, G.A., Manson, J.E., Stampfer, M.J., Rosner, B., Willett, W.C., and Speizer, F.E. (1992). *Am. J. Clin. Nutr.* **55**, 1018–1023.

Crawford, M.A. (1968). *Lancet* **i**, 1329–1333.

Dabelea, D., Hanson, R.L., Lindsay, R.S., Pettitt, D.J., Imperatore, G., Gabir, M.M., Roumain, J., Bennett, P.H., and Knowler, W.C. (2000a). *Diabetes* **49**, 2208–2211.

Dabelea, D., Knowler, W.C., and Pettitt, D.J. (2000b). *J. Matern. Fetal Med.* **9**, 83–88.

Daniel, M., Rowley, K.G., McDermott, R., Mylvaganam, A., and O'Dea, K. (1999). *Diabetes Care* **22**, 1993–1998.

Despres, J.P., Moorjani, S., Lupien, P.J., Tremblay, A., Nadeau, A., and Bouchard, C. (1990). *Arteriosclerosis* **10**, 497–511.

DNCT (1997). *Diabetes Care* **20**, 1078–1080.

Dvorak, R.V., DeNino, W.F., Ades, P.A., and Poehlman, E.T. (1999). *Diabetes* **48**, 2210–2214.

Eastman, R.C., Silverman, R., Harris, M., Javitt, J.C., Chiang, Y.P., and Gorden, P. (1993). *Diabetes Care* **16**, 1095–1102.

Egger, G., and Swinburn, B. (1997). *BMJ* **315**, 477–480.

Elmslie, J.L., Mann, J.I., Silverstone, J.T., Williams, S.M., and Romans, S.E. (2001). *J. Clin. Psychiatry* **62**, 486–491.

Eriksson, K.F., and Lindgarde, F. (1991). *Diabetologia* **34**, 891–898.

Fagot-Campagna, A., Pettitt, D.J., Engelgau, M.M., Burrows, N.R., Geiss, L.S., Valdez, R., Beckles, G.L., Saaddine, J., Gregg, E.W., Williamson, D.F., and Narayan, K.M. (2000). *J. Pediatr.* **136**, 664–672.

Fagot-Campagna, A., Narayan, K.M., and Imperatore, G. (2001). *BMJ* **322**, 377–378.

Fajans, S.S., Bell, G.I., Bowden, D.W., Halter, J.B., and Polonsky, K.S. (1994). *Life Sci.* **55**, 413–422.

Fang, J., Madhavan, S., and Alderman, M.H. (1997). *Ethn. Dis.* **7**, 55–64.

Feskens, E.J., and Kromhout, D. (1989). *Am. J. Epidemiol.* **130**, 1101–1108.

Flegal, K.M., Carroll, M.D., Kuczmarski, R.J., and Johnson, C.L. (1998). *Int. J. Obes. Relat. Metab. Disord.* **22**, 39–47.

Fujimoto, W.Y., Bergstrom, R.W., Boyko, E.J., Kinyoun, J.L., Leonetti, D.L., Newell-Morris, L.L., Robinson, L.R., Shuman, W.P., Stolov, W.C., and Tsunehara, C.H. (1994). *Diabetes Res. Clin. Pract.* **24** Suppl, S43–S52.

Garg, A., Bantle, J.P., Henry, R.R., Coulston, A.M., Griver, K.A., Raatz, S.K., Brinkley, L., Chen, Y.D., Grundy, S.M., and Huet, B.A. (1994). *JAMA* **271**, 1421–1428.

Gaster, B., and Hirsch, I.B. (1998). *Arch. Intern. Med.* **158**, 134–140.

Goodpaster, B.H., Kelley, D.E., Wing, R.R., Meier, A., and Thaete, F.L. (1999). *Diabetes* **48**, 839–847.

Haffner, S.M., and Miettinen, H. (1997). *Am. J. Med.* **103**, 152–162.

Haffner, S.M., Stern, M.P., Hazuda, H.P., Rosenthal, M., Knapp, J.A., and Malina, R.M. *Diabetes Care* **9**, 153–161.

Halle, M., Berg, A., Garwers, U., Baumstark, M.W., Knisel, W., Grathwohl, D., Konig, D., and Keul, J. (1999). *Metabolism* **48**, 641–644.

Hammersley, M.S., Meyer, L.C., Morris, R.J., Manley, S.E., Turner, R.C., and Holman, R.R. (1997). *Metabolism* **46**, 44–49.

Harris, M.I., Flegal, K.M., Cowie, C.C., Eberhardt, M.S., Goldstein, D.E., Little, R.R., Wiedmeyer, H.M., and Byrd-Holt, D.D. (1998). *Diabetes Care* **21**, 518–524.

Helmrich, S.P., Ragland, D.R., Leung, R.W., and Paffenbarger, R.S. (1991). *N. Engl. J. Med.* **325**, 147–152.

Hopper, J.L. (1999). *Diabetologia* **42**, 125–127.

Hotamisligil, G.S., Peraldi, P., Budavari, A., Ellis, R., White, M.F., and Spiegelman, B.M. (1996). *Science* **271**, 665–668.

Hu, F.B., Sigal, R.J., Rich-Edwards, J.W., Colditz, G.A., Solomon, C.G., Willett, W.C., Speizer, F.E., and Manson, J.E. (1999). *JAMA* **282**, 1433–1439.

Hu, F.B., Leitzmann, M.F., Stampfer, M.J., Colditz, G.A., Willett, W.C., and Rimm, E.B. (2001a). *Arch. Intern. Med.* **161**, 1542–1548.

Hu, F.B., Manson, J.E., Stampfer, M.J., Colditz, G., Liu, S., Solomon, C.G., and Willett, W.C. (2001b). *N. Engl. J. Med.* **345**, 790–797.

IDF (1997). International Diabetes Federation Task Force on Diabetes Health Economics, Brussels.

Jackson, A.A. (2000). *Adv. Exp. Med. Biol.* **478**, 41–55.

Kahn, S.E., Beard, J.C., Schwartz, M.W., Ward, W.K., Ding, H.L., Bergman, R.N., Taborsky, G.J., and Porte, D. (1989). *Diabetes* **38**, 562–568.

Kahn, S.E., Larson, V.G., Beard, J.C., Cain, K.C., Fellingham, G.W., Schwartz, R.S., Veith, R.C., Stratton, J.R., Cerqueira, M.D., and Abrass, I.B. (1990). *Am. J. Physiol.* **258**, E937–E943.

Kahn, S.E., Prigeon, R.L., McCulloch, D.K., Boyko, E.J., Bergman, R.N., Schwartz, M.W., Neifing, J.L., Ward, W.K., Beard, J.C., and Palmer, J.P. (1993). *Diabetes* **42**, 1663–1672.

Kahn, S.E., Prigeon, R.L., Schwartz, R.S., Fujimoto, W.Y., Knopp, R.H., Brunzell, J.D., and Porte, D. (2001). *J. Nutr.* **131**, 354S–360S.

Kaprio, J., Tuomilehto, J., Koskenvuo, M., Romanov, K., Reunanen, A., Eriksson, J., Stengard, J., and Kesaniemi, Y.A. (1992). *Diabetologia* **35**, 1060–1067.

Kelley, D.E., and Goodpaster, B.H. (2001). *Med. Sci. Sports Exerc.* **33**, S495–S501; discussion S528–S529.

Kerr, P. (2000). "ANZDATA Registry Report", Adelaide.

King, H., Aubert, R.E., and Herman, W.H. (1998). *Diabetes Care* **21**, 1414–1431.

Kliewer, S.A., Sundseth, S.S., Jones, S.A., Brown, P.J., Wisely, G.B., Koble, C.S., Devchand, P., Wahli, W., Willson, T.M., Lenhard, J.M., and Lehmann, J.M. (1997). *Proc. Natl Acad. Sci. USA* **94**, 4318–4323.

Kriska, A. (2000). *Sports Med.* **29**, 147–151.

Kriska, A.M., Pereira, M.A., Hanson, R.L., de Courten, M.P., Zimmet, P.Z., Alberti, K.G., Chitson, P., Bennett, P.H., Narayan, K.M., and Knowler, W.C. (2001). *Diabetes Care* **24**, 1175–1180.

Lardinois, C.K., Starich, G.H., Mazzaferri, E.L., and DeLett, A. (1987). *J. Am. Coll. Nutr.* **6**, 507–515.

Leaf, A. (1999). *Circulation* **99**, 733–735.

Liebl, A., Neiss, A., Spannheimer, A., Reitberger, U., Wagner, T., and Gortz, A. (2001). *Dtsch Med. Wochenschr.* **126**, 585–589.

Livingstone, M.B., Prentice, A.M., Strain, J.J., Coward, W.A., Black, A.E., Barker, M.E., McKenna, P.G., and Whitehead, R.G. (1990). *BMJ* **300**, 708–712.

Long, B. (1985). *Cognit. Ther. Res.* **9**, 471–478.

Ludwig, D.S., Peterson, K.E., and Gortmaker, S.L. (2001). *Lancet* **357**, 505–508.

Lundgren, H., Bengtsson, C., Blohme, G., Isaksson, B., Lapidus, L., Lenner, R.A., Saaek, A., and Winther, E. (1989). *Am. J. Clin. Nutr.* **49**, 708–712.

Lynch, J., Smith, G.D., Hillemeier, M., Shaw, M., Raghunathan, T., and Kaplan, G. (2001). *Lancet* **358**, 194–200.

Mann, J.I. (2000). *Br. J. Nutr.* **83** Suppl 1, S169–S172.

Mann, J.I., Hendricks, D.A., Truswell, A.S., and Manning, E. (1970). *Lancet* **i**, 870–872.

Manson, J.E., Rimm, E.B., Stampfer, M.J., Colditz, G.A., Willett, W.C., Krolewski, A.S., Rosner, B., Hennekens, C.H., and Speizer, F.E. (1991). *Lancet* **338**, 774–778.

Manson, J.E., Nathan, D.M., Krolewski, A.S., Stampfer, M.J., Willett, W.C., and Hennekens, C.H. (1992). *JAMA* **268**, 63–67.

Marshall, J.A., Hamman, R.F., and Baxter, J. (1991). *Am. J. Epidemiol.* **134**, 590–603.

Marshall, J.A., Hoag, S., Shetterly, S., and Hamman, R.F. (1994). *Diabetes Care* **17**, 50–56.

Mather, H.M., Chaturvedi, N., and Fuller, J.H. (1998). *Diabet. Med.* **15**, 53–59.

Mattes, R.D. (1996). *Physiol. Behav.* **59**, 179–187.

McDevitt, R.M., Poppitt, S.D., Murgatroyd, P.R., and Prentice, A.M. (2000). *Am. J. Clin. Nutr.* **72**, 369–377.

McKeigue, P.M., Shah, B., and Marmot, M.G. (1991). *Lancet* **337**, 382–386.

Medici, F., Hawa, M., Ianari, A., Pyke, D.A., and Leslie, R.D. (1999). *Diabetologia* **42**, 146–150.

Meyer, K.A., Kushi, L.H., Jacobs, D.R., Slavin, J., Sellers, T.A., and Folsom, A.R. (2000). *Am. J. Clin. Nutr.* **71**, 921–930.

Meyer, K.A., Kushi, L.H., Jacobs, D.R., and Folsom, A.R. (2001). *Diabetes Care* **24**, 1528–1535.

Muggeo, M. (1998). *Diabet. Med.* **15** Suppl 4, S60–S62.

Narayan, K.M., Gregg, E.W., Fagot-Campagna, A., Engelgau, M.M., and Vinicor, F. (2000). *Diabetes Res. Clin. Pract.* **50** Suppl 2, S77–S84.

Naughton, J.M., O'Dea, K., and Sinclair, A.J. (1986). *Lipids* **21**, 684–690.

Neel, J.V. (1962). *Am. J. Hum. Genet.* **14**, 353–362.

Neel, J.V. (1999). *Nutr. Rev.* **57**, S2–S9.

NIDDK (2001). "Diabetes Prevention Project". National Institute of Health, Bethesda.

O'Brien, J.A., Shomphe, L.A., Kavanagh, P.L., Raggio, G., and Caro, J.J. (1998). *Diabetes Care* **21**, 1122–1128.

O'Dea, K. (1984). *Diabetes* **33**, 596–603.

O'Dea, K. (1992). *Diabetes Metab. Rev.* **8**, 373–388.

O'Dea, K., Traianedes, K., Chisholm, K., Leyden, H., and Sinclair, A.J. (1990). *Am. J. Clin. Nutr.* **52**, 491–494.

Okada, K., Hayashi, T., Tsumura, K., Suematsu, C., Endo, G., and Fujii, S. (2000). *Diabet. Med.* **17**, 53–58.

O'Loughlin, J. (1999). *Can. Med. Assoc. J.* **161**, 152–153.

Orchard, T.J. (1994). *Diabetes Care* **17**, 326–338.

Pan, X.R., Li, G.W., Hu, Y.H., Wang, J.X., Yang, W.Y., An, Z.X., Hu, Z.X., Lin, J., Xiao, J.Z., Cao, H.B., Liu, P.A., Jiang, X.G., Jiang, Y.Y., Wang, J.P., Zheng, H., Zhang, H., Bennett, P.H., and Howard, B.V. (1997). *Diabetes Care* **20**, 537–544.

Pavan, L., Casiglia, E., Braga, L.M., Winnicki, M., Puato, M., Pauletto, P., and Pessina, A.C. (1999). *J. Hypertens.* **17**, 749–756.

Pelikanova, T., Kohout, M., Valek, J., Base, J., and Kazdova, L. (1989). *Metabolism* **38**, 188–192.

Pettitt, D.J., and Knowler, W.C. (1998). *Diabetes Care* **21** Suppl 2, B138–B141.

Poppitt, S.D., and Prentice, A.M. (1996). *Appetite* **26**, 153–174.

Poppitt, S.D., Eckhardt, J.W., McGonagle, J., Murgatroyd, P.R., and Prentice, A.M. (1996). *Physiol. Behav.* **60**, 1063–1070.

Poulsen, P., Vaag, A., and Beck-Nielsen, H. (1999). *BMJ* **319**, 151–154.

Prigeon, R.L., Kahn, S.E., and Porte, D. (1995). *Metabolism* **44**, 1259–1263.

Proietto, J., Nankervis, A.J., Traianedes, K., Rosella, G., and O'Dea, K. (1992). *Diabetes Res. Clin. Pract.* **17**, 217–226.

Purnell, J.Q., Kahn, S.E., Albers, J.J., Nevin, D.N., Brunzell, J.D., and Schwartz, R.S. (2000). *J. Clin. Endocrinol. Metab.* **85**, 977–982.

Reaven, G.M. (1998). *Diabetologia* **41**, 482–484.

Rosenbloom, A.L., Joe, J.R., Young, R.S., and Winter, W.E. (1999). *Diabetes Care* **22**, 345–354.

Rowley, K.G., Best, J.D., McDermott, R., Green, E.A., Piers, L.S., and O'Dea, K. (1997). *Clin. Exp. Pharmacol. Physiol.* **24**, 776–781.

Schaefer, E.J., Augustin, J.L., Schaefer, M.M., Rasmussen, H., Ordovas, J.M., Dallal, G.E., and Dwyer, J.T. (2000). *Am. J. Clin. Nutr.* **71**, 746–751.

Schneider, S.H., Amorosa, L.F., Khachadurian, A.K., and Ruderman, N.B. (1984). *Diabetologia* **26**, 355–360.

Seidell, J.C. (1997). *Horm. Metab. Res.* **29**, 155–158.

Seidell, J.C. (2000). *Br. J. Nutr.* **83** Suppl 1, S5–S8.

Selby, J.V., Ray, G.T., Zhang, D., and Colby, C.J. (1997). *Diabetes Care* **20**, 1396–1402.

Sheth, T., Nair, C., Nargundkar, M., Anand, S., and Yusuf, S. (1999). *Can. Med. Assoc. J.* **161**, 132–138.

Shobhana, R., Rama Rao, P., Lavanya, A., Williams, R., Vijay, V., and Ramachandran, A. (2000). *Diabetes Res. Clin. Pract.* **48**, 37–42.

Sorensen, T.I. (2000). *Diabetes Care* **23** Suppl 2, B1–B4.

Spielman, R.S., and Nussbaum, R.L. (1992). *Nat Genet* **1**, 82–83.

Stanner, S.A., Bulmer, K., Andres, C., Lantseva, O.E., Borodina, V., Poteen, V.V., and Yudkin, J.S. (1997). *BMJ* **315**, 1342–1348.

Stratton, I.M., Adler, A.I., Neil, H.A., Matthews, D.R., Manley, S.E., Cull, C.A., Hadden, D., Turner, R.C., and Holman, R.R. (2000). *BMJ* **321**, 405–412.

Stubbs, R.J., Johnstone, A.M., O'Reilly, L.M., Barton, K., and Reid, C. (1998). *Int. J. Obes. Relat. Metab. Disord.* **22**, 980–987.

Tudor-Locke, C.E., Bell, R.C., and Meyers, A.M. (2000). *Can. J. Appl. Physiol.* **25**, 466–492.

Tuomilehto, J., Lindstrom, J., Eriksson, J.G., Valle, T.T., Hamalainen, H., Ilanne-Parikka, P., Keinanen-Kiukaanniemi, S., Laakso, M., Louheranta, A., Rastas, M., Salminen, V., and Uusitupa, M. (2001). *N. Engl. J. Med.* **344**, 1343–1350.

UKPDS-33 (1998a). *Lancet* **352**, 837–853.

UKPDS-38 (1998b). *BMJ* **317**, 703–713.

Usui, K., Yamanouchi, K., Asai, K., Yajima, M., Iriyama, A., Okabayashi, N., Sakakibara, H., Kusunoki, M., Kakumu, S., and Sato, Y. (1998). *Diabetes Res. Clin. Pract.* **41**, 57–61.

Uusitupa, M., Louheranta, A., Lindstrom, J., Valle, T., Sundvall, J., Eriksson, J., and Tuomilehto, J. (2000). *Br. J. Nutr.* **83** Suppl 1, S137–S142.

van-Dam, R.M., Boer, J.M., Feskens, E.J., and Seidell, J.C. (2001). *Diabetes Care* **24**, 1454–1459.

Vinicor, F. (1994). *Diabetes Care* **17** Suppl 1, 22–27.

Visscher, T.L., and Seidell, J.C. (2001). *Annu. Rev. Public Health* **22**, 355–375.

Wannamethee, S.G., Shaper, A.G., and Alberti, K.G. (2000). *Arch. Intern. Med.* **160**, 2108–2116.

Wei, M., Gibbons, L.W., Mitchell, T.L., Kampert, J.B., Lee, C.D., and Blair, S.N. (1999). *Ann. Intern. Med.* **130**, 89–96.

Whitaker, R.C., and Dietz, W.H. (1998). *J. Pediatr.* **132**, 768–776.

WHO (1997). "Obesity: Preventing and Managing the Global Epidemic". WHO, Geneva.

Yajnik, C.S. (2001). *Nutr. Rev.* **59**, 1–9.

Yamanouchi, K., Nakajima, H., Shinozaki, T., Chikada, K., Kato, K., Oshida, Y., Osawa, I., Sato, J., Sato, Y., and Higuchi, M. (1992). *J. Appl. Physiol.* **73**, 2241–2245.

Yamanouchi, K., Shinozaki, T., Chikada, K., Nishikawa, T., Ito, K., Shimizu, S., Ozawa, N., Suzuki, Y., Maeno, H., and Kato, K. (1995). *Diabetes Care* **18**, 775–778.

Yudkin, J.S. (1995). *J. Intern. Med.* **238**, 21–30.

Yudkin, J.S. (1996). *Diabet. Med.* **13**, S16–S18.

# Cardiovascular diseases

10

K. Srinath Reddy

## Introduction

One of the most perceptible and pervasive changes that affected human society in the late 20th century has been the accelerated health transition that has propelled non-communicable diseases (NCDs) to the forefront of global public health challenges. In particular, cardiovascular diseases (CVDs) have emerged as the principal cause of death and disability in most regions of the world (Murray and Lopez, 1996; Reddy and Yusuf, 1998; Yusuf et al., 2001a,b; Reddy, 2001, 2002). As these advancing epidemics threaten to overwhelm health care systems in the developing countries through their mounting demands and also disrupt development through premature mortality and prolonged morbidity in mid-life, effective strategies for CVD prevention over the lifespan become imperatives for early attention and urgent action. Nutrition is a major determinant of the process and pace of these epidemics and warrants a key position in the multisectoral matrix of global CVD prevention.

## Burdens of CVD: global and regional estimates

According to the World Health Organization, 30% of all global deaths in 1998, accounting for 15.3 million lives lost that year, were due to CVD. Both men and women experienced these burdens, with CVD contributing to 28% of deaths in the former and 34% of deaths in the latter (WHO, 1999). The low- and middle-income countries contributed 78% of all CVD deaths and 86.3% of disability adjusted life year (DALY) loss attributed to CVD that year. Although this is largely due to the larger populations in those countries, the rise in proportional mortality rates, of CVD deaths as a fraction of all deaths, portends a growing burden of CVD in these countries (Yao et al., 1993; Yusuf et al., 2001a). Coronary heart disease (CHD) and stroke are the dominant CVDs, with rheumatic heart disease (RHD) contributing to the disease burdens only in the

**Table 10.1** Regional differences in burden of cardiovascular disease (1990) (from Murray and Lopez, 1996)

| Region | Population (millions) | CVD mortality (000's) | Coronary mortality (000's) | Cerebrovascular mortality (000's) | DALYs lost (000's) |
| --- | --- | --- | --- | --- | --- |
| Developed regions | 1144.0 | 5328.0 | 2678.0 | 1447.9 | 39 118 |
| Developing regions | 4123.4 | 9016.7 | 2469.6 | 3181.2 | 108 802 |

DALYs, disability adjusted life years.

countries in an early stage of health transition. CHD and stroke vary across the world in their relative burdens (Murray and Lopez, 1996). In 1990, the developing countries accounted for over two-thirds of all stroke deaths and about half of all coronary deaths in the world (Table 10.1).

CVD-related deaths also occur at a younger age in the developing countries, as anticipated by their current stage of health transition. Of the CVD-related deaths that occurred in these countries in 1990, about 46.7% occurred under the age of 70 years, whereas the corresponding proportion in the industrially advanced countries was only 22.7% (Murray and Lopez, 1996; Reddy and Yusuf, 1998). As these epidemics advance in the developing countries, the social gradient too is moving from the rich to the poor as the dominant victims. Although this phenomenon is at present only seen in some regions, depending on their level of health transition, other regions too are likely to witness it as their CVD epidemics mature (Pais *et al.*, 1996; Reddy and Yusuf, 1998; InterAmerican Heart Foundation, 2000).

# Projected CVD burdens in 2020

Most available estimates compare the 1990 baseline against projections for 2020, which are based on demographic and econometric models. The burdens of CVD will rise in all parts of the world, as populations age. The Global Burden of Disease study estimates that the developing countries will experience a 137% rise in men and a 120% rise in women, between 1990 and 2020, in the mortality attributable to CHD (Murray and Lopez, 1996; Yusuf *et al.*, 2001a). The developed countries will witness a much smaller rise (48% in men and 29% in women, respectively). Similarly, stroke mortality would exhibit 124% and 107% increases in men and women, respectively, in the developing countries, during this period. The corresponding elevations in the developed countries would be 56% in men and 28% in women. The world, as a whole, would experience a 100% and 80% rise in CHD mortality in men and women, respectively, as well as 106% and 78% elevations in stroke mortality (Table 10.2).

According to the Global Burden of Disease study, a 55% rise would occur in CVD attributable DALY loss, between 1990 and 2020, in the developing countries (Murray and Lopez, 1996). This would be in contrast to a 14.3% reduction in the proportion of CVD attributable DALY loss during the same period in the developed countries (including

**Table 10.2** Percentage rise in cardiovascular disease mortality 1990–2020 (from Murray and Lopez, 1996)

| | CHD | | Stroke | |
|---|---|---|---|---|
| | **Men** | **Women** | **Men** | **Women** |
| Developed countries | 48 | 29 | 56 | 28 |
| Developing countries | 137 | 127 | 124 | 107 |
| World | 100 | 80 | 106 | 78 |

**Table 10.3** Contribution of cardiovascular disease to DALY loss (% of total) (derived from Murray and Lopez, 1996)

| Region | CVD DALY loss (as % of total DALY loss) | |
|---|---|---|
| | **1990** | **2020** |
| World | 10.8 | 14.7 |
| Developed countries | 25.7 | 22.0 |
| Developing countries | 8.9 | 13.8 |

DALY, disability adjusted life year.

**Table 10.4** Developing countries: cardiovascular disease profile 2020 AD (based on projections by global burden of disease study, Murray and Lopez, 1996)

| | | Estimated deaths in 2020 (million) | Proportion of deaths between 30 and 69 years (%) | Persons dying in middle age (million) |
|---|---|---|---|---|
| Coronary heart disease (heart attacks) | Men | 4.3 | 54 | 3.3 |
| | Women | 3.5 | 27 | |
| Cerebrovascular disease (strokes) | Men | 3.2 | 52.7 | 2.5 |
| | Women | 2.7 | 28 | |
| Inflammatory and rheumatic heart disease | Men | 0.6 | 62.6 | 0.6 |
| | Women | 0.4 | 44.4 | |

both established market economies and former socialist economies) (Table 10.3). The gap would widen further if the former socialist economies, which are facing a resurgence in CVD, are excluded. In India, CVD-related deaths are expected to rise from 24.2% in 1990 to 41.8% of total deaths in 2020. Thus the increasing burden of CVD would be mostly borne by the developing countries in the next two decades (Murray and Lopez, 1996; Reddy, 2002).

The high burdens of mid-life deaths would continue to haunt the developing countries, even as the CVD epidemics advance to claim a higher share of the global disease burden (Table 10.4). It has been projected that 6.4 million deaths would occur due to

CVD in the developing countries in 2020 in the age group 30–69 years (Murray and Lopez, 1996; Reddy, 2002).

These projections do not directly factor in the likely rise in population levels of cardiovascular risk factors, though developmental patterns in the econometric models probably account for some such change. If these risk factors rise rapidly (as is likely from the combined effects of industrialization, urbanization, and globalization), the global dimensions of the future CVD epidemic may be even larger than is presently envisioned.

# Health transition and CVD: determinants and directions

The variations across time and geographical regions, in the overall CVD burden as well as the diversity in relative burdens of different diseases within the CVD spectrum, are best explained by the model of health transition. The model, which has been modified since its original description by Omran, explains the changes in the health status of populations as well as the extent of different CVDs on the basis of progressive developmental pattern influencing the determinants of health and patterns of disease (Omran, 1971; Olshansky and Ault, 1986; Pearson *et al.*, 1993). Such an evolutionary perspective, which has historical validity and predictive value, is superior to static cross-sectional views which afford only fleeting glimpses of an epidemic in motion.

Countries in the earliest phases of epidemiologic transition have a large burden of rheumatic heart disease as well as infectious and nutritional cardiomyopathies. Hypertension emerges as a public health problem in the next phase, as salt consumption rises, and adds hemorrhagic stroke and hypertensive heart disease to the burdens of rheumatic heart disease. As countries advance further in their demographic and socioeconomic transition, these are largely replaced by thrombotic strokes and coronary heart disease, with increased fat intake and rising blood lipids contributing to atherothrombotic vascular disease (Pearson *et al.*, 1993). Although a decline in the burden of rheumatic heart disease is evident in regions experiencing rapid health transition, it is still an important problem in regions that are at an early stage of demographic and developmental transition. The transition to the atherothrombotic phase of the epidemic may be preceded by a sharp fall in the burden of hemorrhagic strokes. The recent decline in CVD mortality, reported from South Korea, reflects such a fall in the contribution from hemorrhagic strokes while thrombotic stroke and coronary heart disease burdens have just begun to rise (Suh, 2001). Large developing countries may have different regions in different phases of health transition with urban areas usually experiencing higher CVD burdens at this stage. This phenomenon is evident in Latin America, parts of Africa, China, and India (Reddy and Yusuf, 1998). The risk factors for cardiovascular diseases also vary regionally and are themselves in transition (Reddy, 2002).

Most of the developed countries have entered the phase of delayed degenerative disease, where cardiovascular diseases remain the leading contributors to death and disability, but mostly manifest at a late age and with an overall decline in mortality. The task before the developing countries is to shorten the phase of large and escalating cardiovascular disease burdens in mid-life and rapidly transit to the phase of delayed and stable cardiovascular disease burdens.

There are several factors, which explain the recent emergence and underlie the projected escalation of the CVD epidemic in the developing countries (Pearson *et al.*, 1993; Reddy and Yusuf, 1998; Yusuf *et al.*, 2001a,b; Reddy, 2002). Firstly, there has been a global surge in life expectancy, especially more so in the developing countries. As a greater proportion of the population survives into older decades, many more individuals are exposed to risk factors of CVD for sufficient duration for clinical consequences to manifest. This epidemiologic transition, due to changing demographic profiles and a decline in the competing causes of death due to infectious and nutritional disorders, characterizes the advent of the CVD epidemic along with those of other chronic diseases. This has been clearly demonstrated in urban China, where mortality attributable to CVD increased from 86.2 per 100 000 (12.1% of total deaths) in 1957 to 214.3 per 100 000 (35.8% of all deaths) in 1990 (Yao *et al.*, 1993).

Secondly, delayed industrialization and recent urbanization have been associated with alteration in living habits, with deleterious changes in diet, physical activity, and tobacco addiction. These environmental changes lead to acquisition or accretion of risk factors. The increased "dose" of risk factor exposure, coupled to longer duration of exposure due to demographic changes, leads to enhanced risk of CVD. In China, the Sino-MONICA study demonstrated that the body mass index (BMI), hypertension, and blood cholesterol levels in the population of age group 35–64 years rose from 1984–86 to 1988–89 (Yao *et al.*, 1993).

There are also possible adverse effects of poor childhood nutrition (Barker *et al.*, 1993), which, if conclusively proven, would have an enormous impact on the developing countries, which still have a substantial fraction of the population which was underweight at birth. The possibility of such programming or as yet unascertained genetic factors may underlie the enhanced susceptibility of some ethnic groups, e.g., South Asian migrants, to CHD (Enas and Mehta, 1995; Yusuf *et al.*, 2001a). The excess risk in these groups may be explained by gene–environment interactions or fetal programming, but public health action must focus on the environmental changes which trigger the expression of susceptibility.

# Dynamics of the CVD epidemic in developing countries

Although the determinants of health transition in the developing countries are similar to those that charted the course of the epidemics in the developed countries, their dynamics are different. The compressed time frame of transition in the developing countries imposes a large double burden of communicable and noncommunicable diseases. Unlike the developed countries where urbanization occurred in prospering economies, urbanization in developing countries occurs in settings of high poverty levels and international debt, restricting resources for public health responses. Organized efforts at prevention began in developed countries when the epidemic had peaked and often accelerated a secular downswing whereas the efforts in the developing countries are commencing when the epidemic is on the upswing. Strategies to control CVD in the developing countries must be based on recognition of these similarities and differences. Principles of prevention must be based on the evidence gathered in developed countries but interventions must be context-specific and resource-sensitive (Reddy, 2001, 2002).

## Tracking the epidemic: risk behaviors to risk factors to events

Today's risk behaviors are tomorrow's risk factors and today's risk factors are tomorrow's events. The natural history of major CVDs plays out the effects of cumulative exposures to biologic risk factors which result from dominant risk behaviors (diet, inactivity, tobacco) which operate from the early years of life. The conventional risk factors may have been underestimated, in terms of their impact, due to (a) regression dilution bias, (b) lag time effect, (c) dichomotous divisions of risk factors which actually operate in a continuum, and (d) unquantitated exposures (Yusuf *et al.*, 2001a,b).

The "lag time" effect of risk factors on CVD means that present mortality rates are the effect of exposure to risk factors in past decades. Present public health strategies, which intend to reduce future CVD burdens, must focus on current levels of risk behaviors, biologic risk factors (which relate principally to those behaviors) as well as the proximate social determinants of those risk behaviors and risk factors. Inappropriate nutrition, reduced physical activity and tobacco consumption are among the behaviors most associated with an increased risk of CVD, whereas overweight, central obesity, high blood pressure, dyslipidemia, and diabetes are among the risk factors which principally contribute to the manifestation of that risk.

A rise in total fat intake and decline in carbohydrate consumption (especially the complex variety), excess energy intake coupled with micronutrient deficiencies, reduced physical activity with energy–activity mismatch leading to obesity as well as excess salt intake characterize the nutrition transition that is becoming increasingly well documented in many developing countries (Drewnowski and Popkin, 1997). The falling price of vegetable fat in the international market and the rising price of dietary fiber (fruit and vegetables) in the domestic markets are economic factors propelling this change. The proportion of Chinese citizens consuming >30% fat as an energy source in their daily diet rose steeply across all income classes between 1989 and 1993. The forces of urbanization and globalization which shift production from the small farmer to the large corporation, distribution from the shopkeeper to the supermarket, consumption from fresh to processed foods and supply from local to export markets are the dynamos of this change in dietary patterns (Lang, 1997). Worldover, food is becoming part of a "common culture" that reflects the dominant forces in globalization.

Although nutrition is an essential need, tobacco is an entirely avoidable external agent which contributes greatly to the risk of CVD. The proportion of all deaths attributable to tobacco is estimated to rise in India, from 1.4% in 1990 to 13.3% in 2020 and from 9.2% to 16.0% in China during the same period. The overall global escalation would be from 6.0% to 12.3% over these 30 years (WHO, 1996). Of the 10 million lives that would be lost globally in 2025, due to tobacco, 7 million would be from the developing countries. The declining tobacco consumption patterns and the tactical, albeit limited, retreat of the tobacco industry in the developed countries are accompanied by aggressive marketing and rising consumption patterns in the developing countries and CVD would be the largest contributor to these tobacco-related deaths.

Recent reports from many developing countries chronicle rising rates of sedentariness, overweight, high blood pressure dyslipidemia, diabetes, and tobacco consumption in their populations (Reddy and Yusuf, 1998; InterAmerican Heart Foundation, 2000; Yusuf *et al.*, 2001a). These presage a sharp rise in future CVD events, unless effective public health interventions to prevent, recognize, and reduce risk factors are urgently introduced and implemented.

The prevalence of hypertension varies according to the definition of hypertension used in different studies. Recent surveys in China and India confirm the higher urban prevalence of hypertension compared to rural (Reddy, 1996). The overall prevalence in China, with threshold values of 140/90 mmHg, was 12.5% in adults aged 35–64 years. Recent Indian studies estimate a prevalence of adult hypertension in India to be 27.3% in an urban setting and 12.2% in a rural setting. Based on these estimates, the number of adults with hypertension in India and China together would exceed 100 million. Prevalence estimates of hypertension in adults in sub-Saharan Africa are in the range of 10–15% with figures as high as 20% in some large studies. The number of hypertensive adults in this region, according to these studies, has been estimated to be between 10 and 20 million (Cooper *et al.*, 1998; Fuentes *et al.*, 2000). Prevalence of hypertension, in a national survey of adults in Mexico in 1993, was found to be 26.6% (Arroyo *et al.*, 1999).

The developing countries are currently contributing to three-quarters of the global burden attributable to diabetes. The anticipated rise in the number of diabetics in the world from 135 million in 1995 to 300 million in 2025 would principally be related to a sharp rise in diabetes prevalence in the developing countries, exemplified by a 195% rise in India (King *et al.*, 1998). This, in turn, would impact adversely on the CVD attributable burden of disease in the developing countries. Although urban diabetes prevalence rates are three- to fourfold higher than rural prevalence rates in most parts of India, urban prevalence of glucose intolerance (diabetes or impaired glucose tolerance) rose in urban Madras (Chennai) from 16.9% in 1988–89 to 20.7% in 1994–95 (Ramachandran *et al.*, 1997). Increase in body mass index as well as central obesity contribute to the rising rates of glucose intolerance. Both of these, in turn, are determined by changing patterns of diet and physical activity.

In most developing countries, at present, urban populations have higher levels of cardiovascular risk factors, which are related to diet and physical activity (overweight, hypertension, dyslipidemia and diabetes) whereas tobacco consumption is more widely prevalent in rural population (Reddy, 1993). This suggests that tobacco consumption is more influenced by education and is the earliest risk factor to demonstrate a reversal of the social gradient. The other risk factors are influenced by more complex social interactions affecting diet and exercise and their social gradients reverse relatively slowly. This variation indicates the need for specifically targeted prevention programs addressing the needs of different social groups. It also offers an opportunity for policy-linked social engineering to influence the dynamics of an advancing epidemic at an early stage.

## Ethnic diversity: variations in the theme

Although the pathways of CVD appear common to all regions of the world, there are differences in populations which are mediated by ethnicity, just as there are differences in individuals mediated by genetic influences. Ethnicity transcends racial designations or genotypic groupings. It represents the conglomeration of cultural practices, lifestyle patterns, social influences, religious pursuits and racial characteristics that shapes the distinctive identity of a community. Ethnicity, therefore, extends beyond race and, although culturally distinctive, is also open to adaptation and alteration (Reddy, 1998).

Ethnic diversity in CVD has been noted at all stages of the CVD epidemic, whether in terms of the dominant stroke profile or the relative burdens of CHD and stroke or interpopulation differences in CHD rates at similar levels of economic development. The Seven Countries Study initially portrayed these differences clearly and provided variability in total blood cholesterol as the best explanation (Keys, 1980). As knowledge about the distribution of coronary risk factors in different populations grew, the interplay of multiple coronary risk factors contributing to variability in coronary disease rates between populations became clear. However, some conundrums have continued to pose challenges to such epidemiologic elucidation. From the "French paradox" to the "Hispanic paradox", from the lower than expected rates in Pima Indians to higher than expected rates in South Asians (based on conventional risk factor levels), there have been several puzzles which have periodically demanded plausible explanations. These ethnic differences have been extensively reviewed recently (Yusuf *et al.*, 2001a,b).

Several factors may contribute to these observed interpopulation differences in the CVD profile. First, countries may be located at different points in the path of epidemiologic transition, with varied life expectancy, diverse demographic profiles and differing contributions from the competing causes of death. Thus the total burden of CVD as well as the composition of the CVD spectrum will vary according to the dynamics of health transition.

Second, environmental factors related to increased or decreased risk of CVD differ widely across populations. These differences are partly culture-specific and partly related to the stage of industrialization. Much of the variability of CVD risk, between and within populations, has been explained by differences in risk factors which are influenced by the environment (lifestyle factors). The greater range of risk factor distributions in interpopulation comparisons demonstrates their association with disease more vividly, even though unconfounded comparisons are difficult in such ecologic studies.

Third, genetic factors explain variance in the risk of incident CVD within populations by providing the basis for differences in individual susceptibility in a shared and relatively homogenous environment. They also contribute to interpopulation differences, due to variable frequencies of one or more genetic determinants of risk in different ethnic groups. Genetic contributions to lipid disorders, obesity, salt sensitivity, insulin resistance, coagulation derangements and endothelial dysfunction are being unraveled and investigated for attributable risk.

Fourth, the "programming" effect of factors promoting selective survival may also determine individual responses to environmental challenges and, thereby, the population differences in CVD. The "thrifty gene" has been postulated to be a factor in promoting selective survival, over generations, of persons who encountered an adverse environment of limited nutritional resources (Reddy, 2001). Although this may have proved advantageous in surviving the rigors of a spartan environment over thousands of years, the relatively recent and rapid changes in environment may have resulted in a metabolic mismatch. Thus the salt-sensitive person whose forefathers thrived despite a limited supply of salt reacts to a salt-enriched diet with high blood pressure. Similarly, an insulin-resistant individual whose ancestors may have survived, because a relative lack of insulin sensitivity in the skeletal muscle ensured adequate blood glucose levels for the brain in daunting conditions of limited calorie intake and demanding physical challenges, may now respond to a high-calorie diet and a sedentary lifestyle with varying degrees of glucose intolerance and hyperinsulinemia.

Yet another postulated "programming factor" which may underlie population differences in CHD is the state of infant nutrition determined by influences *in utero* and in early childhood. An adverse intrauterine growth environment due to poor maternal nutrition may confer a selective survival advantage to the fetus who has been "programmed" for reduced insulin sensitivity. Similarly other physiological mechanisms may be "irreversibly programmed", by the fetal and infant growth environment to confer a survival advantage. However, as the child grows and survives into adulthood, such a programming would result in adverse consequences of high blood pressure, glucose intolerance and dyslipidemia resulting in an increased risk of CVD in later life.

It is only after demographic profiles, environmental factors and possible programming factors are ascertained and adjusted for that differences in gene frequency or expression can be invoked as a probable explanation for interpopulation differences in CVD (Reddy, 1998). The extent to which most chronic diseases, including CVD, occur within and among different populations is determined by genetic–environmental interaction which occurs in a wide and variable array, ranging from the essentially genetic to the predominantly environmental. This is perhaps best illustrated by the knowledge gained from studies in migrant groups, where environmental changes due to altered lifestyles are superimposed over genetic influences. These "natural experiments" have been of great value in enhancing the understanding of why CVD rates differ among racial groups. The classical Ni-Hon-San study of Japanese migrants revealed how blood cholesterol levels and CHD rates rose from Japan to Honolulu and further still to San Francisco, as Japanese communities in the three areas were compared (Robertson *et al*., 1977). The experience gleaned from the study of South Asians, Chinese and Pima Indians further elucidates the complexities of ethnic variations in

CHD (Yusuf *et al.*, 2001a,b). The comparison of Afro-Caribbeans, South Asians and Europeans in UK brought out the sharp differences in central obesity, glucose intolerance, hyperinsulinemia and related dyslipidemia between the three groups despite similar profiles of blood pressure, body mass index and total plasma cholesterol (Chaturvedi *et al.*, 1994). However, urban–rural comparisons within India as well as migrant Indian comparison with their nonmigrant siblings reveal large differences in these conventional risk factors (Reddy, 1993).

Thus, where the environment is common but gene pools differ, the nonconventional risk factors appear to be explanatory of risk variance, whereas when the same gene pool is confronted with different environments, the conventional risk factors stand out in stark relief. Investigation of genetic–environmental interactions in the diverse "ethnic" groups across the world may supply some of the missing pieces of the atherothrombotic puzzle. Identification of characteristic genetic markers of enhanced susceptibility to vascular disease in any ethnic group does not imply that their future lies in gene therapy (involving millions of individuals) but that relevant environmental changes must be specifically targeted in that population. Often, the susceptibility attributed to race may obscure the true association with poverty or inequitable access to health care. Within as well as between ethnic groups, socioeconomic status is a strong determinant of lifestyle practices. Environmental components remain dominant in determining the varied "ethnic" risks for CVD. The mandate of preventive cardiology lies in identifying and addressing the components most relevant to each community at their present and projected levels of development and epidemiologic transition.

# Back to the future: evaluating evidence for initiating interventions

Evidence has been accrued from ecological, observational, and experimental studies, conducted mostly in developed countries, of the principles which underlie CVD risk and of strategies which are likely to be successful in reducing that risk. Prevention must aim at risk reduction across the lifespan and be guided by the following facts. First, risk operates across a continuum for most variables. Second, many more events arise from the "moderate" middle of the distribution than from the "high-risk" tail. Third, risk is multiplied when risk factors coexist, which they often do. Fourth, the majority of CVD events occur in persons with modest levels of multiple risk factors rather than in those with a high level of single risk factor. Fifth, "comprehensive" or "absolute" CVD risk is the best guide for individual interventions, whereas "population-attributable risk" should guide mass interventions, maximizing benefits by bringing about modest distributional shifts. Sixth, a synergistically complementary blend of cost-effective "population-wide" and "high-risk" interventions must extend from primary prevention in children to secondary prevention in older adults (Reddy, 2001, 2002; Yusuf *et al.*, 2001b).

Success of such an approach comes from community-based studies in Finland and Mauritius (Dowsen *et al.*, 1995; Puska *et al.*, 1995) as well as clinical trials employing lifestyle interventions, apart from drug trials. As the evidence from clinical trials reinforces the risk associations identified by observational studies, the "preventive norms" and "clinical norms" move closer, whether it be blood pressure or plasma cholesterol that is under consideration.

The benefits of healthy diet on reducing CVD risk have been well attested by the results of interventions in populations as well as in individuals (Pietinen *et al.*, 1996; De Lorgeril *et al.*, 1999; Sacks *et al.*, 2001). This should provide the basis for global action for CVD prevention utilizing effective strategies to prevent or reduce the CVD risk associated with diet, inactivity, and tobacco.

# Telescoping the transition: pathways for public health action

The model of health transition offers an opportunity to predict the course of the CVD epidemic in many regions of the world and to intervene effectively to alter that course. Developmental and demographic changes will expose more people to the increased risk of CVD but that can be countered by promoting healthy living habits, especially in the area of nutrition and physical activity. Experience of diverse countries (Japan and Southern Europe) suggests that development need not be necessarily accompanied by high burdens of CHD. The burdens of CVD cannot be totally prevented as they will continue to be the major contributors in the elderly. However, opportunities exist for reducing the burdens of mid-life mortality and disability due to CVD, by abbreviating the most dangerous phase of health transition. The challenge of public health in the 21st century, is to telescope the transition in the developing countries to contain these avoidable burdens of CVD. Fortunately, nutrition provides a powerful and practical pathway to meet that challenge. It requires an empowered community and an enlightened policy, catalyzed by an energetic coalition of health professionals, to open up and utilize that pathway for advancing the agenda of global CVD prevention and control.

# References

Arroyo, P., Fernandez, V., Loria, A., *et al.* (1999). Hypertension in urban Mexico: the 1992–93 national survey of chronic disease. *J. Hum. Hypertens.* **13**, 671–675.

Barker, D.J.P., Martyn, C.N., Osmond, C., *et al.* (1993). Growth in utero and serum cholesterol concentrations in adult life. *BMJ* **307**, 1524–1527.

Chaturvedi, N., McKeigue, P.M., and Marmot, M.G. (1994). Relationship of glucose intolerance to coronary risk in Afro-Caribbeans compared with Europeans. *Diabetologia* **37**, 765–772.

Cooper, R., Rotimi, C., Kaufman, J., *et al.* (1998). Hypertension treatment and control in sub-Saharan Africa: the epidemiological basis for policy. *BMJ* **316**, 614–617.

De Lorgeril, M., Salen, P., Martin, J.L., *et al.* (1999). Mediterranean diet, traditional risk factors, and the rate of cardiovascular complications after myocardial infarction: final report of Lyon Diet Heart Study. *Circulation* **99**, 779–785.

Dowsen, G.K., Gareeboo, H., George, K., *et al.* (1995). Changes in population cholesterol concentrations and other cardiovascular risk factor levels after five years of non-communicable disease intervention programme in Mauritius. *BMJ* **311**, 1255–1259.

Drewnowski, A., and Popkin, B.M. (1997). The nutrition transition: new trends in the global diet. *Nutr. Rev.* **55**, 31–43.

Enas, E.A., and Mehta, J. (1995). Malignant coronary artery disease in young Asian Indians. Thoughts on pathogenesis, prevention and therapy. *Clin. Cardiol.* **18**, 131–135.

Fuentes, R., Ilmaniemi, N., Laurikainen, E., *et al.* (2000). Hypertension in developing economies: a review of population-based studies carried out from 1980 to 1998. *J. Hypertens.* **18**, 521–529.

InterAmerican Heart Foundation (2000). "Heart Disease and Stroke in the Americans 2000". InterAmerican Heart Foundation, Dallas, TX.

Keys, A. (1980). "Seven Countries – a Multivariate Analysis of Death and Coronary Heart Disease". Harvard University Press, Boston.

King, H., Aubert, R.E., and Herman, W.H. (1998). Global burden of diabetes, 1995–2025. Prevalence, numeric estimates and projections. *Diabetes Care* **21**, 1414–1431.

Lang, T. (1997). The public health impact of globalisation of food trade. *In* "Diet, Nutrition and Chronic Disease" (P.S. Shetty, and K. McPherson, eds.), pp. 173–187. Wiley, Chichester.

Murray, C.J.L., and Lopez, A.D. (1996). "Global Health Statistics. Global Burden of Disease and Injury Series". Harvard School of Public Health, Boston, MA.

Olshansky, S.J., and Ault, A.B. (1986). The fourth stage of the epidemiologic transition: the age of delayed degenerative diseases. *Millbank Mem. Fund Q.* **64**, 355–391.

Omran, A.R. (1971). The epidemiologic transition: a key of the epidemiology of population change. *Milbank Mem. Fund Q.* **49**, 509–538.

Pais, P., Pogue, J., Gerstein, H., *et al.* (1996). Risk factors for acute myocardial infarction in Indians: a case control study. *Lancet* **348**, 358–363.

Pearson, T.A., Jamison, D.T., Trejo-Gutierrez, H., and Jamison, D.T. (eds.) (1993). "Disease Control Priorities in Developing Countries", pp. 577–599. Oxford University Press, New York.

Pietinen, P., Vartianinen, E., Seppanen, R., *et al.* (1996). Changes in diet in Finland from 1972 to 1992: impact on coronary heart disease risk. *Prev. Med.* **25**, 243–250.

Puska, P., Tuomilehto, J., Aulikki, N., and Enkki, V. (1995). "The North Karelia Project. 20 Years Results and Experiences". National Public Health Institute, Helsinki.

Ramachandran, A., Snehlatha, C., Latha, E., *et al.* (1997). Rising prevalence of NIDDM in an urban population in India. *Diabetologia* **40**, 232–237.

Reddy, K.S. (1993). Cardiovascular disease in India. *World Health Stat.* **46**, 101–107.

Reddy, K.S. (1996). Hypertension control in developing countries: generic issues. *J. Hum. Hypertens.* **10**, S33–S38.

Reddy, K.S. (1998). Ethnic diversity: the new challenge of preventive cardiology. *CVD Prevention* **1**, 6–8.

Reddy, K.S. (2001). Neglecting cardiovascular disease is unaffordable. *Bull. World Health Organ.* **79**, 984–985.

Reddy, K.S. (2002). Cardiovascular diseases in the developing countries: dimensions, determinants, dynamics and directions for public health action. *Public Health Nutr.* **5**, 2317.

Reddy, K.S., and Yusuf, S. (1998). Emerging epidemic of cardiovascular disease in developing countries. *Circulation* **97**, 569–601.

Robertson, T.L., Kato, H., Rhoads, G.G., *et al.* (1977). Epidemiologic studies of coronary heart disease and stroke in Japanese men living in Japan, Hawai and California. Incidence of myocardial infarction and death from coronary heart disease. *Am. J. Cardiol.* **39**, 239–249.

Sacks, F.M., Svetkey, L.P., Vollmer, W.M., *et al.* (2001). Effects on blood pressure of reduced dietary sodium and the dietary approaches to stop hypertension (DASH) diet. *N. Engl. J. Med.* **344**, 3–10.

Suh, I. (2001). Cardiovascular mortality in Korea: a country experiencing epidemiologic transition. *Acta Cardiol.* **56**, 75–81.

WHO (1996). "Tobacco or Health: First Global Status Report". World Health Organization, Geneva.

WHO (1999). "The World Health Report 1999 Making a Difference". World Health Organization, Geneva.

Yao, C., Wu, W., and Wu, Y. (1993). The changing pattern of cardiovascular disease in China. *World Health Stat. Q.* **46**, 113–118.

Yusuf, S., Reddy, S., Ounpuu, S., and Anand, S. (2001a). Global burden of cardiovascular diseases. Part I: General considerations, the epidemiological transition, risk factors, and impact of urbanization. *Circulation* **104**, 2746.

Yusuf, S., Reddy, S., Ounpuu, S., and Anand, S. (2001b). Global burden of cardiovascular diseases. Part II: Variations in cardiovascular disease by specific ethnic groups and geographic regions and prevention strategies. *Circulation* **104**, 2855.

# The nutrition transition in China: a new stage of the Chinese diet

**11**

*Shufa Du, Bing Lu, Fengying Zhai, and Barry M. Popkin*

## Introduction

China represents one of the more rapidly developing countries in the world. In the past two decades, the annual growth rate of the gross domestic product (GDP) was more than 8%; the highest rate in recent world history (World Bank, 2001). China has achieved remarkable economic progress and high levels of education. Annual income per capita is now almost 20 times greater than 20 years ago (State Statistical Bureau, 2001), reaching $400 in rural areas and $850 in urban areas in 1999 (Fig. 11.1). As a result, the proportion of the population considered to be poor decreased sharply from 20% in 1978 to lower than 5% in 1999. The proportion of the population with an income below $1 a day declined from 80% in 1978 to 12% in 1998 (World Bank, 2001). Only one-third of all adults were able to read or write in 1978. By 1998, illiteracy among 15–25 year-olds was about 7% (World Bank, 2001).

Along with these economic shifts, and many related social changes, has come a rapid evolution of the Chinese diet. The Chinese cuisine has one of the oldest histories. By the third century BC, there was a complex theory of cuisine and gastronomy developed for China. The starting point for modern Chinese cuisine is the cultivation and consumption of cereals (Legge, 1885). Yi Yin, a famous cook and prime minister, developed the standards that are still followed. These stress the mastery of cooking techniques and the harmony of flavors (Chen Qiyou, 1984; Knechtges, 1986). Foods are classified by nature (hot, cold, temperate, cool) and their flavor (salty, sour, sweet, bitter, acrid). The absence of excessive oil, other higher fat ingredients, and cooking options from this traditional cuisine, and even from the regional cuisines that emerged during the Ching and Manchu dynasties, is surprising. The excessive use of meat in the overall diet and the heavy additions of oils in modern dishes are new dimensions.

The Nutrition Transition
ISBN: 0-12-153654-8

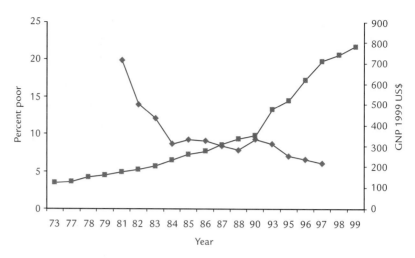

**Figure 11.1** Income and poverty trends in China (from World Bank: World Development Indicators, 2001). ◆, Poverty (%); ■, GNP.

There appears to be no ancient precedent for the current "westernization" of the Chinese diet.

The classic Chinese diet includes cereals (usually rice in the south; wheat and wheat products in the north) and vegetables with few animal foods. In rural areas, residents did not usually consume animal food, except when guests visited the family or there was a large festival (e.g., spring festival). Typically, such a diet is low fat, low-energy density, high in carbohydrates and high in dietary fiber. It is a diet that many scholars consider most healthful when adequate levels of intake are achieved (Campbell and Chen, 1994; Campbell *et al.*, 1998).

Earlier research by these authors has shown rapid changes in the diets and body composition of Chinese adults during the 1980–91 period (Popkin *et al.*, 1993, 1995). As the classic eating pattern shifts, intake of cereals and many lower-fat mixed dishes are being replaced. Animal foods are becoming popular and the consumption of edible oils is also quickly increasing. Most recently, Western fast food companies have entered China (Watson, 1997). For example, no restaurants sold western fast foods in Beijing in 1985; there are now more than 100 McDonald's or Kentucky Fried Chicken restaurants in Beijing. It is fashionable to eat at these restaurants.

There are five clear stages of the nutrition transition; that is, of dietary and body composition patterns in human history: collecting food, famine, receding famine, degenerative diseases and behavioral change (Popkin, 1993). This chapter shows that China is transforming very rapidly from the pattern of the present receding famine stage to that of diet-related degenerative diseases.

This shift in the composition of diet and body composition has been accompanied by many positive and some negative changes. Infectious diseases and hunger, important causes of death in the 1950s, no longer affect most of the population. Although malnutrition and nutrition deficiency diseases are still problems that should not be overlooked, the burden is shifting to diet-related degenerative diseases with a rapid increase in the prevalence of obesity. Mortality, particularly infant and child mortality, and fertility are declining, and life expectancy has reached high levels. Heart diseases, cerebrovascular diseases and cancer are now the major sources of mortality. Respiratory diseases are rapidly receding in importance.

# Subjects and methods

## Dietary data

Data were obtained from three sources. The first source, the State Statistics Bureau (SSB), has had a national random sampling framework since 1952, which was clustered by urban/rural areas and economic levels. A national representative sample was drawn from this framework. SSB has two survey teams: the Urban Survey Team and the Rural Survey Team. The two teams are in charge of the urban and rural area surveys, respectively, and collect data such as economic, occupation, population, marriage, and diet each year. The survey design is similar to a longitudinal survey, but about 20% of the households in the sampling communities would be changed each year. In this study, data from 1952 to 2000 were used to analyze the long-term transitions in diet and nutrition in China. Not every year's data before 1978 were available and data after 1992 did not include the total consumption of urban and rural residents.

The second data source was the China National Nutrition Survey (CNNS) which was conducted as three rounds of a national nutrition survey in 1959, 1982, and 1992. Unfortunately, since no computer files of data in 1959 were available; data from 1982 and 1992 were used in this chapter. CNNS used a multistage, cluster sampling method to draw the sample. In 1982, about 1500 persons in each of 178 communities were surveyed; the sample size was 238 134. Dietary data were collected using a five-consecutive days weighing method. In 1992, 30 households in each of 960 communities were surveyed and the sample size was 100 201. Dietary data were collected by a combination of the weighing method and three consecutive 24-hour recalls.

The third data source was the China Health and Nutrition Survey (CHNS), a longitudinal survey designed to examine the effects of the health, nutrition, and family planning policies and programs implemented by the national and local governments and to observe how the social and economic transformation of Chinese society is affecting the health and nutritional status of its population. The survey originally covered eight provinces, and now includes nine, that vary substantially in geography, economic development, public resources, and health indicators. A multistage, random-cluster process was used to select the sample surveyed in each of the provinces. In 1989, 190 communities including about 3800 households and 16 000 subjects were surveyed; they were followed up in 1991, 1993, 1997 and 2000. Three consecutive days of 24-hour recall and detailed household food consumption data were collected (Popkin *et al.*, in press). These three days were randomly allocated, from Monday to Sunday, and are almost equally balanced across the seven days of the week for each sampling unit. Household food consumption was determined by examining changes in inventory, from the beginning to the end of each day, in combination with a weighing and measurement technique.

### Physical activity data

The CHNS collected detailed data on occupation, work character, labor force, work time and other items related to physical activities. Physical activity was classified into three categories: light, moderate, and vigorous (Bell *et al.*, 2001). The proportion of ownership of television (TV) sets was also analyzed to reflect the shifts in physical activities.

### Anthropometric data

Data from both CNNS and CHNS were used. Both surveys measured height and weight in an elaborate way and these methods were described in Du *et al.* (2001a) and Ge *et al.* (1996). The World Health Organization's (WHO) cutoff points for body mass index (BMI) were used to define underweight (BMI < 18.5) and overweight (BMI ≥ 25). Overweight and obesity (BMI ≥ 30) categories are combined for two reasons. The proportion of BMI ≥ 30 was very low (only 1.5% in 1992) and a recent international group from the WHO-Pacific Region has recommended that a lower BMI cutoff for overweight of 23 and obesity of 25 should be used in Asia (Inoue and Zimmet, 2000).

### Mortality and causes of death data

These data came from the Annual Death Report from the Ministry of Health of China. China has a fairly complete death registration system that appears to be of reasonable quality. In rural areas, village clinics collect death data (including decedant's name, gender, age, death date and time, causes of death and diagnostic hospital, etc.) and report to town hospitals, which totals each village's data. In urban areas, anti-epidemic stations at the district level collect all death data from hospitals, clinics, and neighborhoods (the lowest government unit in a city). All data from anti-epidemic stations are submitted to the Ministry of Health. Diseases are classified according to the WHO's International Classification of Disease, Injuries, and Causes of Death, version 9 (ICD-9). Death data before 1973 were not used since they were not complete and the classification varied slightly from ICD-9.

## Results

### Food consumption pattern

The shift in the Chinese diet follows a classic westernization pattern. The economic progress, linked in part to liberalization of food production controls and the introduction of a free market for food and food products, are linked to these important shifts in diet (Guo *et al.*, 1999). Focus was placed on shifts in key, separate components of the Chinese diet.

## Cereals

### The long term

In the past, China was an autarkic agriculture country. Over 80% of the population lived in rural areas. They worked on farms and their main income came from foods they produced. However, this status has been changing in the last 50 years and this change is considered historic. There are really five different stages of change (Fig. 11.2). First, was the shift from an independent China, free of war, between 1949 and 1957. After a long period of civil wars and anti-Japanese aggression, famine was widespread, mortality was very high, and many people died young. China in 1949 was like a wasteland, but people received hope from the new government. Farmers got their lands, and workers got their jobs; economics began to recover, and food products began to increase. Limited by the poor agriculture mode and poor land sources, food production was inadequate and low cereal consumption patterns existed (Fig. 11.2).

In the second period, there was a sharp decrease in food consumption from 1957 to 1962 during the famine linked with the Great Leap Forward. The causes and consequences of the famine during this period are not well documented, but it is clear that a large-scale famine occurred and there was a major regression in the Chinese economy during this period (Piazza, 1986). In 1962, cereal intake reached the level of consumption of 1949, only 165 kg per capita, per year.

The third period, between 1962 and 1979, was one of strong recovery. During this period, per capita intake of cereals increased steadily from 165 kg to 195 kg. This was an annual per capita increase of only 1.8 kg.

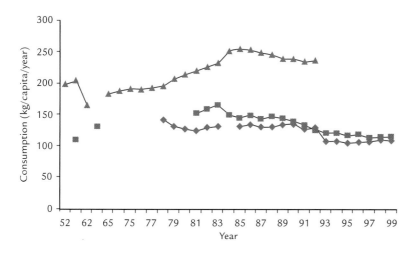

**Figure 11.2** Consumption of cereals and vegetables (data from State Statistical Bureau, China Statistical Yearbook, 1952–2000). ◆, vegetables (rural); ■, vegetables (urban); ▲, cereals.

The fourth or reform period of 1979 to 1985 came after the liberalization of food production when the annual economic growth rate was over 10%. During this period, China began to import cereals from the United States and other countries. As a result, per capita intake of cereals increased by 60 kg within 6 years, 10 kg each year, or a 27.4 g increase each day.

After this rapid growth, further economic improvement led to a shift in energy requirements. The structure of the Chinese diet shifted and cereal consumption began to slowly decline; this is the fifth period presented in Popkin *et al.* (1993).

Large cultural, economic, and communications differences existing between urban areas and rural areas are linked with different cereal intake patterns. Urban cereal intake decreased slowly before 1979 and rapidly thereafter. In 1999, the intake of cereals by urban residents was only 84.9 kg per capita. This was almost half of the intake of cereals in 1979, or one-third of that for rural residents in 1999.

**The short term**

Both CNNS and CHNS data showed that intake of cereals decreased considerably during the past two decades in both urban and rural areas and among all income groups (Table 11.1). During the eight-year period from 1989 to 1997, the total intake of cereals decreased by 127 g, per capita, per day (67 g for urban residents and 161 g for rural residents). The decrease in the low-income group was the highest: 196 g per capita, compared with their counterparts in mid- and high-income groups (86 g and 85 g, respectively). However, there remains an inverse relationship between income and cereal intake. For example, in 1997, the intake in low-, mid- and high-income groups was 615 g, 556 g and 510 g per capita, respectively.

The shift away from coarse grain consumption such as millet, sorghum and corn, is a key component of this change. CHNS data showed a 38 g decrease in refined cereals

**Table 11.1** Shift in consumption in the Chinese diet (China Health and Nutrition Study, 1989–1997) for adults, ages 20 to 45

| Food | Mean intake (g/capita/day) | | | | | | | | | | | |
| --- | --- | --- | --- | --- | --- | --- | --- | --- | --- | --- | --- | --- |
| | Urban | | Rural | | Low income | | Mid income | | High income | | Total | |
| | 1989 | 1997 | 1989 | 1997 | 1989 | 1997 | 1989 | 1997 | 1989 | 1997 | 1989 | 1997 |
| Total grains | 556 | 489 | 742 | 581 | 811 | 615 | 642 | 556 | 595 | 510 | 684 | 557 |
| Coarse | 46 | 25 | 175 | 54 | 226 | 68 | 98 | 43 | 78 | 30 | 135 | 46 |
| Refined | 510 | 465 | 567 | 527 | 585 | 546 | 544 | 513 | 517 | 479 | 549 | 511 |
| Fresh vegetables | 309 | 311 | 409 | 357 | 436 | 356 | 360 | 357 | 335 | 325 | 377 | 345 |
| Fresh fruit | 14.5 | 35.9 | 14.9 | 16.7 | 5.5 | 8.0 | 13.2 | 18.1 | 26.1 | 37.5 | 14.8 | 21.7 |
| Meat and meat products | 73.9 | 96.6 | 43.9 | 57.6 | 36.3 | 40.2 | 57.5 | 63.9 | 66.5 | 96.2 | 53.3 | 67.8 |
| Poultry and game | 10.6 | 15.5 | 4.1 | 11.7 | 4.1 | 7.0 | 6.6 | 10.2 | 7.7 | 20.3 | 6.1 | 12.7 |
| Eggs and egg products | 15.8 | 31.6 | 8.5 | 19.6 | 6.0 | 13.9 | 10.6 | 21.7 | 15.8 | 31.5 | 10.8 | 22.7 |
| Fish and seafood | 27.5 | 30.5 | 23.2 | 26.9 | 11.8 | 16.4 | 28.7 | 26.0 | 33.4 | 40.1 | 24.6 | 27.9 |
| Milk and milk products | 3.7 | 4.0 | 0.2 | 0.9 | 0.8 | 0.1 | 0.2 | 1.4 | 3.5 | 3.6 | 1.3 | 1.7 |
| Plant oil | 17.2 | 40.4 | 14.0 | 35.9 | 12.9 | 32.1 | 15.8 | 37.1 | 16.4 | 41.5 | 15.0 | 37.1 |

between 1989 and 1997, but an even larger decrease in coarse cereal consumption of 89 g. In CNNS data, the intake of refined cereals in 1992 was similar to that in 1982, but the intake of coarse cereals decreased by 59 g per capita, per day.

## Vegetables and fruits

### The long term
Figure 11.2 presents a long-term shift in household vegetable consumption. Urban residents' intake, which was slightly higher than that of rural residents, decreased steadily before 1997 and increased slightly thereafter. Among rural residents, there was a sharp decrease from 1992 to 1993, a smaller decline from 1993 to 1995 and then a slight increase.

### Short term
The intake of vegetables decreased between 1989 and 1997. In contrast, the intake of fruits, which are much more expensive than vegetables, showed an increase. CHNS data showed that the urban residents' intake of vegetables did not change from 1989 to 1997, but the intake of fruits in 1997 was 2.5 times that of 1989 (Table 11.1). As a result, the total intake of vegetables and fruits in urban areas during this period increased. The intake of vegetables of rural residents decreased 52 g per capita, per day (409 g in 1989 to 357 g in 1997), whereas the intake of fruits increased by 1.8 g per capita, per day during the same period. As a whole, total intake of vegetables and fruits decreased from 391.8 g per capita per day in 1989 to 366.7 g per capita, per day in 1997. The largest decrease occurred in the low-income group, where the intake decreased from 441.5 g to 364 g, or 77.5 g per capita, per day.

## Animal foods

### Long term
In the past 50 years, annual consumption of animal foods more than tripled from a very low level of consumption of 11 kg per capita in 1952 to 38 kg per capita in 1992 (Fig. 11.3). Urban residents' intake increased to 65.3 kg per capita in 1999. There was a slow rate of increase prior to 1979 but thereafter, it was much higher. From 1952 to 1979, intake increased by only 5.6 kg (0.2 kg annually), but it increased by 21 kg (1.6 kg annually) between 1979 and 1992. Of the subcomponents, meat and meat products increased from 8.4 kg to 20.3 kg, poultry and game from 0.6 kg to 2.3 kg, fish from 3.2 kg to 7.3 kg and eggs from 2.0 kg to 7.8 kg per capita, per year.

Meat and meat products were the main sources of animal foods, but the proportion decreased from 76% to 58% in rural areas and from 57% to 44% in urban areas. The proportions of other sources increased, but at a very low level. For example, the proportion of fish, as an animal food, increased from 11% to 16% in rural areas but there was no change in urban areas (22%); poultry increased from 3% to 10% in rural areas and from 6% to 12% in urban areas.

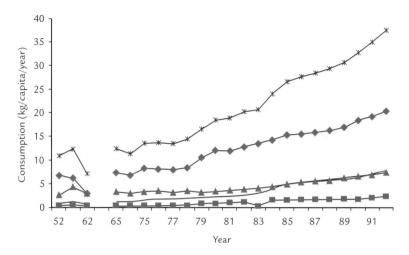

**Figure 11.3** Consumption of animal foods (data from State Statistical Bureau, China Statistical Yearbook, 1952–2000). ◆, meat; ■, poultry; ▲, fish; ——, eggs; ✱, animal.

### Short term
Urban residents' intake of animal foods per capita, per day in 1997 was higher than for rural residents (178.2 g for urban vs. 116.7 g for rural) and also showed a larger increase (46.7 g vs. 36.8 g) from 1989 to 1997. The amount and growth of intake of animal foods was positively associated with income levels. Intake in the low-income group was 77.6 g per capita, per day in 1997, an increase of 18.6 g, whereas it was 123.2 g and 19.6 g in the mid-income group; and 191.7 g and 64.8 g per capita, per day for the high-income group. The intake level and the increase in the high-income group from 1989 to 1997 was almost three times those in the low-income group.

## The composition of energy in the diet

### Long term
Figure 11.4 presents the long-term shifts in the proportion of energy from each macronutrient component; trends of energy intake were similar to those of cereals. Total energy intake increased before 1985; then began to decrease. Total energy intake was 2270 kcal (9.50 MJ) in 1952, 2440 kcal (10.21 MJ) in 1982, and 2328 kcal (9.74 MJ) in 1992. Among the energy components, there was little change in the proportion of energy from protein during this period, but the proportion of protein from animals increased considerably. Only 3.1% of protein came from animal foods in 1952 and this increased to 18.9% in 1992; intake of fat doubled in this time period (28.3 g vs. 58.3 g). Sources of energy changed remarkably; energy from fat increased two times (11% vs. 22%), energy from carbohydrates decreased from 77% to 66%, and energy from animal foods increased from 4.9% to 9.3%.

### Short term
Data from the CHNS show the shift away from carbohydrates to fat in the diet. Energy from carbohydrates (Table 11.2) decreased to 59.8% in 1997 from 68.7% in 1989 for

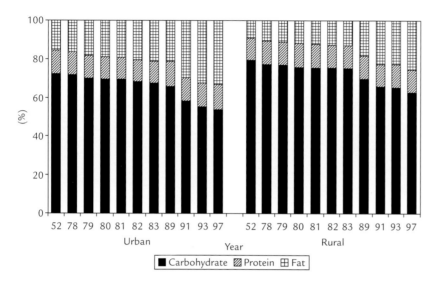

**Figure 11.4** The proportion of energy from macronutrient sources, 1952–1997 (data from State Statistical Bureau, China Statistical Yearbook, 1978–1983 and China Health and Nutrition Survey, 1989–1997).

**Table 11.2 Shifts in energy sources in the Chinese diet for adults, ages 20 to 45 (China Health and Nutrition Survey, 1989–1997)**

| | Energy from fat (%) | | | | Energy from carbohydrates (%) | | | |
|---|---|---|---|---|---|---|---|---|
| | 1989 | 1991 | 1993 | 1997 | 1989 | 1991 | 1993 | 1997 |
| Urban | 21.4 | 29.7 | 32.0 | 32.8 | 65.8 | 58.0 | 55.0 | 53.3 |
| Rural | 18.2 | 22.5 | 22.7 | 25.4 | 70.0 | 65.6 | 65.2 | 62.1 |
| Low income | 16.0 | 19.3 | 19.7 | 23.0 | 72.9 | 69.2 | 68.6 | 64.5 |
| Mid income | 20.3 | 25.2 | 25.5 | 27.1 | 67.5 | 62.6 | 62.2 | 60.3 |
| High income | 21.5 | 30.0 | 31.5 | 31.6 | 65.4 | 57.5 | 55.4 | 54.8 |
| Total | 19.3 | 24.8 | 25.5 | 27.3 | 68.7 | 63.2 | 62.1 | 59.8 |

all residents, and to only 53.3% from 65.8% in 1989 among urban residents, the lowest for any group. Energy from fat increased sharply from 19.3% in 1989 to 27.3% in 1997. The shift toward a high fat diet is shown more pointedly by examining those with low and high fat diets and higher animal fat diets from 1989 to 1997 (Table 11.3). The proportion of adults with a high fat diet increased by 2.5 times (14.7% vs. 38.5%) within these eight years. Over 60% of urban residents consumed more than 30% of energy from fat in 1997. The proportion of diets with a fat energy less than 10% declined considerably (18.4% to 3.1%) over this same eight-year period.

## Physical activity

Energy expenditure at work and the proportion of TV set ownership were used to measure changes in daily physical activities. Large changes in technology in the workplace

**Table 11.3** Shifts in consumption of total and saturated fat for adults, ages 20 to 45 (China Health and Nutrition Survey, 1989–1997)

|  | Percentage with energy from animal fat <10% | | | | Percentage with energy from fat ≥30% | | | | Percentage with energy from animal fat ≥10% | | | |
|---|---|---|---|---|---|---|---|---|---|---|---|---|
|  | 1989 | 1991 | 1993 | 1997 | 1989 | 1991 | 1993 | 1997 | 1989 | 1991 | 1993 | 1997 |
| Urban | 13.1 | 2.6 | 2.1 | 1.9 | 19.8 | 51.4 | 58.4 | 60.1 | 49.8 | 64.7 | 69.9 | 68.9 |
| Rural | 21.0 | 10.4 | 8.9 | 3.6 | 12.1 | 23.0 | 23.1 | 29.5 | 33.3 | 41.4 | 44.3 | 39.3 |
| Low income | 30.4 | 16.9 | 13.1 | 5.8 | 9.3 | 14.3 | 14.2 | 21.4 | 26.2 | 32.5 | 33.6 | 32.1 |
| Mid income | 14.8 | 5.4 | 6.1 | 2.7 | 16.2 | 31.1 | 31.4 | 35.5 | 42.8 | 50.6 | 53.2 | 42.6 |
| High income | 10.1 | 1.5 | 1.1 | 1.3 | 18.5 | 51.4 | 56.1 | 54.6 | 47.8 | 63.7 | 69.6 | 61.1 |
| Total | 18.4 | 7.9 | 6.8 | 3.1 | 14.7 | 32.0 | 33.7 | 38.5 | 38.8 | 48.7 | 52.0 | 48.0 |

**Table 11.4** Activity distribution among adults, ages 20 to 45 years (China Health and Nutrition Survey, 1989, 1997)

|  |  | Light (%) | | Vigorous (%) | |
|---|---|---|---|---|---|
|  |  | 1989 | 1997 | 1989 | 1997 |
| Urban | Male | 32.7 | 38.2 | 27.1 | 22.4 |
|  | Female | 36.3 | 54.1 | 24.8 | 20.8 |
| Rural | Male | 19.0 | 18.7 | 52.5 | 59.9 |
|  | Female | 19.3 | 25.5 | 47.4 | 60.0 |

**Table 11.5** The proportion of ownership of TV sets in China (%) (China Health and Nutrition Survey, 1989–1997)

|  | 1989 | 1993 | 1997 |
|---|---|---|---|
| Urban | 84.6 | 90.1 | 94.0 |
| Rural | 55.2 | 75.0 | 85.8 |
| Total | 64.7 | 79.6 | 88.5 |

and in leisure activities are linked with rapid declines in physical activity. Economic activities are shifting toward the service sector, particularly in urban areas (Popkin, 1998). The proportion of urban adults (male and female) working in occupations where they participate in vigorous activity patterns has decreased, and increased where the activity pattern is light. In rural areas, however, there has been a shift toward increased physical activity linked to holding multiple jobs and more intensive effort. For rural women, there is a shift toward a larger proportion engaged in more energy intensive work but there are also proportions where light effort is increasing. In contrast, for rural men there is a small decrease in the proportion engaged in light work effort. The results are presented in Table 11.4.

Television set ownership increased considerably during this eight-year period, especially in rural areas and among lower income groups (Table 11.5). Clearly TV

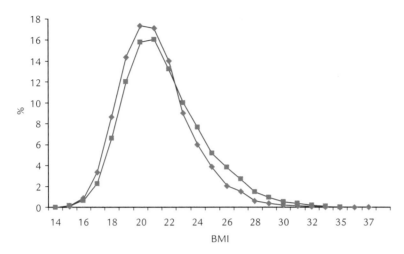

**Figure 11.5** Shift in the distribution of BMI for Chinese adults aged 20–45 years, CHNS89–97 (from Bell *et al.*, 2001). ♦, 1989; ■, 1997.

ownership represents a major potential source of inactivity. In 1997, close to 90% of Chinese households owned TV sets.

## Body composition

There has been a profound rightward shift in the body mass index (BMI) distribution of Chinese adults particularly at levels of BMI from 23 to 30 as shown in Fig. 11.5. Overweight and obesity were rare in 1982; only 3.5% of adults in the younger age (20–45 years of age) range had a BMI above 25 and only 0.2% were classified as being obese. These rates increased fourfold to 14.1% and 1.3%, respectively, in 1997. Compared with rural areas, the prevalence was much higher in urban areas (20.9% vs. 14.2%), especially in large cities. In 1992, more than 40% of urban residents in Beijing were overweight and obese, which would be a serious public health problem (Ge, 1996). In the past 15 years, there has been almost a one percentage point per year (0.93 percentage point annually) increase in the prevalence rate or an additional 12 million overweight and obese cases each year.

At the same time, there is still a meaningful proportion of adults facing chronic undernutrition and having a low BMI as shown in Table 11.6; the prevalence of undernutrition was 5.8% in 1997. During the period 1982 to 1992, this proportion decreased by 0.4 each year, and by 0.2 between 1992 and 1997 (using our CHNS and CNNS data).

## Morbidity

Blood pressure data from the CHNS show a modest increase in hypertension between 1991 and 1997 among adults, aged 30–65 years. Hypertension is greater among males and urban residents, which is not surprising, given the greater obesity found in urban

**Table 11.6** Trends of BMI distribution for 20- to 45-year-old adults (China Health and Nutrition Survey, 1989–1997)

| | BMI <18.5 (%) | | | | BMI ≥25 (%) | | | |
|---|---|---|---|---|---|---|---|---|
| | 1989 | 1991 | 1993 | 1997 | 1989 | 1991 | 1993 | 1997 |
| Urban | 7.8 | 7.8 | 7.7 | 6.2 | 10.6 | 12.1 | 12.7 | 18.7 |
| Rural | 8.3 | 8.4 | 7.3 | 5.6 | 8.4 | 9.9 | 10.2 | 13.7 |
| Male | 7.4 | 7.3 | 6.2 | 5.5 | 6.4 | 8.2 | 9.1 | 14.5 |
| Female | 8.7 | 9.1 | 8.6 | 6 | 11.5 | 12.7 | 12.6 | 16.2 |
| Low Income | 6.9 | 9.8 | 7.4 | 6 | 6.3 | 6.6 | 9.5 | 10.9 |
| Mid Income | 10 | 8.1 | 7.7 | 6.3 | 9.1 | 11.7 | 10 | 14.7 |
| High Income | 7.5 | 6.7 | 7.2 | 4.5 | 10.7 | 13.6 | 13.5 | 19.6 |
| Total | 8.1 | 8.2 | 7.5 | 5.8 | 10.3 | 10.6 | 10.9 | 15.4 |

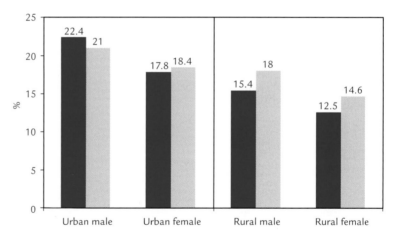

**Figure 11.6** Trends in the prevalence of hypertension, adults aged 30–65 years, CHNS 1991 (■) and 1997 (▨).

areas. Interestingly, the prevalence of hypertension in males in urban areas decreased slightly from 1991 to 1997 (the difference was not statistically significant), whereas the prevalence increased among all other groups, especially in rural males (Fig. 11.6).

## Mortality of degenerate chronic diseases

The overall death rate decreased between 1974 and 1984, with no major clear reduction from 1984 to 1990 and then rose in urban areas. It increased by 34.7 per 100 000 during this latter period (553.4 vs. 588.1). These results are presented in Fig. 11.7. This shift is noteworthy as it seems to be concurrent with the increase in diet-related noncommunicable diseases related to the circulatory system and cancer. The 1999 specific mortality of infection and parasite diseases in rural areas, for example, was one-seventh of the 1974 rate (58.2 vs. 8.0 per 100 000) but the mortality of diabetes in urban areas increased fivefold in 1999 compared to 1974 (15.4 vs. 3.4 per 100 000).

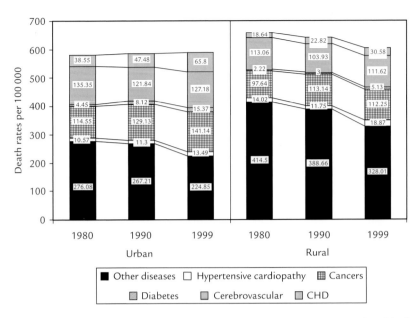

**Figure 11.7** Trends in the causes of mortality in China, 1980–99 (data from Ministry of Health of China: Annual Statistical Reports of Death, Injuries and Cause of Death in China, 1979–2000).

# Discussion

In the half century since Chinese independence, there have been three major periods related to the stages of the nutrition transition. Before 1985, the country was transformed from one facing famine and extreme food shortages to one where the food supply addressed basic needs. Food intake of key food types (cereals, vegetables, animal foods) as well as total energy intake increased. Continuing the shift toward a reduction of malnutrition between 1985 and 1990, food diversity increased considerably, total energy began to decrease, and animal food intake increased considerably, as did the proportions of poultry, eggs, and milk. After 1990, China entered a later stage of the transition as obesity began to increase, energy density of the diet increased considerably, and cereal intake decreased considerably. Diet-related noncommunicable diseases began to increase rapidly.

### What is the basis of stating a new stage of the nutrition transition was reached?

First, the overall 1999 death rates among urban residents increased to a higher rate than in the early 1970s. The main reason was that mortality increased from diet-related degenerative diseases such as cardiovascular diseases, diabetes and cancers. Mortality rates of rural residents are still improving but we expect these rates will also shift upward in the next several decades. Farmers have become richer in many regions of the country and the rural diet is following the same shift toward animal products that urban areas followed, i.e., reduced carbohydrate and increased edible oil and total fat. Adult obesity in rural areas is beginning to increase. Cancer and cardiovascular disease (CVD) will soon become the major sources of adult and total mortality in rural China.

Second, China is facing both challenges of malnutrition and overnutrition. In past decades, the government tried its best to solve the malnutrition problem and made great progress. However, the prevalence of malnutrition is still very high: 35% of pre-school children were stunting; 20% of preschool children, 22% of school children and adolescents, and 8% of adults were suffering from undernutrition (Du *et al.*, 2001b). On the other hand, the prevalence of overweight and obesity has risen to a relatively high degree. Although details on overweight status among Chinese children were not presented, other studies have shown large increases in overweight among preschool children, older children, and teens (Du *et al.*, 1999; Wang *et al.*, in press).

For example, based on the cutoff points of BMI for overweight and obesity from the International Obesity Task Force (IOTF), 15% (28% in urban areas) of children aged 2–6 years and 8% (12% in urban areas, 11 times that of 15 years ago) of children and adolescents aged 7–17 years were overweight and obese (Du *et al.*, 2001b).

The research by Doak *et al.* (2000) highlights this shift in the distribution of under- and overnutrition in a different way. Her research identified households in which overweight and underweight coexist, and explored causative household levels. In China, the prevalence of such households was 8% (Doak *et al.*, 2000).

Third, marked shifts in the Chinese diet have been shown. Unlike other East Asian countries, such as South Korea (which has actively promoted its traditional diets), China seems to be rapidly relinquishing its traditional diets (Kim *et al.*, 2000). South Korea has used mass media and other government programs to encourage retention of their high-vegetable, low-fat traditional cuisine.

The level of fat intake in South Korea is even lower than in China, although China's GNP was less than 1/14 of the GNP in South Korea in 1996. Starting in the 1990s, people in China obtained more than 20% of energy from fat whereas South Koreans still consumed less than 20% of energy from fat in 1995 (Kim *et al.*, 2000). In China, edible oil intake increases unabated as does the intake of other animal products (Drewnowski and Popkin, 1997).

Also, there has recently been a rapid increase in food consumption from away-from-home sources (Popkin *et al.*, in press). In 1989 only 0.4% of all energy was con-sumed at restaurants and stalls in China, but by 1997, over 7.4% of energy came from restaurants and food stalls. Some scholars feel that increased away-home food consumption is a contributing factor to increased overweight and obesity (Binkley *et al.*, 2000).

## Why did the prevalence of overweight and obesity and diet-related noncommunicable disease mortality rise so quickly?

The ongoing demographic and economic transition in China is promoting changes in diet and lifestyle, as in other developing countries (Popkin, 1993, 1998; Caballero and Rubinstein, 1997). The shifts in diet and activity have certainly been implicated in the increase in obesity (Paeratakul *et al.*, 1998). Traditional diets are shifting to high-fat and high-energy density diets. China is experiencing the nutrition transition much sooner and at a much lower level of GNP than the United States and Western European countries (Drewnowski and Popkin, 1997). The increase in energy density of the food consumed in the Chinese diet was over 10% during the 1989 to 1997 period (Popkin *et al.*, in press); reports showed energy density was probably responsible for the increase of energy intake and obesity (Bell *et al.*, 1998; Hill and Peters, 1998; Rolls *et al.*, 1999).

This chapter has shown a large increase in fat from animal sources. Over two-thirds of urban Chinese consume over 10% of their energy from animal fat. These animal food sources are predominantly high-fat pork and pork products with less lower fat and healthier poultry and fish.

Other types of change that might be linked to future accelerations of the diet are less clear. Other work shows large increases in the speed of consumption changes (Guo *et al.*, 2000). Media exposure might be a critical element in this shift. A less clear effect is the role of the rapid increase in away-from-home consumption; it represents a small proportion of the diet, but it is clear that this will increase rapidly. Today, all provinces and almost all large cities have either a McDonald's or a Kentucky Fried Chicken outlet and the spread in many areas is astounding (Watson, 1997).

Physical activities in daily life have been reduced due to advances in technology and transportation (Bell *et al.*, 2001). A large proportion of the people live a sedentary life and this trend will continue. Also, the large shifts in ownership of TV sets and the equally large reduction in physical activity at work are important. People spend more time watching TV, playing electronic games, and working with the computer.

Urbanization plays an important role in the rapid transition found in China. Its role in shifting occupational patterns and other dimensions of physical activity, as well as access to a different more processed, higher fat and sugar diet is important (Drewnowski and Popkin, 1997; Popkin, 1999; Holmboe-Ottesen, 2000). Moreover, the proportion of the population that resides in urban areas has grown.

A further issue is the potentially greater vulnerability for noncommunicable diseases that persons residing in rural areas face due to early fetal and infant malnutrition (Barker *et al.*, 1993; Barker, 1997; Hoffman *et al.*, 2000a,b,c). In past decades, there were very high rates of low birth weight and stunting among Chinese children, all of which could have enhanced the likelihood of later obesity and other chronic diseases (Popkin *et al.*, 1996). As they grow, the metabolic balance (that served well in conditions of undernutrition) may become maladaptive, leading to the development of abnormal lipid profiles, altered glucose and insulin metabolism, and obesity (Barker *et al.*, 1993; Hoffman *et al.*, 2000 a,b,c).

Today, diet-related noncommunicable diseases represent the major causes of mortality in China. By 1995, the economic costs of undernutrition and overnutrition were of similar magnitude in China and diet-related noncommunicable disease costs will predominate in 2025. The economic cost of diet-related noncommunicable diseases exceeded 2.1% of the GDP in China in 1995 (B.M. Popkin, S. Horton, S. Kim, A. Mahal and S. Jin, unpublished results). The question is whether the public health system, faced with such massive increases in costs from these noncommunicable diseases, can rise to the challenge and create the coordinated effort needed to address China's emerging problems.

## Acknowledgments

This analysis was conducted while Shufa Du was a postdoctoral fellow at the Carolina Population Center, University of North Carolina at Chapel Hill. Shufa Du and Bing Lu received funding from the Fogarty International Center, NIH. Also we thank the National Institutes of Health (NIH) (R01-HD30880 and R01-HD38700) for financial support for the analysis. We wish to thank Ms Frances L. Dancy for administrative assistance, Tom Swasey for graphics support, and Ms Zhihong Wang and Ms Hongfei Hao for research assistance.

## References

Barker, D.J. (1997). *Br. Med. Bull.* **53**, 96–108.

Barker, D.J., Gluckman, P.D., Godfrey, K.M., Harding, J.E., Owens, J.A., and Robinson, J.S. (1993). *Lancet* **341**, 938–941.

Bell, E.A., Castellanos, V.H., Pelkman, C.L., Thorwart, M.L., and Rolls, B.J. (1998). *Am. J. Clin. Nutr.* **67**, 412–420.

Bell, C., Ge, K., and Popkin, B.M. (2001). *Int. J. Obes. Relat. Metab. Disord.* **25**, 1079–1086.

Binkley, J.K., Eales, J., and Jekanowski, M. (2000). *Int. J. Obes. Relat. Metab. Disord.* **24**, 1032–1039.

Caballero, B., and Rubinstein, S. (1997). *Arch. Latinoam Nutr.* **47** Suppl 1, 3–8.

Campbell, T.C., and Chen, J. (1994). *Am. J. Clin. Nutr.* **59**, 1153S–1161S.

Campbell, T.C., Parpia, B., and Chen, J. (1998). *Am. J. Cardiol.* **82**, 18T–21T.

Chen, Q. (ed.) (1984). "Lü Shi Chun Qiu Jiao Shi", Vol. 14. Xuelin Publishing House, Shanghai, China.

Doak, C., Adair, L., Monteiro, C., and Popkin, B.M. (2000). *J. Nutr.* **130**, 2965–2980.

Drewnowski, A., and Popkin, B.M. (1997). *Nutr. Rev.* **55**(2), 31–43.

Du, S. (1999). *In* "The Dietary and Nutritional Status of Chinese Population – Children and Adolescents (1992 National Nutrition Survey)" (K. Ge, and F. Zhai, eds.), Vol. 2, pp. 12–34. People's Medical Publishing House, China.

Du, S., Zhai, F., and Ge, K. (2001a). *J. Hyg. Res.* **30**, 339–342.

Du, S., Lu, B., Wang, Z., Zhai, F., and Popkin, B.M. (2001b). *J. Hyg. Res.* **30**, 221–225.

Ge, K. (1996). *J. Hyg. Res.* **25** Suppl, 1–8 (in Chinese).

Ge, K., Zhai, F., and Yan, H. (eds.) (1996). " The Dietary and Nutritional Status of Chinese Population (1992 National Nutrition Survey)". People's Medical Publishing House, China.

Guo, X., Popkin, B.M., Mroz, T.A., and Zhai, F. (1999). *J. Nutr.* **129**, 994–1001.

Guo, X., Mroz, T.A., Popkin, B.M., and Zhai, F. (2000). *Econ. Dev. Cult. Change* **4**, 737–760.

Hill, J.O., and Peters, J.C. (1998). *Science* **280**, 1371–1374.

Hoffman, D.J., Sawaya, A.L., Coward, A., Wright, A., Martins, P.A., de Nascimento, C., Tucker, K., and Roberts, S.B. (2000a). *Am. J. Clin. Nutr.* **72**, 1025–1031.

Hoffman, D.J., Sawaya, A.L., Verreschi, I., Tucker, K.L., and Roberts, S.B. (2000b). *Am. J. Clin. Nutr.* **72**, 702–707.

Hoffman, D.J., Roberts, S.B., Verreschi, I., Martins, P.A., de Nascimento, C., Tucker, K.L., and Sawaya, A.L. (2000c). *J. Nutr.* **130**, 2265–2270.

Holmboe-Ottesen, G. (2000). *Tidsskr Nor Laegeforen.* **120**, 78–82.

Inoue, S., and Zimmet, P. (2000) "The Asia-Pacific Perspective: Redefining Obesity and its Treatment". Health Commun, Sydney, Australia.

Kim, S., Moon, S., and Popkin, B.M. (2000). *Am. J. Clin. Nutr.* **71**, 44–53.

Knechtges, D.R. (1986). *J. Am. Orient. Soc.* **106**, 49–63.

Legge, J. (1885). "The Li Ki in The Sacred Books of China, Part 3", The Royal Regulations, Sect. III/14, Oxford.

Paeratakul, S., Popkin, B.M., Ge, K., Adair, L.S., and Stevens, J. (1998). *Int. J. Obes. Relat. Metab. Disord.* **22**, 424–432.

Piazza, A. (1986). "Food Consumption and Nutritional Status in the PRC". Westview Special Studies on China, Boulder, CO.

Popkin, B.M. (1993). *Pop. Dev. Rev.* **19**, 138–157.

Popkin, B.M. (1998). *Publ. Health Nutr.* **1**, 5–21.

Popkin, B.M. (1999). *World Dev.* **27**, 1905–1916.

Popkin, B.M., Ge, K., Zhai, F., Guo, X., Ma, H., and Zohoori, N. (1993). *Eur. J. Clin. Nutr.* **47**, 333–346.

Popkin, B.M., Paeratakul, S., Zhai, F., and Ge, K. (1995). *Am. J. Publ. Health* **85**(5), 690–694.

Popkin, B.M., Richards, M.K., and Monteiro, C. (1996). *J. Nutr.* **126**, 3009–3016.

Popkin, B.M., Lu, B., and Zhai, F. (2002). *Publ. Health Nutr.* (in press).

Rolls, B.J., Bell, E.A., Castellanos, V.H., Chow, M., Pelkman, C.L., and Throwart, M.L. (1999). *Am. J. Clin. Nutr.* **69**, 863–871.

State Statistical Bureau (2001). "China Statistical Yearbook 2000". China Statistics Press, China.

Wang, Y., Monteiro, C., and Popkin, B.M. (2002). *Am. J. Clin. Nutr.* (in press).

Watson, J.L. (ed.) (1997). "Golden Arches East: McDonald's in East Asia", pp. 1–256. Stanford University Press, Stanford.

World Bank (2001). "World development indicators 2001". World Bank, Washington, DC.

# Trends in under- and overnutrition in Brazil

*Carlos A. Monteiro, Wolney L. Conde, and Barry M. Popkin*

## Introduction

The process known as nutrition transition refers to major cyclical changes in the nutritional profile of human populations, produced by modifications in both dietary and nutrient expenditure patterns, and basically determined by an interplay of economic, demographic, environmental, and cultural changes occurring in the society (Popkin, 1993).

Outstanding changes in economic, demographic, environmental, and cultural factors have been registered in the last quarter of the 20th century in most developing countries, but the impact of these changes on the nutritional profile of their populations is still to be fully assessed (Popkin *et al.*, 1995; Popkin, 1998; Popkin and Doak, 1998). The relative burden of disease, represented by under- and overnutrition, the pace of the transition process among children, adolescents and adults, and the distinct effects on the social classes are still unclear in these countries.

Brazil is placed in a privileged position concerning the description of the nutrition transition process. First, demographic, socioeconomic, environmental, and cultural changes have been impressive in Brazil in the last quarter of the 20th century (Iunes, 2000; Patarra, 2000; Ibge, 2001). Second, in Brazil the availability of repeated nationally representative cross-sectional surveys provides a basis for the careful understanding of secular trends of the nutritional profile of its population. Third, Brazil has continental dimensions (it is the fifth largest country in the world) and great economic differences between the least-developed northern regions and the most-developed southern regions; this makes it possible to stage the process of the nutrition transition at different levels of economic development. Fourth, the strong uneven income distribution across the country permits the dynamics of the nutrition transition among the relatively poorer and richer social strata to be individualized and compared within each region.

The Nutrition Transition
ISBN: 0-12-153654-8

This chapter complements and updates previous analyses on specific aspects of the nutrition transition in Brazil (Monteiro *et al.*, 1992, 1994, 1995, 2000a,b,c,d, 2001; Mondini and Monteiro, 1994; Monteiro and Conde, 1999).

# Methods

## Populations and sampling

Data used in this section come from four successive nationwide surveys undertaken in Brazil in 1975, 1989, 1996, and 1997 (Estudo Nacional da Despesa Familiar, 1975; Pesquisa Nacional sobre Saúde e Nutrição, 1989; Pesquisa Nacional sobre Demografia e Saúde, 1996; Pesquisa sobre Padrões de Vida, 1997). The four surveys were executed by, or with the support of, the federal agency in charge of national statistics in Brazil (the Instituto Brasileiro de Geografia e Estatística) using similar probabilistic, census-based, multistage, stratified, clustering sampling procedures (Ibge/UNICEF, 1982; Ibge/UNICEF, 1992; Bemfam, 1997; Ibge, 1998). The most recent survey, undertaken in 1997, was restricted to the northeastern and southeastern regions of Brazil. Therefore, to allow proper comparisons, all trend analyses presented in this section will consider only the sample of households studied by the four surveys in those two regions. The northeastern and southeastern regions are, respectively, the least and the most economically developed regions in the country (1995 per capita gross domestic product (GDP) of US$ 1728 and US$ 4913, respectively) (Lavinas and Magina, 1996). Together, these two regions also concentrate 70% of the total Brazilian population (28% and 42%, respectively, according to the demographic census of 2000). The number of sampled households in these two regions was: (a) 36 105 in 1975, (b) 14 602 in 1989, (c) 8922 in 1996, and (d) 11 033 in 1997. In the 1975, 1989, and 1997 surveys, all individuals living in the households were eligible for nutritional assessment through anthropometry (weight and height measurements), but in 1996, this assessment was restricted to children under five years of age. To avoid age groups where the assessment of the nutritional status through anthropometry poses more difficulties, our trend analyses are focused on three age groups:

1. 1–4-year-old individuals – hereafter called the young child group – studied in 1975, 1989, and 1996;
2. 10–17-year-old individuals – hereafter called the old child/adolescent group – studied in 1975, 1989, and 1997;
3. Individuals aged 20 or more years – hereafter called the adult group – also studied in 1975, 1989, and 1997.

The coverage of the anthropometrical exams was very high in the four surveys among all age groups (from 91% to 99%). The absolute number of young children, older children and adolescents, and adults examined by each survey, pregnant women excluded, is shown in Table 12.1.

**Table 12.1** Number of individuals studied in four anthropometric surveys by age groups and region. Brazil: 1975–1997

| Year of the survey | Region | Age group | | |
| --- | --- | --- | --- | --- |
| | | 1–4 years | 10–17 years | Over 20 years |
| 1975 | Northeast | 7798 | 15 870 | 33 582 |
| | Southeast | 7335 | 18 414 | 44 449 |
| 1989 | Northeast | 1290 | 2894 | 6919 |
| | Southeast | 890 | 2250 | 7097 |
| 1996 | Northeast | 1141 | – | – |
| | Southeast | 645 | – | – |
| 1997 | Northeast | – | 1678 | 4559 |
| | Southeast | – | 1305 | 4838 |

## Data collection

The four surveys adopted similar processes for collecting anthropometrical data. Weight and height measurements were obtained at the households by pairs of trained and standardized interviewers. Weight was measured using calibrated portable scales (mechanical in 1975 and microelectronic in the subsequent surveys) with the sampled individuals wearing light clothes and no shoes. Recumbent length was obtained from children less than two years of age using a horizontal stadiometer; height was obtained in older children and adults using inextensible tapes in bare-footed individuals, with the head held in the Frankfort plane. The age of all individuals was calculated based on birth certificates or equivalent documents. The economic status of the studied individuals was assessed through the direct collection of family income data in 1975, 1989, and 1997 whereas the 1996 survey used an inventory of goods in the household (radio, TV set, video player, refrigerator, vacuum cleaner, washing machine, and car).

## Indicators and data analysis

Height-for-age and weight-for-height indices expressed as z-scores of the international growth reference (HAZ and WHZ, respectively) were used to assess children's nutritional status; stunted, wasted and underweight children corresponded to $HAZ < -2$, $WHZ < -2$ and $WHZ > 2$, respectively (WHO, 1995). Body mass index (BMI) or the weight in kg divided by the height in meters squared ($kg/m^2$), was used to assess the nutritional status of both adolescents and adults (WHO, 1995). Underweight and overweight adolescents corresponded to BMI below the 5th centile or above the 95th centile, respectively, of a gender and age-specific BMI reference distribution built upon the whole national sample of adolescents studied in 1989 using the LMS method (Cole, 1990). Underweight adults corresponded to $BMI < 18.5 \, kg/m^2$ and obese adults to $BMI \geqslant 30.0 \, kg/m^2$ (WHO, 1995).

Time-trend analyses consider changes in the prevalence (and correspondent 95% confidence intervals) of:

1. stunted, wasted, and overweight young children;
2. underweight and overweight old child/adolescents;
3. underweight and obese adults.

Time-trend analyses also consider changes in mean z-scores (and correspondent 95% confidence intervals) of young child HAZ and WHZ, old child/adolescent, and adult BMI z-scores as well as shifts in the distribution curves of these variables. BMI z-scores for adolescents were calculated with reference to the previously mentioned gender and age-specific BMI distribution built on the whole national sample of older children and adolescents studied in 1989. The BMI z-score for adults was calculated, in an analogous way, with reference to a gender and age-specific BMI distribution built on the whole national sample of adults studied in 1989. The analyses will be performed firstly for the combined northeastern and southeastern populations (hereafter referred to as a proxy of the Brazilian population); separately for each region; and finally for region-specific quartiles relative to the per capita family income (1975, 1989, and 1997) or the number of goods in the household (1996).

All statistical analyses of this study were carried out using STATA (Stata Corp., 1997). All estimates accounted for the sampling weights and the sampling design effects on standard errors (and confidence intervals) resulting from the complex, stratified, clustered, sample design employed by each survey. Estimates of adult underweight and adult obesity were age-adjusted by the direct method to the gender-specific age distribution observed in the last survey in order to control for ageing trends across the surveys, existing in the case of the adult population. Statistical significance of changes over time in child, adolescent, and adult nutritional status was assessed by grouping the individual data files of each survey in one single data file and running linear or logistic regression analyses in which the continuous or discrete nutritional status indicators were the dependent variable and the survey year was the independent variable (age group was a control variable for all analyses involving the adult population). Tests for linear trends in the logistic models were calculated by unfactoring the independent variable (the survey year).

# Results

## Trends in young children

Figures 12.1 and 12.2 display HAZ and WHZ distributions for the 1–4-year-old Brazilian children studied in 1975, 1989, and 1996 (z-scores relative to the international growth reference). The distributions refer to combined genders since no relevant difference was found between time-trends in boys and girls. The HAZ curve shifts progressively toward the right (higher values) throughout the three surveys whereas the WHZ curve shifts slightly toward the right from 1975 to 1989 but then remains

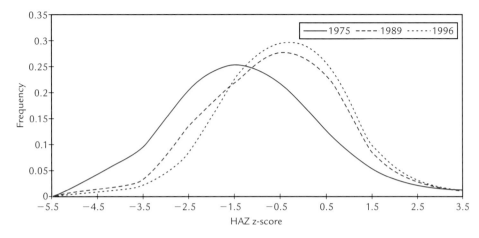

**Figure 12.1** Height-for-age distribution in 1–4-year-old children. Brazil: 1975–1996.

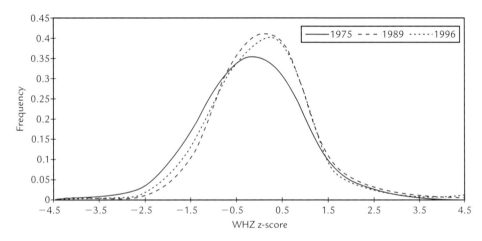

**Figure 12.2** Weight-for-height distribution in 1–4-year-old children. Brazil: 1975–1996.

relatively unchanged to 1996. In the three successive surveys (1975, 1989, and 1996) the average child HAZ increased from $-1.33$ to $-0.69$ and then to $-0.47$ ($P < 0.0001$ for linear trend), whereas the average child WHZ increased from $-0.17$ to $+0.06$ ($P < 0.0001$) and then stabilized near zero ($+0.02$ in 1996). Although improving throughout the surveys, the final average child HAZ achieved at the last 1996 survey ($-0.47$; 95% CI: $-0.41$; $-0.53$) remains significantly negative (i.e., below the international growth reference) indicating that child stunting is still present in the population. The average WHZ is significantly negative in 1975 ($-0.17$; 95% CI: $-0.19$; $-0.15$) but positive and close to zero in the two most recent (1989 and 1996) surveys indicating the control of child wasting in the population.

Table 12.2 presents time-trends in gender combined child stunting, child wasting, and child overweight. The prevalence of each event in each survey is given with correspondent 95% confidence intervals. Trends are presented for the entire country, for each region, and, within each region, for extreme income groups (the 25% poorest and

**Table 12.2** Secular trends in the prevalence (%) of stunted, wasted, and overweight 1–4-year-old children by region and income group. Brazil: 1975–1996

| Region and income group | Stunted[a] | | | Wasted[b] | | | Overweight[c] | | |
|---|---|---|---|---|---|---|---|---|---|
| | 1975 | 1989 | 1996 | 1975 | 1989 | 1996 | 1975 | 1989 | 1996 |
| Northeast | 47.1 | 29.9 | 19.0 | 4.1 | 1.8 | 2.6 | 2.9 | 1.5 | 2.7 |
| | (45.9–48.4)[d] | (27.3–32.6) | (16.6–21.5) | (3.6–4.7) | (1.0–2.5) | (1.6–3.6) | (2.5–3.3) | (0.8–2.2) | (1.8–3.7) |
| 25% poorest | 60.8 | 42.4 | 28.8 | 5.0 | 2.6 | 3.4 | 2.4 | 1.2 | 2.3 |
| | (58.3–63.2) | (37.4–47.5) | (25.0–32.5) | (3.9–6.0) | (0.9–4.2) | (1.8–5.0) | (1.7–3.2) | (0.1–2.3) | (1.0–3.6) |
| 25% richest | 26.2 | 8.6 | 2.4 | 2.8 | 1.0 | 0.0 | 3.3 | 2.8 | 6.9 |
| | (24.0–28.4) | (4.9–12.3) | (0.3–5.1) | (2.0–3.6) | (0.0–2.2) | – | (2.5–4.1) | (0.8–4.7) | (2.1–11.6) |
| Southeast | 22.7 | 8.0 | 4.8 | 5.0 | 1.3 | 1.5 | 3.7 | 4.5 | 5.2 |
| | (21.7–23.8) | (5.7–10.3) | (3.1–6.5) | (4.4–5.5) | (0.2–2.4) | (0.5–2.5) | (3.1–4.0) | (2.7–6.3) | (3.4–6.9) |
| 25% poorest | 39.9 | 17.3 | 7.2 | 6.5 | 2.0 | 1.9 | 2.9 | 2.1 | 4.0 |
| | (37.7–42.1) | (11.6–22.9) | (4.3–10.2) | (5.4–7.7) | (0.0–4.5) | (0.3–3.4) | (2.1–3.7) | (0.0–4.6) | (1.8–6.2) |
| 25% richest | 6.0 | 3.4 | 3.0 | 2.5 | 0.9 | 1.2 | 6.8 | 10.3 | 8.6 |
| | (4.8–7.3) | (0.4–7.3) | (0.6–6.5) | (1.6–3.3) | (0.0–2.8) | (1.2–3.7) | (5.3–8.3) | (4.8–15.8) | (2.8–14.4) |
| **Brazil** | 34.3 | 18.2 | 11.4 | 4.6 | 1.5 | 2.0 | 3.3 | 3.1 | 4.0 |
| | (33.5–35.1) | (16.5–20.0) | (9.9–12.8) | (4.2–5.0) | (0.9–2.2) | (1.3–2.7) | (3.0–3.6) | (2.1–4.1) | (3.0–5.1) |

[a] Height-for-age $< -2$ z-scores of the international growth reference.
[b] Weight-for-height $< -2$ z-scores of the international growth reference.
[c] Weight-for-height $> 2$ z-scores of the international growth reference.
[d] 95% confidence intervals are given in parentheses.

the 25% richest children). For the entire country, stunting decreases continuously throughout the surveys (34.3%, 18.2%, and 11.4%, respectively; $P < 0.0001$ for linear trend) while wasting decreases in the first period (from 4.6% to 1.5%; $P < 0.0001$) and remains low and relatively constant in the second period (2.0% in 1996). Similar patterns of changes (i.e., strong continuous reductions in stunting throughout the three surveys and apparent control of wasting by 1989) are seen in all regional and income strata. The prevalence of young child overweight for the entire country is relatively low and does not change significantly throughout the three surveys: 3.3%, 3.1% and 4.0%, respectively. Higher rates of child overweight are seen among the higher income children from the more-developed southeastern region but these rates also do not change significantly throughout the three surveys (i.e., 6.8%, 10.3%, and 8.6%, respectively).

Changes in stunting affect in a complex way the regional and social distribution of this event in the population. The regional gap in child stunting is actually increased throughout the surveys because the pace of the stunting decline in the more-developed region exceeds that observed in the less-developed region. The income gap in child stunting increases in the less-developed region but decreases in the more-developed region due to a more favorable trend among the poorest children. In both regions, child wasting tends to be more common among lower income families, whereas overweight tends to be more common among higher income families. However, this pattern of association with income does not essentially change throughout the surveys.

The relative importance of problems associated with child underfeeding (mostly stunting in Brazil) and child overfeeding (overweight) clearly changed throughout the

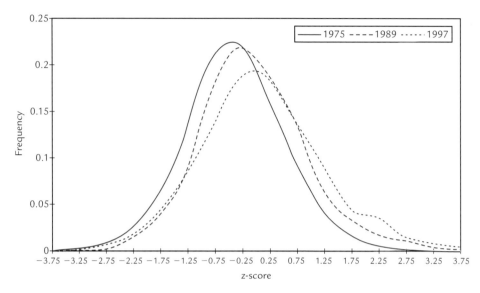

**Figure 12.3** BMI distribution in older children and adolescents. Brazil: 1975-1997.

surveys. For instance, there were 10 cases of child stunting to one case of overweight in 1975, countrywide, whereas, in 1996, this ratio was reduced to 3:1. Changes were more pronounced in the more-developed southeastern region, where the ratio of six cases of stunting to one case of overweight was replaced by an equilibrium between the two events. Still more dramatic was the change among the higher income children from the least-developed region, where eight cases of stunting to one case of overweight was reversed to almost three cases of overweight to one case of stunting. Yet, it should be noted that, in 1996, the average child living in the country's least-developed region was still seven times more susceptible to stunting than to overweight (and twelve times more susceptible to stunting if he/she belonged to the lower income group).

## Trends in old children and adolescents

Figure 12.3 shows BMI z-score distributions from the 10–17-year-old individuals (old child/adolescents) studied in 1975, 1989, and 1997 (BMI z-score relative to the gender and age-specific total BMI distribution in 1989). Distributions refer to combined genders since trends did not differ by gender. A clear, progressive shift toward higher z-score values is seen throughout the three surveys. The average old child/adolescent BMI z-score in the three successive surveys was: $-0.39$, $-0.04$, and $+0.11$, respectively ($P < 0.0001$ for linear trend).

Table 12.3 presents time-trends for the prevalence of underweight and overweight for gender combined old child/adolescents (BMI below the 5th or above the 95th centile of the adolescent BMI reference mentioned previously). The prevalence of both underweight and overweight in each survey is given with correspondent 95% confidence intervals. Trends are again presented for the entire country, for each region, and

**Table 12.3** Secular trends in the prevalence (%) of underweight and overweight in older children and adolescents by region and income group. Brazil: 1975–1997

| Region and income group | Underweight[a] | | | Overweight[b] | | |
|---|---|---|---|---|---|---|
| | 1975 | 1989 | 1997 | 1975 | 1989 | 1997 |
| Northeast | 8.9 | 4.9 | 5.9 | 1.0 | 2.5 | 4.6 |
| | (8.4–9.4)[c] | (4.1–5.8) | (4.4–7.4) | (0.8–1.1) | (1.9–3.1) | (3.3–5.8) |
| 25% poorest | 10.5 | 6.0 | 3.4 | 0.7 | 1.4 | 2.5 |
| | (9.3–11.7) | (4.1–7.8) | (1.0–5.9) | (0.4–1.1) | (0.5–2.4) | (0.2–4.9) |
| 25% richest | 8.3 | 5.5 | 4.5 | 1.5 | 4.5 | 7.2 |
| | (7.5–9.2) | (3.9–7.2) | (2.1–6.9) | (1.2–1.9) | (3.1–6.0) | (4.4–10.1) |
| Southeast | 8.2 | 3.9 | 5.3 | 2.5 | 7.3 | 12.9 |
| | (7.8–8.7) | (2.9–4.9) | (3.8–6.8) | (2.3–2.8) | (5.9–8.6) | (10.6–15.2) |
| 25% poorest | 10.5 | 5.9 | 8.2 | 0.9 | 5.0 | 5.3 |
| | (9.4–11.4) | (3.3–8.6) | (4.4–11.9) | (0.6–1.3) | (2.4–7.5) | (2.5–8.2) |
| 25% richest | 5.9 | 2.9 | 5.0 | 4.9 | 10.7 | 13.5 |
| | (5.2–6.7) | (1.1–4.7) | (1.8–8.2) | (4.3–5.6) | (7.3–14.0) | (8.9–18.1) |
| **Brazil** | 8.5 | 4.3 | 5.6 | 1.8 | 5.3 | 9.2 |
| | (8.2–8.8) | (3.6–5.0) | (4.5–6.6) | (1.7–2.0) | (4.5–6.2) | (7.8–10.6) |

[a] BMI values lower than the gender and age-specific 5th centile in the 1989 survey.
[b] BMI values higher than the gender and age-specific 95th centile in the 1989 survey.
[c] 95% confidence intervals are shown in parentheses.

for the extreme income groups within each region. For the entire country, underweight decreases significantly in the first period (from 8.5% to 4.3%; $P < 0.0001$) but not in the second period (5.6% in 1997), whereas overweight increases continuously throughout the three surveys (1.8%, 5.3%, and 9.2%; $P < 0.0001$ for linear trend).

Similar patterns of change (i.e., significant reductions in underweight in the first period and continuous increases in overweight throughout the three surveys) are seen in all region and income strata. These changes do not essentially alter either the direct association between level of regional development or individual income and risk of old child/adolescent overweight nor the inverse association observed with underweight.

Time changes, however, do alter the relative importance of under- and overweight for the adolescent population. In 1975, the risk of underweight for the whole adolescent population exceeded the risk of overweight by almost five times whereas, in 1997, overweight exceeds underweight (by 1.6 times). Similar changes in the relative importance of under- and overweight were observed in all region and income strata.

## Trends in adults

Figures 12.4 and 12.5 display gender-specific BMI z-score distributions of Brazilian adults, 20 years of age or older, studied in 1975, 1989, and 1997 (BMI z-score relative to the gender and age-specific total adult BMI distribution in 1989). The BMI distribution for men shifts progressively toward the right (higher BMI values) throughout the three surveys and the average BMI z-score increases from −0.31 to +0.02 and then to +0.27 ($P < 0.0001$ for linear trend). In the case of women,

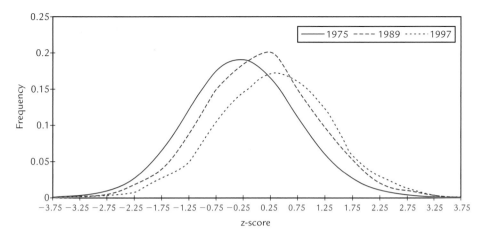

**Figure 12.4**  BMI distribution in adult males. Brazil: 1975–1997.

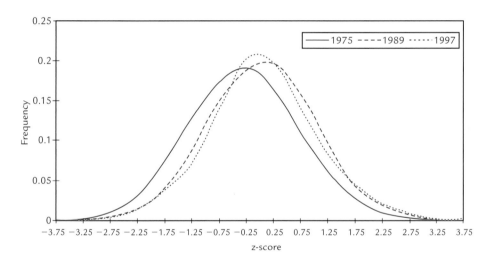

**Figure 12.5**  BMI distribution in adult females. Brazil: 1975–1997.

BMI clearly shifts to the right from 1975 to 1989 (average z-scores of $-0.31$ to $+0.04$, respectively; $P < 0.0001$) but then stabilizes in the following period (average z-score of $+0.04$ in 1996).

Tables 12.4 and 12.5 present time-trends in the age-adjusted prevalence of underweight and obesity among adults (BMI $< 18.5\,\text{kg/m}^2$ or $\geqslant 30\,\text{kg/m}^2$, respectively). The prevalence of each event in the three successive surveys is given with corresponding 95% confidence intervals. Time-trends are once more presented for the entire country, for each region, and for extreme income groups within each region. Since trends in the adult population differ by gender, results are presented separately for males and females.

Trends of underweight and obesity in men are clearly opposite. For the whole population, the prevalence of underweight declines throughout the three surveys from

**Table 12.4** Secular trends in the prevalence (%) of underweight and obesity in male adults by region and income group. Brazil: 1975–1997

| Region and income group | Underweight[a] | | | Obese[b] | | |
|---|---|---|---|---|---|---|
| | 1975 | 1989 | 1997 | 1975 | 1989 | 1997 |
| Northeast | 7.9 | 5.2 | 4.2 | 1.2 | 2.4 | 4.4 |
| | (7.5–8.4) | (4.4–5.9) | (3.3–5.1) | (1.1–1.4) | (1.9–3.0) | (3.5–5.3) |
| 25% poorest | 7.8 | 4.8 | 5.5 | 0.7 | 0.8 | 1.8 |
| | (6.8–8.7) | (3.4–6.2) | (3.1–8.0) | (0.4–0.9) | (0.4–1.2) | (0.9–2.7) |
| 25% richest | 7.5 | 3.5 | 2.6 | 2.5 | 5.1 | 8.4 |
| | (6.7–8.3) | (2.2–4.8) | (1.6–3.5) | (2.1–3.0) | (3.6–6.7) | (6.3–10.5) |
| Southeast | 8.7 | 4.8 | 2.9 | 2.9 | 5.8 | 8.4 |
| | (8.3–9.1) | (4.1–5.5) | (2.2–3.6) | (2.7–3.2) | (5.0–6.6) | (7.2–9.6) |
| 25% poorest | 13.0 | 7.7 | 3.3 | 1.6 | 2.9 | 3.8 |
| | (12.1–14.0) | (6.2–9.2) | (1.9–4.7) | (1.2–1.9) | (2.1–3.7) | (2.2–5.3) |
| 25% richest | 4.1 | 2.9 | 2.0 | 5.4 | 8.2 | 10.2 |
| | (3.5–4.7) | (1.7–4.2) | (0.9–3.1) | (4.7–6.0) | (6.1–10.4) | (7.6–12.7) |
| **Brazil** | 8.3 | 5.0 | 3.5 | 2.1 | 4.1 | 6.4 |
| | (7.9–8.7) | (4.2–5.7) | (2.8–4.3) | (1.9–2.3) | (3.5–4.8) | (5.3–7.4) |

[a] Body mass index $< 18.5 \, \text{kg/m}^2$.
[b] Body mass index $\geq 30 \, \text{kg/m}^2$.
Prevalences are age-adjusted according to the age distribution in the 1997 surveys; 95% confidence intervals in parentheses.

**Table 12.5** Secular trends in the prevalence (%) of underweight and obesity in female adults by region and income group. Brazil: 1975–1997

| Gender, region and income group | Underweight[a] | | | Obese[b] | | |
|---|---|---|---|---|---|---|
| | 1975 | 1989 | 1997 | 1975 | 1989 | 1997 |
| Northeast | 16.0 | 9.5 | 7.6 | 4.1 | 7.8 | 12.5 |
| | (15.4–16.6) | (8.5–10.5) | (6.6–8.7) | (3.9–4.4) | (6.9–8.7) | (11.1–13.8) |
| 25% poorest | 17.6 | 11.2 | 9.6 | 3.1 | 5.2 | 7.7 |
| | (16.3–18.9) | (9.0–13.3) | (6.7–12.4) | (2.5–3.6) | (3.8–6.7) | (5.2–10.2) |
| 25% richest | 12.4 | 6.1 | 5.6 | 6.7 | 9.8 | 14.5 |
| | (11.4–13.3) | (4.6–7.7) | (4.1–7.1) | (6.0–7.4) | (7.9–11.6) | (12.1–16.8) |
| Southeast | 10.8 | 5.4 | 5.4 | 7.8 | 14.0 | 12.3 |
| | (10.3–11.2) | (4.6–6.1) | (4.5–6.3) | (7.5–8.2) | (12.8–15.2) | (11.0–13.6) |
| 25% poorest | 13.9 | 6.4 | 8.9 | 6.1 | 11.2 | 14.1 |
| | (12.9–14.8) | (5.1–7.6) | (6.8–11.1) | (5.5–6.7) | (9.5–13.0) | (11.4–16.9) |
| 25% richest | 6.8 | 4.3 | 3.1 | 7.9 | 14.4 | 8.9 |
| | (6.1–7.5) | (2.9–5.8) | (1.9–4.3) | (7.2–8.7) | (11.8–17.0) | (6.7–11.2) |
| **Brazil** | 13.4 | 7.5 | 6.5 | 6.0 | 10.9 | 12.4 |
| | (12.9–13.9) | (6.6–8.3) | (5.6–7.5) | (5.7–6.3) | (9.9–12.0) | (11.0–13.7) |

[a] Body mass index $< 18.5 \, \text{kg/m}^2$.
[b] Body mass index $\geq 30 \, \text{kg/m}^2$.
Prevalences are age-adjusted according to the age distribution in the 1997 survey; 95% confidence intervals in parentheses.

8.3% to 5.0% (1975 to 1989) and then to 3.5% (1997) whereas obesity increases from 2.1% to 4.1% and then to 6.4% ($P < 0.0001$ for linear trend in both cases), respectively. Similar trends of continuous reductions in underweight and increases in obesity are observed for most region and income strata of the adult male population.

Clear trends toward decreasing underweight and increasing obesity also exist among women, but only from 1975 to 1989. In this period, underweight declines among all women from 13.4% to 7.5% ($P < 0.0001$) while obesity increases from 6.0% to 10.9% ($P < 0.0001$). Additionally, much lower, and nonsignificant reductions in female underweight (from 7.5% to 6.5%) and additional increases in obesity (from 10.9% to 12.4%) occur from 1989 to 1997.

The region and income stratification confirms the general tendency toward the reduction in female underweight (particularly in the first period) and the tendency toward the increase in female obesity (only in the first period). However, trends in female obesity from 1989 to 1997 strongly differ according to region and income level. In this period, female obesity increased significantly in the less-developed region (from 7.8% to 12.5%) whereas it tended to decline in the more developed region (from 14.0% to 12.3%). Within the less-developed region, obesity showed minor, nonsignificant increases among lower income women (from 5.2% to 7.7%) but major, significant increases among higher income women (from 9.8% to 14.5%). Within the more-developed region, obesity tended to increase among lower income women (from 11.2% to 14.1%) but decline significantly among higher income women (from 14.4% to 8.9%). Obesity also increased significantly among the intermediate income groups from the less-developed region and tended to decrease among the intermediate income groups from the more-developed region (data not shown).

The recent trends described for female obesity profoundly changed the regional and income distribution of this event in Brazil. In 1997, contrary to what was observed in 1975 and 1989, the average woman from the less-developed region was no longer less exposed to obesity than her counterpart living in the more-developed region. Still in 1997, in the more developed region, the lower income women (and no longer the higher income) were the group most vulnerable to obesity. Actually, in 1997, lower income women in the more-developed region were significantly more susceptible than higher income women to both underweight (8.9% vs. 3.1%, $P < 0.05$) and obesity (14.1% vs. 8.9%, $P < 0.0001$). This simultaneous higher vulnerability of the lower income women to both underweight and obesity is also seen when the whole BMI distributions of lower and higher income women are compared (Fig. 12.6).

The relative importance of underweight and obesity was clearly changed throughout the surveys in both men and women. In 1975, for the whole country, there were two to four cases of adult underweight to one case of obesity whereas, in 1996, there were almost two obese adults to one underweight adult. This pattern of excessive underweight being replaced by excessive obesity was found in most region and income strata of the country. Two exceptions were: (1) lower income adults from the less-developed region, particularly males, for whom underweight remained more frequent than obesity, even in 1996, and (2) the higher income adults from the more-developed region, for whom obesity was already more frequent than underweight in 1975.

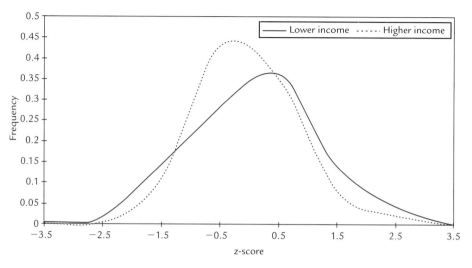

**Figure 12.6** BMI distribution in Brazilian women from the southeastern region: lower versus higher income group in 1997.

## Discussion

Brazil, along with other middle-income countries in Latin America, Asia, and the Middle East, is far advanced in the processes involving the demographic, economic, environmental, and cultural transitions. Although Brazil has almost doubled its total population in the last three decades (from 93 million in 1970 to 170 million in 2000) population growth has been continuously declining: from near 3% per year in the 1960s to less than 1.5% in the 1990s. Impressive reduction in fertility rates – 5.8 births per woman in 1970 to only 2.3 in 1999 – and the consequent decline in birth rates – 40.8 per thousand inhabitants in 1970 and 21.2 in 1999 – were decisive for lowering population growth. The strong decline in fertility and birth rates, combined with changes in age-specific mortality rates, more than doubled the proportion of Brazilians over 60 years of age (from 4% in 1970 to 10% in 1999). Another relevant component of the demographic transition in the period was the continuous rural–urban migration that reduced the country's rural population (from 41 million in 1970 to 32 million in 2000) and resulted in more than 80% of the total Brazilian population living in cities (the urbanization rate increased from 56.0% in 1970 to 81.2% in 2000). The expansion of the Brazilian GDP and the increase in the average family income (particularly in the 1970s, when both the GDP and family income were doubled) were also relevant in the period from 1970 to 1999. No less important was the continuous expansion in occupations within the services sector and, to a lesser extent, within industry, to the detriment of agricultural occupations. Finally, it is also important to recognize the great expansion that occurred during the period in the public infrastructure and essential services (communications, transport, energy supply, water supply, health care and education) and also the higher public access to durable goods (cars, refrigerators, TV sets and other household assets) (Ibge, 2001).

However, a known, undesirable characteristic of the Brazilian society, i.e., the enormous interpersonal and interregional concentration of wealth, did not improve in the period from 1970 to 1999. For instance, during this period, the 10% richest individuals in the country had an average income 15–20 times higher than the poorest 40%. In the less-developed northeastern region, where the average income is 2–3 times lower than in the more-developed southeastern region, the richest 10% had an average income up to 25 times higher than the poorest 40%. The same concentrated distribution pattern exists concerning people's access to the public infrastructure and services. For instance, in 1999, only 34% of the country's lower income households were served by both water supply and sanitation services whereas the same coverage to the higher income households was 86%. This gap between lower and higher income households was still larger in the less-developed northeastern region (20% and 67%, respectively) than in the more developed southeastern region (68% and 97%, respectively) (Ibge, 2001).

Carefully designed and adequately implemented nationwide probabilistic surveys conducted at three moments within the period from 1975 to 1997 indicated that the nutritional profile of the Brazilian population responded to the intense demographic, economic, environmental, and cultural changes that occurred in the country. Clear declining trends in undernutrition were documented for young children, old children and adolescents, and adults throughout the country and among all regional and income strata. Fortunately, there was no evidence that undernutrition (stunting and wasting) in young children, in any regional or income strata, had been replaced by obesity. However, increasing trends in overweight or obesity were simultaneous to the decreasing trends in undernutrition for older children and adolescents, male adults, and women in the less-developed region. An interesting situation was documented for women living in the more developed region of the country. Earlier trends (1975–1989) in undernutrition and obesity for this group were similar to that described earlier for the other population groups, i.e., declining trends for undernutrition and increasing trends for obesity, but recent trends (1989–1997) pointed to a stability of both undernutrition and obesity. In the particular case of obesity, the observed stability resulted from increasing disease rates among the lower income women and decreasing rates among the higher income women.

In most situations, regional and social gaps in undernutrition, unfavorable to the less-developed region and to lower income individuals in general, were kept unchanged or even increased throughout the surveys. An auspicious exception to this occurred with the evolution of undernutrition among young children from the more-developed region, where the gap in both child stunting and child wasting between lower and higher income groups was substantially reduced. The association between income and overweight/obesity remained positive throughout the surveys among all age, region, and income groups with the single exception of adult females living in the more developed southeastern region. In this particular group of women, a slight positive association between income and obesity, existing in 1975, was reversed in 1997 into a significant negative association. Since the negative association between income and undernutrition for this group was not changed throughout the surveys, lower income women of the southeastern region are, in 1997, significantly more susceptible than the higher income women to both undernutrition and obesity.

The relative importance of under- and overnutrition was perhaps the characteristic that most changed throughout the surveys. In 1975, cases of undernutrition in children, adolescents, and adults predominated over cases of overweight/obesity. The only exception to this occurred in the higher income stratum, within the more-developed southeastern region, where undernutrition and overweight/obesity were in equilibrium. However, in 1997, cases of overweight/obesity were more common than undernutrition among all higher income individuals (children, adolescents, and adults) from both regions and also among lower income women from the more-developed southeastern region.

The declining trends in undernutrition among young Brazilian children and the relatively low and stable prevalence of overweight in this group agree with trends reported for most developing countries in the same period (de Onis *et al.*, 1993; de Onis and Blössner, 2000; Martorell *et al.*, 2000a). In the United States, an increase in overweight among young children has been demonstrated for girls, but not boys (Ogden *et al.*, 1997). Reports on trends in undernutrition among older children, adolescents and adults are rare, in both the developed and the developing countries, and usually not based on comparable representative surveys, which precludes an adequate comparison with the results presented here. The systematic increase in overweight documented in older children and adolescents in Brazil agrees with trends observed in a few developed countries that count with repeated population-based studies on this age group (WHO, 1998; Troiano and Flegal, 1998) and also with trends documented in China (Wang *et al.*, 2001). A recent report on 12–15-year-old school children suggests that adolescent obesity might also be increasing in Taiwan (Chu, 2001). The increasing trends in adult obesity observed before 1997 in Brazilian males and before 1989 in Brazilian females agree with trends reported by the various population-based studies undertaken in the developed countries and the few in developing countries (WHO, 1998; Popkin and Doak, 1998; Martorell *et al.*, 2000b). However, the trends in female obesity observed from 1989 to 1997 in the more-developed southeastern region of Brazil (i.e., increasing obesity rates in lower income groups and decreasing rates in higher income groups) were not described for any developing country. Actually, an extensive review of studies in both the developing and the developed countries conducted by the International Obesity Task Force (WHO, 1998) identified a single setting, two Finnish provinces, where declining obesity in adults (also women from higher socioeconomic status) had been well documented (Pietinen *et al.*, 1996). The scarcity of studies relative to changes over time in the social distribution of both under- and overnutrition, and also in the ratio between the two (under-/overnutrition) in both the developing and the developed countries, makes the comparison of the present results very difficult. One review of studies on young child overweight in developing countries identified that, in one determined point in time, countries with higher rates of wasting tended to have lower rates of overweight and vice versa but no data on time-trends were provided for the individual countries (de Onis and Blössner, 2000).

The identification of the specific variables and mechanisms responsible for the changes documented in the nutritional profile of the Brazilian population is a complex task. In this respect we should refer to the plausibility of hypotheses rather than strict hypotheses verification. Elsewhere, we have demonstrated that reductions in young child undernutrition in Brazil could be attributed to a moderate increase in family income, combined with an exceptional expansion in the public provision of health, sanitation, and education services. Both these factors were facilitated by favorable demographic changes which included the rapid urbanization of the country and substantial declines in fertility rates (Monteiro *et al.*, 1992, 2000b). The same factors could explain at least part of the reduction in undernutrition among old child/adolescents and adults described in the present study.

The worldwide trend towards increased obesity has been attributed, in both the developed and the developing countries, to rapid declines in energy expenditures related to shifts toward much less physically demanding occupations and sedentary leisure activities. Equally important for many countries may have been the shift toward a much higher fat, energy-dense diet. In developing countries in particular, marked increases in urbanization and income, coupled with the increased penetration of the Western culture, certainly favored shifts in diet and physical activity conducive to obesity (Popkin, 1998). All these factors are probably underlying the increase in obesity indicators documented in Brazilian old child/adolescents and adults. As in most countries, there is no specific secular trend information in Brazil on patterns of physical activity, although the expansion of the services sector of the economy is in line with increasingly less physically demanding occupations. Individuals employed by the services sector increased from 29% in 1970 to 55% in 1999, whereas those employed in agriculture declined from 55% to 25% (Ibge, 2001). The enormous increase in the proportion of Brazilian households with TV sets (24% in 1970 and 88% in 1999) could indicate trends toward more sedentary leisure activities and higher exposure to the Western diet and lifestyles. Secular trend data on dietary intake in Brazil from 1975 to 1987 – only available at the family level and restricted to metropolitan areas of the country – point to an increase of 2–7 percentage points in the proportion of energy relative to fat intake (Mondini and Monteiro, 1994). The relative stability of overweight observed among Brazilian children below 5 years of age is consistent with the relatively higher energy requirements of this group and the higher capacity of self-regulation of the energy intake observed in younger children (Birch and Deysher, 1986; Birch *et al.*, 1991).

It is difficult to explain the interruption of the increase in female obesity observed from 1989 to 1997 in the more-developed southeastern region of Brazil, and even harder to explain the reversal in the obesity prevalence documented specifically among the higher income women. Data from the last metropolitan food expenditure survey conducted in Brazil in 1996 indicate that the proportion of energy relative to fat intake had further increased in the relatively poorer cities of the northeastern region (from 23% in 1987 to 25% in 1996) but remained stable (about 30%) in the richer cities of the southeastern region (Monteiro *et al.*, 2000d). A more disaggregated analysis of these data by income levels will be necessary to assess how changes in diet might explain recent trends of obesity in Brazil. Patterns of leisure time physical activity were assessed for the first time in the country by the national survey of 1997. In this survey, the practice of regular physical exercise among women, although incipient, was more frequent in the more-developed southeastern region than in the less-developed northeastern region (9.8% and 5.5%, respectively) and much more frequent in higher income than in lower income women (18.0% and 1.3%, respectively).

Regardless of the immediate determinants involved with the decline in obesity from 1989 to 1997, governmental public health policies are unlikely to have contributed significantly to it since only recently have the health authorities in Brazil chosen the control of obesity as a real priority (Ministério da Saúde, 2000). Elsewhere, we defended the possibility that the intense informal education work done by the Brazilian mass media vehicles – focused on combating sedentary lifestyles and promoting better food habits – could be one of the factors responsible for the decline of obesity among the higher income, and better educated, women's population from the southeastern region (Monteiro *et al.*, 2000a). The findings of the 1989 national survey, disclosed in 1992, showed that obesity, and not undernutrition, was the main nutritional problem of the adult population in Brazil. Since then, several major TV networks and leading newspapers and magazines have produced, on an almost weekly basis, extensive information on the health consequences of obesity and the importance of avoiding energy-dense diets and increasing physical activity. Part of the media (particularly TV programs targeted to the female population) has also been engaged in promoting a, sometimes unrealistic, thin image for women.

To conclude this chapter on the description of the nutrition transition in Brazil, it is necessary to say that in July 1999, after a long and productive process of consultations with relevant parts of the civil society (e.g., scholars, professional and scientific associations, workers unions, and representatives of private companies, among others) and relevant governmental bodies, the Brazilian Ministry of Health approved a new national food and nutrition policy that is more in line with the contemporaneous nutritional profile disclosed by the last nationwide survey (Ministério da Saúde, 2000). The main goal of this new policy is the promotion, protection and support of eating practices and lifestyles conducive to optimum nutritional and health status for all rather than the exclusive control of nutritional deficiencies. Its main features are the formulation of evidence-based priorities and the acknowledgment that intersector work is essential to assure the control of most nutritional problems. This new policy has assured continual resources to combat nutritional deficiencies where they still exist, particularly through well-targeted, integrated interventions but it has also initiated courageous actions, with a great potential to prevent nutritional disorders due to over- or wrong-feeding (e.g., obligatory nutritional labeling of any processed food commercialized in the country, the regulation of health claims in foods, and the inclusion of a 70% minimum of fresh or minimally processed foods in the multimillion dollar national school feeding program) (Ministério da Saúde, 2001). The publicity of soft drinks and other nonhealthy foods during TV broadcastings directed to children and adolescents is under study and may also be regulated in the near future. Large-scale changes in the curriculum of the public primary and secondary schools are also being implemented to promote healthier eating habits and lifestyles among teachers and students. Another positive characteristic of the new policy is the stimulus to form partnerships with local governments and nongovernmental organizations. The best example in this case is perhaps the series of local initiatives, started in cities of the São Paulo state, but now spread throughout the country, to promote and support physical activities in schools, work places and every available public space in the community (Matsudo, 1997). Although not yet fully evaluated, it is certain that the recent food and nutrition policy established in Brazil will be an important source of information to all individuals and institutions concerned with the development of policies and programs consistent with the new nutritional profile found in the developing countries.

# References

Bemfam (1997). "Pesquisa Nacional sobre Demografia e Saúde 1996". Sociedade de Bem Estar Familiar, Rio de Janeiro.

Birch, L.L., and Deysher, M. (1986). *Appetite* **7**, 323–331.

Birch, L.L., Johnson, S.L., Graciela Andresen, M.S., Peters, J.C., and Schulte, M.C. (1991). *N. Engl. J. Med.* **324**, 232–235.

Chu, N.-F. (2001). *Int. J. Obes.* **25**, 170–176.

Cole, T.J. (1990). *Eur. J. Clin. Nutr.* **44**, 45–60.

de Onis, M., and Blössner, M. (2000). *Am. J. Clin. Nutr.* **72**, 1032–1039.

de Onis, M., Monteiro, C.A., Akre, J., and Clugston, G. (1993). *Bull. WHO* **71**, 703–712.

Ibge (1998). "Pesquisa sobre padrões de vida 1996–1997". Instituto Brasileiro de Geografia e Estatística, Rio de Janeiro.

Ibge (2001). "Síntese de indicadores sociais 2000". Instituto Brasileiro de Geografia e Estatística, Rio de Janeiro.

Ibge/UNICEF (1982). "Perfil estatístico de crianças e mães no Brasil: aspectos nutricionais, 1974–75". Instituto Brasileiro de Geografia e Estatística, Rio de Janeiro.

Ibge/UNICEF (1992). "Perfil estatístico de crianças e mães no Brasil: aspectos de saúde e nutrição de crianças no Brasil, 1989". Instituto Brasileiro de Geografia e Estatística, Rio de Janeiro.

Iunes, R.F. (2000). *In* "Velhos e novos males da saúde no Brasil: a evolução do país e de suas doenças" (C.A. Monteiro, ed.), 2nd edn. aumentada, pp. 33–60. Hucitec/Nupens-USP, São Paulo.

Lavinas, L., and Magina, M. (coordinators) (1996). "Atlas regional das desigualdades. Banco de dados com indicadores sócio-econômicos por R.F. e macrorregiões". IPEA/DIPES, Rio de Janeiro.

Martorell, R., Kettel Khan, L., Hughes, M.L., and Grummer-Strawn, L.M. (2000a). *Int. J. Obes.* **24**, 959–967.

Martorell, R., Kettel Khan, L., Hughes, M.L., and Grummer-Strawn, L.M. (2000b). *Eur. J. Clin. Nutr.* **54**, 247–252.

Matsudo, V.K.R. (1997). *World Health* **50**, 16–17.

Ministério da Saúde (2000). "Política nacional de alimentação e nutrição". Ministério da Saúde, Brasília.

Ministério da Saúde (2001). "Estratégia nacional para promoção da alimentação saudável e da atividade física. Fase 1". Ministério da Saúde, Brasília.

Mondini, L., and Monteiro, C.A. (1994). *Rev. Saúde Públ.* **28**, 433–439.

Monteiro, C.A., and Conde, W.L. (1999). *In* "Progress in Obesity Research" (G. Ailhaud, and B. Guy-Grand, eds.), pp. 665–671. John Libbey/8th International Congress on Obesity.

Monteiro, C.A., Benicio, M.H.D'A., Iunes, R.F., Gouveia, N.C., Taddei, J.A.A.C., and Cardoso, M.A. (1992). *Bull. WHO* **70**, 657–666.

Monteiro, C.A., Benicio, M.H.D'A., and Gouveia, N.C. (1994). *Ann. Hum. Biol.* **21**, 381–390.

Monteiro, C.A., Mondini, L., Medeiros de Souza, A.L., and Popkin, B.M. (1995). *Eur. J. Clin. Nutr.* **49**, 105–113.

Monteiro, C.A., Benicio, M.H.D'A., Conde, W.L., and Popkin, B.M. (2000a). *Eur. J. Clin. Nutr.* **54**, 342–346.

Monteiro, C.A., Benicio, M.H.D'A., and Freitas, I.C.M. (2000b). *In* "Velhos e novos males da saúde no Brasil: a evolução do país e de suas doenças" (C.A. Monteiro, ed.), 2nd edn. aumentada, pp. 393–420. Hucitec/Nupens-USP, São Paulo.

Monteiro, C.A., Benicio, M.H.D'A., and Popkin, B.M. (2000c). *Rev. Bras. Nutr. Clin.* **15**, 253–260.

Monteiro, C.A., Mondini, L., and Costa, R.B.L. (2000d). *In* "Velhos e novos males da saúde no Brasil: a evolução do país e de suas doenças" (C.A. Monteiro, ed.), 2nd edn. aumentada, pp. 359–369. Hucitec/Nupens-USP, São Paulo.

Monteiro, C.A., Conde, W.L., and Popkin, B.M. (2001). *J. Nutr.* **131**, 881s–886s.

Ogden, C.L., Troiano, R.P., Briefel, R.R., Kuczmarski, R.J., Flegal, K.M., and Johnson, C.L. (1997). *Pediatrics* **99**, 1–11.

Patarra, N.L. (2000). *In* "Velhos e novos males da saúde no Brasil: a evolução do país e de suas doenças" (C.A. Monteiro, ed.), 2nd edn. aumentada, pp. 61–78. Hucitec/Nupens-USP, São Paulo.

Pietinen, P., Vartiainem E., and Mannisto, S. (1996). *Int. J. Obes.* **20**, 114–120.

Popkin, B.M. (1993). *Popul. Dev. Rev.* **19**, 138–157.

Popkin, B.M. (1998). *Public Health Nutr.* **1**, 5–21.

Popkin, B.M., and Doak, C. (1998). *Nutr. Rev.* **56**, 95–103.

Popkin, B.M., Paeratakul, S., and Ge, K. (1995). *Obes. Res.* **3**, 145s–153s.

Stata Corp. (1997). Stata statistical software: release 5.0. College Station, TX: Stata Corporation.

Troiano, R.P., and Flegal, K.M. (1998). *Pediatrics* **101**, 497–504.

Wang, Y., Monteiro, C.A., and Popkin, B.M. (2002). *Am. J. Clin. Nutr.* (in press).

WHO (1995). "Physical Status: The Use and Interpretation of Anthropometry". Report of a WHO Expert Committee (Technical Report Series 854). World Health Organization, Geneva.

WHO (1998). "Obesity: Preventing and Managing the Global Epidemic". Report of a WHO Consultation on Obesity. World Health Organization, Geneva.

# Policy implications

**13**

Benjamin Caballero and Barry M. Popkin

The countries in transition face a very different set of circumstances than did higher-income countries who began their epidemiological transition and faced a period with a high level of nutrition-related noncommunicable diseases (NR-NCD) in the first half of the 20th century. First and foremost, NR-NCD are not the only problem of these countries. Protein-energy malnutrition and single- or multiple-micronutrient deficiencies are still endemic in several parts of the developing world. The pace of the nutrition transition is such that in most countries undergoing this transition, the protracted problems of undernutrition overlap with the emerging threat of overnutrition and diet-related chronic diseases. To these contrasting situations, many countries must add the burden of infectious diseases such as malaria and HIV. Developing a comprehensive public health policy to address these issues, usually with limited resources, is perhaps the most difficult challenge for developing countries today.

There is some consensus that prevention is the only viable strategy to reduce the burden of NR-NCD in developing countries. A traditional medical treatment approach is not realistic under the conditions of most developing country health systems. The US is a clear example on how medical care for chronic diseases can demand an enormous fraction of the health care budget. There is little expectation that the limited health care budgets of most developing countries will be able to provide continuing care to the increasing number of persons with diabetes, hypertension, and cardiovascular diseases. In addition, debilitating chronic diseases reduce work capacity, thus constraining economic growth and creating a vicious circle of poverty and inadequate health care.

The burden of NR-NCD on the national economy can be substantial, and its impact can be felt in economies as varied as China's or India's. In China, the overall cost of health care and lost work output due to premature death associated with NR-NCD was estimated as a minimum of 2.2% of the GDP for 1995. In India, that figure was 1.1% (Popkin et al., 2001). In contrast the costs of undernutrition are decreasing in these countries and in 1995 were less than the costs of overnutrition for China and equal for India.

The Nutrition Transition
ISBN: 0-12-153654-8

# Constraints to NR-NCD prevention strategies in the developing world

Countries currently in transition face unique challenges in confronting chronic non-communicable diseases, compared to countries that experienced that transition earlier in the 20th century. As noted above, NR-NCD in developing countries emerge in conditions in which poverty and undernutrition are still widespread, where there are high rates of low birth weight and stunting, and within a health care system often fragmented, underfunded, and frequently focused on treatment rather than prevention.

## Poverty and undernutrition

The association between poverty and health outcomes has been documented in numerous studies. But as pointed out above, this and other factors operate in a unique way in populations in transition. First, urban dwelling is frequently associated with a widening of the gap between rich and poor (Menon *et al.*, 2000), with the potential to exacerbate health risks associated with income. Second, improvements in socioeconomic status, which could in other contexts result in improvement in health status, may in fact increase the risk for NR-NCD, for example, by leading to more consumption of saturated and total fat, or to a more sedentary lifestyle (television watching). A closer look at the data on NR-NCD burden in developing regions indicates that for the poorest segment of the population in countries in transition, communicable diseases are still the more serious threat to health (Gwatkin *et al.*, 1999); however as Monteiro and his collaborators have shown in a series of studies, the burden of NR-NCDs is rising rapidly for the poor, and not only in Brazil but also in other countries is already greater for the poor than the rich (Monteiro *et al.*, 2000, 2002). Consistent with this, data on stunting showed a larger socioeconomic differential in urban than in rural areas (Menon *et al.*, 2000). Longitudinal data from several countries also indicate that the burden of NR-NCD is rapidly shifting to the poor (Berrios *et al.*, 1990; Grol *et al.*, 1997; Guo *et al.*, 2000; Monteiro *et al.*, 2002).

## Low birth weight and childhood malnutrition

As discussed in Chapter 7, the possibility that early malnutrition results in a life-long increase in risk for adult NCD is of obvious importance for the developing world. This concept, initially based on descriptive epidemiological studies by Barker (1992), has been supported by data from a number of other cohorts (Phipps *et al.*, 1993; Phillips *et al.*, 1994; Adair *et al.*, 2001). Thus, efforts to reduce the prevalence of childhood stunting in developing country populations would constitute an effective prevention approach for NCD. Similarly, the possible role of breast feeding in reducing the risk for diabetes (Pettitt *et al.*, 1999) and hypertension (Singhai *et al.*, 2001) in the adult makes breastfeeding promotion another potentially important intervention for the prevention of NCD.

## Limited health care infrastructure

In many developing countries, the health care system is poorly funded, frequently segmented and focused on treatment rather than prevention. Few developing countries have even begun to recognize the magnitude of NR-NCD. A recent WHO survey showed that many countries have not yet formulated policies or plans for the prevention and control of noncommunicable diseases (WHO, 2001a). The percentages ranged from 13% in the African region to 59% in European countries. Other studies have also shown that only a few countries have started pilot activities in this area focused on prevention (Doak, 2002). One important consequence of this is the lack of stable surveillance systems that could allow a better understanding of the magnitude of the problem and its national or regional characteristics.

# Approaches to prevention of NR-NCD

There is general consensus that the three major modifiable factors responsible for the increase in noncommunicable diseases are smoking, diet, and physical activity. A discussion of the first factor is beyond the scope of the present work, but it may be mentioned that efforts to introduce smoking cessation programs in the developing world have encountered mixed success. In some cases, powerful economic interests and aggressive marketing by tobacco companies have limited the actual impact of these programs.

In the developed world, where NR-NCD have been major public health problems for decades, several community-based prevention interventions have been developed and evaluated. One frequently cited as an example of success is the North Karelia Project, initiated in 1972 in that region of Finland (Puska, 1981). A number of other interventions and demonstration projects have been implemented in the US and Europe. Efforts to implement similar NCD prevention programs in developing countries were undertaken by the WHO and its regional offices. The Interhealth program, initiated in 1986 by the World Health Organization (Interhealth, 1991), aimed at introducing health promotion and maintenance interventions at the community level, and involved some 12 countries, but initially only three were in the developing world (Mauritius, China, and Chile). A number of similar programs were launched in Latin America (Cuba, Chile, Central America, and Argentina) with the assistance of the WHO regional office. Others are being launched independently by the countries themselves (e.g. Cointinho *et al.*, 2002).

The rapid shift in the stage of the nutrition transition towards the pattern of NR-NCD creates unique conditions for the implementation of prevention strategies. Issues like early malnutrition, poverty, and degree of urbanization, which are major determinants of the stage of the transition, vary widely across developing countries, and are critical elements to define the best type of preventive strategy. In general, most of the prevention approaches used in the developed world would be unworkable in developing countries, due to cost or cultural limitations. The optimal mix of primary and secondary prevention has also not been adequately identified, an important issue for countries that already have high rates of one or more NR-NCD. The complex issue is that a number of developing countries, including lower income ones such as Egypt, face similar situations. The opposite situation may occur in most countries in transition, where NR-NCD still affect a smaller proportion of the population, or predominate only in urban areas. Thus, interventions targeted at the general population have a better potential for success.

A prevention strategy aimed at delivering simple, inexpensive measures to large numbers of people may require substantial modifications to the traditional health care delivery system. These programs also make extensive use of community resources, such as the media, the school system, churches, and other community institutions. On the other hand, narrowly targeted interventions for high-risk groups can also be cost-effective, but they should complement rather than replace population-wide programs. The appropriate endpoints for primary prevention programs must also be identified. Some of the more simple indicators, such as body mass index, may not be appropriate for certain types of interventions, but at the same time more specific biochemical indicators may be impractical or too expensive.

# Program and policy options

Each country will require its own combination of integrated set of activities, across a variety of sectors, to promote healthier dietary and physical activity patterns. There are several new, innovative programs emerging from several developing countries, such as Brazil (Cointinho *et al.*, 2002). Other efforts have recently been reviewed (Doak, 2002; Zhai *et al.*, 2002). These interventions usually involve activities in several settings, such as schools, the workplace, and community organizations. The focus includes changes in food production policy, marketing, and other macroeconomic efforts. All this requires active involvement in the legislative process.

## Improvements of diets

As the Finnish experience has shown, successful food policy can shift the prices and availability of the foods one wishes to promote and demote in the diet in ways that radically can shift eating patterns. The relative and absolute prices of high and low saturated fats, salt and many other elements of the Finnish diet were affected by taxation, import controls, and shifts in agricultural research subsidies, among others. In every country in transition, the costs and availability of hundreds of food products are affected by government policies. The Finnish experience was the first to show that promotion of a healthy diet can effectively use these same levers of policy. Not only did the Finns affect food prices, they also affected consumer knowledge and attitudes through systematic public education and social marketing efforts. The campaign to reduce salt intake in Finland was one such example that involved health care personnel, and public education in cooperation with the food and catering industry.

And there was legislation to reduce the sodium content of the foods and the creation of new labeling options related to salt intake.

This broad-based macroeconomic incentive system, along with public education, will also be essential for success in developing countries.

Some countries, most notably Brazil, have begun to develop approaches similar to those found in Finland. For example, an intervention to improve dietary patterns in children in Brazil took advantage of the federally funded school lunch program (similar to those existing in several countries), requiring that 70% of the resources be spent on fresh vegetables and fruits. To overcome the problem of convenience and preparation time, usual justifications for the use of processed foods, the intervention engaged local producers, who agreed to prepare their produce (clean, cut, sort, and pack) in order to reduce preparation time at the school. In exchange, local producers would become selected vendors for the school system (Cointinho *et al.*, 2002). It should be noted that this effort resulted from a nationwide consensus-building activity, involving health professionals, consumers, the private sector, and the health authorities at the national, regional and local levels.

## Physical activity

The same type of systematic effort is needed to reduce sedentarism and improve overall physical activity patterns. For instance, city planning, building design and transportation system layout must go hand in hand with efforts across all settings and macro and micro efforts to promote healthy activity patterns. Brazil is again a leader in this effort. *Agita* is a multilevel, community-wide intervention designed to increase the knowledge about benefits and the level of physical activity in Brazil (Matsudo *et al.*, 2002). With a focus on getting all persons to have at least 30 minutes of physical activity of moderate intensity, on most days of the week, they have included promotion of activities in four settings: home, transport, work, and leisure time.

# Surveillance

Surveillance is a critical element of any disease prevention policy, but few countries in transition have developed meaningful surveillance systems. Although there is continuing progress in this regard, data on specific risk factors, longitudinal national surveys, and data on biomarkers of risk in different populations are still scarce. The establishment of national surveillance systems is one approach to overcome those limitations. For instance, one model is that promoted by the WHO for development of NCD surveillance, the "STEPwise" approach. As implied by its name, the program involves progressively more intense data collection, from mortality data and simple survey questionnaires to identify major risk factors, progressing to disease-specific mortality (by verbal autopsy) and anthropometric measurements, and advancing to death rates by death certificate, cause-specific incidence and prevalence, and assessment of biochemical indicators (WHO, 2001b). The use of a standardized protocol would permit comparison of data across countries, as well as sharing resources at the regional level. An approach for assessing the quality of surveillance activities has also been proposed by Silva *et al.* (2001).

Efforts for the prevention of NR-NCD must receive priority consideration by countries in transition. Although in some of these countries the prevalence of NCD has not reached the level of developed countries, the economic cost and burden on the health care system are magnified by the limited health infrastructure in countries in transition. Existing interventions focused on reducing the prevalence of low birth weight, promoting breastfeeding, and reducing chronic malnutrition, may all have a positive impact on adult NR-NCD. Specific programs aimed at providing healthy alternatives to the demand for "better" diets by populations undergoing the nutrition transition are also essential. Critical elements for success would include nutrition education from the early years, community-based health promotion interventions, and market strategies to promote healthier eating habits.

A coherent summary of the rapid shift toward higher rates of NR-NCDs and the need for systematic program and policy preventive options is the Bellagio Declaration (2002). The text of this declaration is provided at the end of this chapter.

# References

Adair, L.S., Kuzawa, C.W., and Borja, J. (2001). Maternal energy stores and diet composition during pregnancy program adolescent blood pressure. *Circulation* **104**, 1034–1039.

Barker, D.J.P. (1992). The effects of nutrition of the fetus and neonate on cardiovascular disease in later life. *Proc. Nutr. Soc.* **51**, 135–144.

Berrios, X., Jadue, L., Zenteno, J., Ross, M.I., and Rodriguez, H. (1990). Prevalence of risk factors for chronic diseases. A study in the general population of the metropolitan area, 1986–1987. *Rev. Med. Chile* **118**, 597–604.

Cointinho, D., Monteiro, C.A., and Popkin, B. (2002). What Brazil is doing to promote healthy diets and active life-styles? *Public Health Nutr.* **5**, 263–267.

Doak, C. (2002). Large scale interventions and programs addressing nutrition related chronic diseases and obesity: examples from fourteen countries. *Public Health Nutr.* **5**, 275–277.

Drewnowski, A., and Popkin, B.M. (1997). The nutrition transition: new trends in the global diet. *Nutr. Rev.* **55**, 31–43.

Grol, M.E.C., Eimers, J.M., Alberts, J.F., Bouter, L.M., Gerstenbluth, I., Halabi, Y., van Sonderen, E., and van den Heuvel, W.J.A. (1997). Alarmingly high prevalence of obesity in Curaçao: data from an interview survey stratified for socioeconomic status. *Int. J. Obes.* **21**, 1002–1009.

Guo, X., Mroz, T.A., Popkin, B.M., and Zhai, F. (2000). Structural changes in the impact of income on food consumption in China, 1989–93. *Econ. Dev. Cult. Change* **48**, 737–760.

Gwatkin, D.R., Guillot, M., and Heuveline, P. (1999). The burden of disease among the urban poor. *Lancet* **354**, 586–589.

Interhealth Steering Committee (1991). Demonstration projects for the integrated control and prevention of noncommunicable diseases: epidemiological background and rationale. *World Health Stat. Q.* **44**, 48–54.

Matsudo, V., Matsudo, S., Andrade, D., Araujo, T., Andrade, E., de Oliveria, L.C., and Braggion, G. (2002). Promotion of physical activity in a developing country: the Agita Sao Paulo experience. *Public Health Nutr.* **5**, 253–261.

Menon, P., Ruel, M., and Morris, S.S. (2000). "Socioeconomic Differentials in Child Stunting are Consistently Larger in Urban than in Rural Areas." International Food Policy Research Institute. http://www.ifpri.org/divs/fcnd/dp.htm

Monteiro, C.A., Benicio, M.H.D'A., Conde, W.L., and Popkin, B.M. (2000). Shifting obesity trends in Brazil. *Eur. J. Clin. Nutr.* **54**, 342–346.

Monteiro, C.A., Conde, W.L., and Popkin, B.M. (2002). Is obesity replacing or adding to under-nutrition? Evidence from different social classes in Brazil. *Public Health Nutr.* **5**, 105–112.

Pettitt, D.J., Forman, M.R., Hanson, R.L., Knowler, W.C., and Bennett, P.H. (1999). Breastfeeding and incidence of non-insulin-dependent diabetes mellitus in Pima Indians. *Lancet* **350**, 166–168.

Phillips, D.I.W., Barker, D.J.P., Hales, C.N., Hirst, S., and Osmond, C. (1994). Thinness at birth and insulin resistance in adult life. *Diabetologia* **37**, 150–154.

Phipps, K., Barker, D.J.P., Hales, C.N., Fall, C.H., Osmond, C., and Clark, P.M.S. (1993). Fetal growth and impaired glucose tolerance in men and women. *Diabetologia* **36**, 225–228.

Popkin, B.M., Horton, S., Kim, S., Mahal, A., and Shuigao, J. (2001). Trends in diet, nutritional status and diet-related noncommunicable diseases in China and India: the economic costs of the nutrition transition. *Nutr. Rev.* **59**, 379–390.

Puska, P. (1981). "The North Karelia Project: Evaluation of a Comprehensive Community Programme for Control of Cardiovascular Diseases in North Karelia, Finland". World Health Organization, Copenhagen.

Puska, P., Pietinen, P., and Uusitalo, U. (2002). Influencing public nutrition for noncommunicable disease prevention: from community intervention to national programme – experiences from Finland. *Public Health Nutr.* **5**, 245–251.

Silva, L.C., Ordunez, P., Rodriguez, P., and Robles, S. (2001). A tool for assessing the usefulness of prevalence studies done for surveillance purposes: the example of hypertension. *Rev. Panam. Salud Publica* **10**, 152–160.

Singhai, A., Cole, T.J., and Lucas, A. (2001). Early nutrition in preterm infants and later blood pressure: two cohorts after randomised trials. *Lancet* **357**, 413–419.

The Bellagio Declaration (2002). *Public Health Nutr.* **5**, 279–280.

WHO (2001a). "Report: Assessment of National Capacity for Non-communicable Disease Prevention and Control, Report of a Global Survey". WHO, Geneva.

WHO (2001b). "Noncommunicable Diseases and Mental Health Cluster. Surveillance of risk factors for noncommunicable diseases. The WHO STEPwise Approach." http://www.who.int/ncd/surveillance

Zhai, F., Dawei, F., Du, S., Ge, K., Chen, C., and Popkin, B. (2002). What is China doing in policy-making to push back the negative aspects of the nutrition transition? *Public Health Nutr.* **5**, 269–273.

# Bellagio Declaration: Nutrition and health transition in the developing world: *the time to act*

*We from Africa, the Middle East, Asia, Europe and the Americas, met as participants in the meeting on the Nutrition Transition and its Implications for Health in the Developing World, held at the Rockefeller Centre at Bellagio, Lake Como, Italy, under the auspices of the International Union of Nutritional Sciences, declare as follows.*

The control and prevention of undernutrition is unfinished work in many countries. At the same time nutrition-related chronic diseases are now the main causes of disability and death, not only globally but also in most developing countries.

Evidence presented at our meeting supports and reinforces evidence already accepted by the World Health Organization and many national governments, and proves that the patterns of disease throughout the developing world are rapidly changing.

Changes in food systems and patterns of work and leisure, and therefore in diets and physical activity, are causing overweight, obesity, diabetes, high blood pressure, cardiovascular disease including stroke, and increasingly cancer, even in the poorest countries. Malnutrition early in life, followed by inappropriate diets and physical inactivity in childhood and adult life, increases vulnerability to chronic diseases.

Evidence from many developing countries discussed at the meeting shows that nutrition-related chronic diseases prematurely disable and kill a large proportion of economically productive people, a preventable loss of precious human capital. This includes countries where HIV/AIDS is a dominant problem. Four out of five deaths from nutrition-related chronic diseases occur in middle and low-income countries. The burden of cardiovascular disease alone, is now far greater in India, and also in China, than in all economically developed countries in the world added together. Low income communities are especially vulnerable to nutrition-related chronic diseases, which are not only diseases of affluence.

Obesity, itself a disease, also predicts more serious diseases. Current rates of overweight and obesity most of all in children, young adults and women, project rapidly increasing disability and premature death from nutrition-related chronic diseases for most developing countries. Phenomenal social and economic changes, on a scale and at a speed unprecedented in history, have resulted in an epidemic of nutrition-related chronic diseases that must be contained.

Prevention is the only feasible approach to nutrition-related chronic diseases. The cost of their treatment and management imposes an intolerable economic burden on developing countries. There is an urgent need for governments, in partnership with all relevant constituencies, to integrate strategies to promote healthful diets and regular physical activity throughout life into all relevant policies and programs including those designed to combat undernutrition.

Chronic diseases are preventable. This has already been demonstrated by successful programs in a few developed countries. Their chief causes are smoking, inappropriate diet and nutrition, and physical inactivity. Exposure to these factors is largely determined by political, economic and commercial policies and practices which reflect decisions made at national and transnational levels.

Effective programs and policies will include not only health promotion and education but community empowerment and action to overcome the environmental, social, and economic constraints to improvement in dietary quality and reduction of sedentarism. Finland and Norway have succeeded in reversing, over a short time span, extremely high levels of nutrition-related chronic diseases through comprehensive food policy and community involvement.

Several examples of innovative and promising approaches in developing countries emerged from the meeting. These include: promotion of daily physical activity through massive community participation as in *Agita São Paulo* in Brazil; protection of healthful aspects of the traditional low-fat high-vegetable diet as in South Korea with a strong support from home economics and dietetic professionals and infrastructure; selective price policies promoting consumption of soy products in China; development of food-based dietary guidelines in several countries based on local disease patterns and available foods. School based programs to promote healthy diets and physical activity are an especially valuable opportunity for action early on which should protect health over the lifespan. Examples are the national school food program in Brazil that provides fresh unprocessed food to school children and the new national physical activity program in Thailand.

Immediate action to control and prevent nutrition-related chronic diseases is not only a public health imperative but also a political, economic, social necessity. Successful programs will be multidisciplinary and intersectoral, and will include government, industry, the health professions, the media and civil society, as well as international agencies, as partners.

We, present at this meeting, pledge ourselves to be part of this process.

*Agreed at the Rockefeller Centre at Bellagio, Lake Como, Italy*
*Thursday 24, August 2001*

*At the meeting in Bellagio papers were presented from Egypt, Morocco, Tanzania and South Africa; Cuba, Mexico, Brazil and Chile; Iran; and India, China, Thailand, Malaysia, and South Korea. Material showing information and trends from Africa, Latin America, the Middle East and Asia was also reviewed. Senior officials from the World Health Organization in Geneva, and from the Food and Agriculture Organization of the United Nations in Rome, were also present at the meeting as observers.*

*The group met at Bellagio responsible for this Declaration proposes to continue to work together, initially as members of the IUNS Task Force on the Nutrition Transition and its Implications for Health in the Economically Developing World, in consultation with UN, international and bilateral agencies, national governments, and other constituencies. Other information on the meeting, slide presentations and papers can be found at:* www.nutrans.org or www.nutritiontransition.org

Barry Popkin, Convenor, University of North Carolina at Chapel Hill, USA
Cecilia Albala, Instituto de Nutricion y Tecnologia de los Alimentos (INTA), Chile
Sabah Benjelloun, Institut Agronomique et Vétérinaire Hassan II, Morocco
Lesley Bourne, Medical Research Council, South Africa

Colleen Doak, University of North Carolina at Chapel Hill, USA

Geoffrey Cannon, Rapporteur, World Health Policy Forum, Switzerland

Osman Mahmoud Galal, High Institute of Public Health, Alexandria University, Egypt

Hossein Ghassemi, Formerly Director, National Study on Food and Nutrition Security in Iran, Iran

Gail Harrison, UCLA School of Public Health, USA

Vongsvat Kosulwat, Institute of Nutrition, Mahidol University, Thailand

Min-June Lee, The Graduate School of Human Environmental Science, South Korea

Tumsifu Maletnlema, Child Growth Promotion Union, Tanzania

Victor Matsudo, CELAFISCS, Brazil

Carlos Monteiro, São Paulo University, Brazil

Denise Coitinho, Ministry of Health, Brazil

Mohd Ismail Noor, Universiti Kebangsaan Malaysia, Malaysia

K. Srinath Reddy, All India Institute of Medical Sciences, India

Juan Rivera, Instituto Nacional de Salud Publica (INSP), Mexico

Arturo Rodriguez-Ojea, Instituto Superior de Ciencias Medicas de La Habana, Facultad de Ciencias Medicas, Cuba

Ricardo Uauy, Instituto de Nutricion y Tecnologia de los Alimentos (INTA), Chile

Hester H. Vorster, Potchefstroom University for CHE, South Africa

Zhai Fengying, Chinese Academy of Preventive Medicine, China

*Observed and acknowledged by*

Pekka Puska, World Health Organization, Geneva

Prakash Shetty, Food and Agriculture Organization of the United Nations, Rome

# Index

Page numbers in *italic* refer to illustrations and tables and those in **bold** refer to main discussions.

Abdominal (central) obesity 137, 148
  cardiovascular disease risk 140
  impaired glucose tolerance/insulin
    resistance 171, 176, 197
  low birth weight relationship 139
  type 2 diabetes risk 140
Acquired immune deficiency syndrome
  *see* AIDS
Additives 62
Adolescents
  Brazilian study 229–230, *230*
  sweetened drinks–obesity relationship
    180–181
Adulteration 61, 62
Afghanistan 38
Africa
  cardiovascular disease 194
  diabetes 130, 137
  famine 30
  fertility trends 80
  hypertension 130
  life expectancy 82
  low birth weight 130
  noncommunicable disease rates 130
  population growth 84, 85, 86
  rural populations 99, 100, 103
  urban populations 99, 103
    mega-cities 104
Agriculture
  agroecosystem management 46
  animal feeding efficiencies **45–46**
  demographic changes *28*
  fertilizer use 29, 31, *31*, 46, 115
  genetic engineering 47–48
  historical development 26, 114–115
  investment 39, **46–48**
  mechanization **30–31**, 32, **115–116**
  modern farming 26, **30–33**
    workforce reduction 14, 31, 32
  new crop varieties 31, 32
  pesticides use 31, 32, 58, 62
  productivity 14, 23, 32–33, *33*, 56
    secular trends 10, 22
    USA post-war expansion 20–21, 22
  research 46–47
  traditional farming 26, **27–30**

AIDS (acquired immune deficiency
  syndrome) 42, 75, 241
  future projections of prevalence 82
  impact on life expectancy 80, **82–83**, *83*,
    90, 91
Ammonia fertilizers 31
Angola 95
Animal feed 45
  soybeans 35
Animal food products 33
  agricultural productivity
    feeding efficiencies **45–46**
    mechanization impact 115
  Chinese consumption trends 206,
    **211–212**, *212*, 217, 219
  demand in developing world 4–5, 39,
    **42–46**
    forcasting intake patterns 44–45
  early agricultural societies 115
  global per capita supply 36
  preagricultural foraging societies
    27, 114
  traditional farming 30
  urban versus rural populations 123
  Western countries' intake 43–44
Argentina
  fertility trends 76
  fetal programming studies 134
Asia
  agricultural mechanization 32
  animal protein consumption 42
  diabetes type 2 137
  fertility trends 80
  low birth weight 130
  obesity 152, 157, 158
  population aging 94
  population growth 85, 86, 88
  rural populations 99, 100, 103
  urban populations 99, 103
    mega-cities 103, 104
Asian bird viruses 43
Australia
  Aboriginal populations
    diabetes type 2 166, 168, 183
    fetal programming studies 132,
      133

  selective insulin resistance hypothesis
    169–170
  fertility trends 76
  food trade disputes 65
Austria 95
Away-from-home food consumption
  160
  China 210
  urban versus rural populations 123

Bangladesh 53
  childhood diabetes 165
  fertility trends 76
  low birth weight 130
  obesity 153, *153*
  population aging 94
  population growth prediction 89
Barley 29, 30
Basal metabolic rate (BMR) 12, 16
Beans 29
Beef
  feed conversion efficiency 45
  global production 35
  hormones in production 64–65
Behavioral dietary change *113*,
  **117–118**
Bellagio Declaration 246, **248–250**
Beriberi 116
Biodiversity 47, 58
Birth to Ten (BTT) study 131, 134, 138
Birth weight 129
  adult obesity relationship 139, 161
  developing world 131
  diabetes during pregnancy 161, 176
  *see also* Fetal programming hypothesis;
    Low birth weight
Blindness
  diabetic retinopathy 182
  vitamin A deficiency 38
Blood lipids
  alterations in children 133
  cardiovascular risk 197
  China 195
  fetal programming hypothesis
    studies in adults 132
    studies in children 136

Blood pressure
 elevation in children 133
 fetal programming hypothesis
  studies in adults **131–132**
  studies in children 133, 134
 *see also* Hypertension
Body fat distribution
 insulin sensitivity 170–171
 *see also* Abdominal (central) obesity
Body fat percentage estimation 148
Body height *see* Height, body
Body mass index (BMI)
 Brazil
  adults 230, *231*, *232*
  children/adolescents 229, *229*
 Chinese nutrition transition study 215, *216*
 insulin sensitivity relationship 170
 mortality relationship 17, *17*, 18, *19*
 obesity 148
 overweight 148
 secular trends 10, *11*, 16
Body size secular trends **9–23**
 labor productivity relationship 16–20
Body weight
 secular trends 10, *11*, 16, 19, *19*
 *see also* Body mass index (BMI)
Bovine spongiform encephalopathy (BSE; mad cow disease) 43, 61
Brand image 53, 54
Brazil
 agricultural resources for population growth 40
 famine 30
 fertility reduction 234, 237
 fetal programming studies 132, 139
 national food and nutrition policy 238, 244, 245
 nutrition transition study **223–239**
  adults 230–233, *231*, *232*
  data collection/analysis 225–226
  older children/adolescents 229–230, *230*
  survey population 224, *225*
  young children 226–229, *227*, *228*
 obesity 153, *153*, 231, *231*, *232*, 233, 235, 236, 237–238
  children/child overweight 160, 227, 228–229, 230, *230*, 235, 236
  low income associations 233, *234*, 235
 physical activity levels 237, 238
 population aging 94
 population growth 89, 234
 soybean production 35
 underweight
  adults 231, *231*, *232*, 233
  child stunting/wasting 227, 228–229, 235, 236
  older children/adolescents 229, 230, *230*, 236
 urbanization 234, 237
Brazilian Amondava 168
Breast feeding 58, 116, 161, 175–176, 242, 246
 urban versus rural populations 123

Buckwheat 30
Bulgaria 59
 population decline 89

Calcium 36
*Campylobacter* 61
Canada
 agricultural mechanization 32
 diabetes in children/adolescents 165
 fertility trends 76
Cancer 58, 61, 118
 China 207
  mortality data 216, 217, *217*, 218
 obesity association 149
Cardiovascular disease 36, 58, 61, 118, **191–201**
 China 207
  mortality data 216, 217, *217*, 218
 developing world **191–192**, *192*
  dynamics of epidemic **195–196**
  ethnicity influences 198–200
  health transition model 194–195, 201
  projections for 2020 **192–194**, *193*
  public health approaches 201
  risk behaviors/risk factors 196–197
  urbanization associations 195–196
 diabetes type 2 166, 171, 182
  influence of intrauterine factors 137, 176
 fetal programming hypothesis 129, 140, 142
 insulin resistance association 137
  studies in adults **131–133**
  studies in children/adolescents **133–136**
 interventions 196, **200–201**
 mortality/morbidity **191–194**, *192*
 obesity association 140, 149
 urban stress relationship 141
Caribbean
 fertility trends 80
 fetal programming studies 134, 135, 136
 mega-cities 104
 obesity in preschool children 157, 158, 159
 population aging 94
 population growth 85–86
 rural populations 100
 urbanization 99, 101, 103
Carp aquaculture 45–46
Cassava 28
Catfish aquaculture 46
Cebu Longitudinal Health and Nutrition Survey (CLHNS) 131, 134–135, *135*, *136*
Central obesity *see* Abdominal obesity
Cereals consumption
 China *209*, **209–211**
  recent trends 210–211, *210*, 217
  traditional diet 206
 early agricultural societies 115
 milled grains 116
 urban versus rural populations 123

Cereals production
 animal feed 45
 global production 33, *33*, 34–35, 36
 historical aspects 28–29
Cheese 118
Chickpeas 29
Children
 Brazil
  overweight 227, 228–229, 230, *230*
  stunting/wasting 227, 228–229
  underweight in older children/ adolescents 229, 230, *230*
 cardiovascular disease precursor changes 133
 diabetes type 2 165
  fetal programming studies **138–139**
  maternal diabetes-related risk 175–176
  sweetened drinks–obesity relationship 180–181
 obesity
  definitions 148–149
  measurement 148
  preschool children **157–159**
  school-age children **159–160**
 physical inactivity 161
 population distribution 91–94, *92*
Chile
 fetal programming studies 133, 134, 135
 Interhealth program interventions 243
Chimpanzee meat eating habits 42
China **205–220**
 agricultural resources for population growth 40, 41
 animal food products consumption 44, 206, **211–212**, *212*
 blood cholesterol levels 195
 cancer 207
 cardiovascular disease 194, 195, 207
 cereals consumption *209*, **209–211**
  recent trends 210–211, *210*
  urban/rural differences 210
 diabetes type 2 166
  lifestyle interventions 168, 169, 173, 175
 diet composition
  diversity **118–119**, *119*
  effect of income 124–125, *125*
  energy sources **212–213**, *213*, *214*, 219
 famine 30, 209
 fat intake 196, 212, 213, *213*, *214*, 219
 fertility trends 76
 fetal programming studies 132, 133, 137, 139
  birth outcome epidemiological data 131
 food production 25, 26, 34, 37, *37*
  fruit 35
  mean rice harvest 33
  traditional farming 27, 28, 29
 fruit consumption 211
 healthcare costs of nutrition-related noncommunicable diseases 241
 hypertension 195, 197, 215–216, *216*
 income/poverty trends 205, *206*
 Interhealth program interventions 243

mortality 208, **216**, *217*
  degenerative chronic diseases 216, 217, *217*
  life expectancy 207
nitrogen fertilizer use 32
nutrition transition study
  anthropometric data 208
  body mass index (BMI) 215, *216*
  data collection 207–208
  dietary intake surveys 207–208
  food consumption patterns 208–213, *209, 210, 211, 212, 213*
  rapidity of disease rate changes 218–220
  stages of transition 206, 217–218
  obesity 152, 171, 195, 207, 215, 217, 218, 219
  physical activity 208, **213–215**, *214*, 219
  population aging 94
  population growth 86, 88
  television ownership **126**, *127*, 219
  tobacco-related deaths 197
  traditional diet 205–206
  traditional farming 29
    stages of change 209–210, *209*
  undernutrition 38, 215
  urbanization 219
  vegetables consumption **211**
  Western food company markets 54
    fast food outlets 206, 219
China Health and Nutrition Survey (CHNS) 207, 210, 212
China National Nutrition Survey (CNNS) 207, 210, 211
Civil war 38, 58
Climate change 58
CODE-2 Study 184
Codex 63–64, 65
Collecting food *see* Foraging
Communications expansion 3
Company mergers 54
Congo
  agricultural resources for population growth 40, 41
  population growth prediction 89
Consumer-driven food safety issues 65
Consuming unit 12
Contamination 2, 61, 62
Corn 29, 30, 47, 123, 124, 210
  animal feed 45
  global mean harvest 33
  historical cultivation 28
Coronary heart disease 117, 118, 191, 192
  developing world 130
    health transition model 194
    projections for 2020 192
  dietary influences 178
  ethnic variability 167, 198
Corporate turnover *52, 53*
Counter-urbanization 99
Cowpeas 29
Croatia 132
Crop rotation 29, 46, 115
Culture 4, 51

Dairy products
  current dietary shifts 120
  global production 35
Deficiency diseases 115, 116
Degenerative diseases *113*, **116–117**
  China 206
  preventive behavioral changes **117–118**
Demographic transition 71, 72
Demographic trends 1, *2*, **71–106**
  data sets 73
  developing world 2, 3
  population aging **91–96**, *92, 93, 95*
  population growth 71, *72*, **73–91**
  productivity-related changes in USA 20–21
  traditional farming impact 27, *28*
  urbanization 72, *73*, *96*, **96–105**, *97*
Denmark 175
Developing world
  agricultural mechanization 32
  animal food products
    consumption 42–43
    demand 4–5, **42–46**
    forcasting intake patterns 44–45
  cardiovascular disease *see* Cardiovascular disease
  characteristic features of diet 2
  demographic change 2, 3
  diabetes prevalence 165–166, 197
  fertility trends 72, 73, *74*, 75, 89
    least-developed regions 78, 80
    transition to low fertility **75–76**, *77*, **78**
  fetal programming *see* Fetal programming hypothesis
  food production 4, 34–35
  low birth weight (intrauterine growth retardation) 129, 130
  mortality (life expectancy) 72, 73, *81, 82*, 195
  noncommunicable diseases 2, 3, 130
  obesity 130, **147–162**, 175
    men **156–157**
    preschool children **157–159**, *158*
    school-age children **159–160**
    social mapping 153–155, *153, 154*
    trends 155–156
    women **150–156**, *151, 152, 153*
  period of receding famine 2
  population aging 93
  population growth 2, 3, 40, 73, 75
    agricultural resources 40, *41*
    least-developed regions 85, 86
    predictions for future *84*, **84–86**, *86, 87, 88*, **88–89**
  population momentum 75
  poverty **4–5**
  prevention strategies for non-communicable diseases 242, 243–244
    diet 244–245
    physical activity 245
    surveillance 245–246
  seasonality of food supply 37

undernutrition 23, **38–39**
  economic impact 39
  micronutrient deficiencies 38–39
  urbanization 3, 72, *96, 97*, 98–99
Diabetes 36, 61, **165–185**
  cardiovascular disease risk 197
  Chinese mortality data 216, 217, *217*
  developing world 130
  fetal programming hypothesis 129, 140, 142
    studies in adults **137–138**
    studies in children **138–139**
  Indian populations 137
  obesity relationship 140, 149
  prevalence in developing world 165–166, 197
Diabetes Prevention Program (DPP) **174–175**
Diabetes type 2
  children/adolescents 180–181
  complications 166, 182
    blood glucose control relationship 183, 184
    cardiovascular disease 166, 171, 176, 182
    nephropathy 166, 171, 182, 183, 184
    neuropathy 166, 171, 182, 183, 184
    public health implications 171
    retinopathy 166, 171, 182, 183, 184
    treatment costs 182–183, 184
  dietary influences **177–182**
    fat intake 177, 178, 181–182
    increased energy density 179–180
    sweetened drinks 180–181
  ethnic variability in prevalence 166–167
  genetic heterogeneity 170
  genetic risk factors 167–168
  health care **182–185**
  hypertension association 174
  insulin resistance 173–174
  intrauterine factors 175–177
    maternal diabetes 175
  lifestyle interventions **168–169**, 172–173
    Diabetes Prevention Program (DPP) **174–175**
  obesity/overweight association 166, 168, 170, 175, 179
  physical inactivity association 168, **171–173**
  prevention at population level 184–185
  screening 185
  socioeconomic factors 166
  thrifty genotype hypothesis **169–170**
Dietary intake
  agriculture mechanization impact 115–116
  cardiovascular disease risk 196, 201
  Chinese nutrition transition study
    data collection 208
    food consumption patterns **208–213**, *209, 210, 211, 212, 213*
  current shifts 1, *2*, **119–122**
    income relationship 120, *120*, 121, *121*, 122
    vegetable fats 120–121

Dietary intake *cont.*
  degenerative disease prevention
      strategies **117–118**, 244–245
  diabetes type 2 influence **177–182**
  diversity improvements 118–119, *119*
  early agricultural societies 115
  foraging societies 114
  income–food choice relationship
      124–126
  industrialization-related changes 117
  migration impact 124
  post-Industrial Revolution 116–117, *117*
  self-report studies 178–179
  urbanization impact 119, 121, **122–124**,
      *123*
  *see also* Food intake (calories per capita)
Diversity of diet 118–119, *119*
Djibouti 95
Draft animals 31
  historical aspects 29
Dreze, Jean 57
Drinking water quality 58
Drought 30

Early nutritional deprivation **129–142**, 148
  *see also* Fetal programming hypothesis
Eastern Europe 82
Economic change 1
  productivity-related in USA 20–21
Eggs 42, 118, 119, 160
  Chinese consumption 211, *212*, 217
  feed conversion efficiency 45
  global production 35
  income-related consumption 125–126
  production targets 56
Egypt
  fertility trends 76
  meat consumption 44
  obesity levels 153, *153*
El Niño Southern Oscillation (ENSO) 30
Elderly people
  population distribution 91–94, *92*
  *see also* Population aging
Energy adaptation maladaptation syndrome
      (ENAMAS) 139
Energy requirement 11–12
  maintenance diet 12
*Escherichia coli* 61
Estonia 89
Ethiopia
  agricultural resources for population
      growth 40
  population growth prediction 89
Ethnicity
  cardiovascular disease risk variations
      198–200
  definitions 166–167
  diabetes type 2 prevalence variations
      166–167
  health attribute comparisons 167
  socioeconomic considerations 167
Europe
  agricultural mechanization 32
  animal protein consumption 42, 43, 44
  demography 40

diabetes treatment costs 184
diet-related health inequalities 57
fertility trends 71, 76, **80**
fetal programming studies 132
food production 34
  dairy products 35
late-eighteenth century chronic
    malnutrition 12, *13*
mean cereal harvest 33
mortality trends 9, *10*, 71, 73, 82
population growth reduction 84, 85, 86
technophysio evolution 10
traditional farming 29, 30
urbanization 99, 100, 101, 103
waste recycling 58–59
Eutrophication 48
Exercise (physical activity levels)
  Brazil 237, 238
  China 208, **213–215**, *214*, 219
  degenerative disease prevention 117, 245
  diabetes management 172–173, 174
  insulin resistance improvement 174
  serum lipid response 174
  weight loss 172

Famine 30, *113*, **114–115**
  China 209, 217
  preindustrial societies 30
Fat fold measurements 148
Fat intake 116, 117, 196, 242
  behavioral dietary change 117, 118
  China 212, 213, *213*, *214*, 219
  coronary heart disease risk 178
  current dietary shifts **119–122**, *120*
    low-income countries 119, 121
  diabetes relationship 177, 178, **181–182**
  dietary diversity relationship 118
  foraging (hunting and gathering)
      societies 27, 114
  income-related consumption 120, *120*,
      121, *121*, 122, 125–126
  meat 116–117
  obesity relationship 179
  urban versus rural populations 123
  vegetable fats 120–121
  Western diets 36, 43
Feed crops 33
  traditional farming 29
Fertility trends 71, 72, 73–74, *74*
  least-developed countries 78, 80
  projections for population growth
      prediction **75–78**, *79*, 83, 89
  transition to low fertility ('fertility
      transition') **75–76**, *77*, **78**, **80**, 90
  Brazil 234
  population aging effect 91, 94
Fertilizer use 31, *31*, 46, 115
  historical aspects 29
Fetal programming hypothesis 129, 199
  coronary heart disease risk 195
  role of overweight/obesity **139–140**
  studies in developing world
    blood lipids 132, 133, 136
    blood pressure 131–132, 133, 134
    cardiovascular disease **131–136**

diabetes **137–139**
  epidemiological data collection
      **130–131**
Fiber intake 2, 116, 117
  agriculture mechanization 116
  behavioral dietary change 117, 118
  foraging (hunting and gathering)
      societies 114
Finland
  animal fat consumption 43
  preventive interventions 243, 244
    cardiovascular disease 200
    diabetes 168–169, 175
Fish 114, 118
  Chinese consumption 211, *212*, 219
  feed conversion efficiency 45–46
  food policy 53–54
  global production
    aquaculture 35
    marine catch 35–36
  preagricultural foraging societies 26
  stocks decline 58
Fishing bans 54
Flood 30
Food corporations turnover *52*, 53, *53*
Food intake (calories per capita)
  European secular trend 13, *13*, 22
  excesses in Western diet 36
  global inequalities 36, **55–58**
    future improvement 41–42
  labor productivity effect **13–16**, *15*
    empirical estimates 15–16
  *see also* Dietary intake
Food policy **53–55**, *55*
  economic framework for food security
      56–57
  food inequalities **55–58**
  governance **60–66**
    multilevel 56
  health goals *63*
    WHO European Region model 62,
      *62*
  institutions **62–66**
Food prices, globalization impact 4
Food production **25–48**, 54, *54*
  agricultural investment **46–48**
  animal products demand in developing
      world 4–5, **42–46**
  current global levels **34–36**
  current per capita food supply 36–37
  data sources 33–34
  foraging societies 25, **26–27**
  future needs **39–42**
  local urban/peri-urban 59–60
  modern farming 26, **30–33**
  traditional farming 26, **27–30**
Food security 56–57, 65
Food-borne infections 61
Foot-and-mouth epizootic 43
Foraging (hunting and gathering) societies
      25, **26–27**, *112*, *113*, **114**
  thrifty genotype hypothesis 169
Former Soviet Union 54
  mortality trends 82
Formula feeding 116

France
body height/body weight 16, 19, *19*
food intake (calories per capita) 13, *13*
late-eighteenth century chronic
malnutrition 12, *13*
energy available for work 14, *15*
meat consumption 43
mortality (life expectancy) 9, *10*,
19–20
Fruit 118, 119, 196, 245
Chinese consumption trends **211**
global production 35
local urban/peri-urban production 59
production targets 56

General Agreement on Tariffs and Trade
(GATT) 57, 60, 62, 63, 64, 65, 66
Agreement on Agriculture 63
Genetic engineering 39, 47–48
Genetic factors 5
cardiovascular disease 199, 200
diabetes **167–168**
Georgia
fertility trends 76
local food production 59
Gestational diabetes 142, 161
Global Burden of Disease Study 192
Global food corporations *52*, 53, *53*
Global food production **34–36**
inequalities 34
Global population growth **39–41**, *40*
Globalization 3–4, **52–53**, 196–197
cultural context 4
Goiter 39
Governance 51, **60–66**
multilevel 56
Greece 43
Green manuring 29
Green Revolution 32
Guatamala
fetal programming studies 131, 132, 133,
134, 139
obesity 156

Harrowing 28
Harvesting 28
Health care infrastructure 20, 243
diabetes impact **182–185**
Health changes (epidemiological transition)
2
Health inequalities
diet-related 55
food policy influences 53, 60–61, *61*
implications of General Agreement on
Tariffs and Trade (GATT) **62–66**
Height, body
morbidity relationship 18
mortality relationship 18, *18*, *19*
secular trends 10, *10*, 17–18, 19, *19*
Herbicides 32
High altitude adaptation 148
High-yielding crop varieties 32, 47
History of food production **25–33**
HIV infection *see* AIDS
Hominid foraging behavior 25–26

Hong-Kong
childhood diabetes 165
fetal programming studies 132
local food production 59
Hormones in meat fattening 64–65
Human capital investment 20
Human Development Index 66
*Human Development Report* 66
Hunting 112
meat composition 116–117
preagricultural foraging societies 26–27
Hybrid seed 47
Hypertension 58, 118
cardiovascular disease risk 197
China 195, **215–216**, *216*
developing world 130
diabetes association 174
ethnic variability 167
health transition model 194
obesity association 149
prevalence 197
urbanization association 170

Impaired glucose tolerance 142, 199
dietary fat influence 178
fetal programming studies 137, 138
lifestyle interventions 168–169
Diabetes Prevention Program (DPP)
**174–175**
prevalence in developing world 197
Income
dietary intake impact 120, *120*, 121,
*121*, 122
China 124–125, *125*
food choice 124–126, *125*, *126*
obesity associations in Brazil 233, *234*,
235
India
agricultural resources for population
growth 40, 41
cardiovascular disease 130, 176, 193, 194
diabetes 130, 137, 138, 139, 166, 176,
183, 197
famine 30
fetal programming studies 131–132, 139
birth outcome epidemiological data
131
food production 34, 35, 37
hypertension 197
insulin resistance syndrome 137, 139,
176
noncommunicable diseases 130
healthcare costs 241
obesity 171
population aging 94
population growth 86, 89
Pune Maternal Nutrition Study 131,
138–139
tobacco-related deaths 197
traditional farming 29
undernutrition 38
Western food company markets 54
Indonesia 53, 116
agricultural resources for population
growth 40, 41

food supply 37
population aging 94
Infectious cardiomyopathy 194
Infectious diseases 4, 80, 114, 241
China 206
mortality data 216
Insulin resistance
body mass index (BMI) relationship
170
central obesity 171
diabetes type 2 173–174
dyslipoproteinemia 174
exercise responsiveness 174
fetal programming hypothesis 137,
139, 141
thrifty genotype hypothesis 169
Insulin resistance syndrome 132, 137, 139,
168, 173–174, 176
Interhealth program 243
Intrauterine factors
diabetes type 2 175–177
*see also* Fetal programming hypothesis
Inuit 27
Iodine deficiency 39
Iowa Women's Health Study 181
Iran 152
Irish potato famine 30
Iron 5, 36, 48
Irrigation 29, 58
mechanization 32
Italy 95

Japan
animal protein consumption 42, 44
children
diabetes 165
obesity 159
demography 40
fertility trends 76
food supply 37
mean rice harvest 33
population aging 94, 95
Japanese migrant groups 199
Jordan, Michael 57

!Kung San 114
Kuwait 159–160

Labor force participation rate
agricultural advances impact 14
UK 15
USA 16, 21
Latin America
cardiovascular disease 194
diabetes 137
fertility trends 80
Interhealth program interventions 243
mega-cities 103, 104
obesity 155, 156
preschool children 157, 158, 159
school-age children 160
population aging 94
population growth rate 85, 89
rural populations 100
urbanization 99, 101, 103

Legumes 46
  global production 35
  historical aspects 28, 29
Leisure-related energy expenditure 23
Lentils 29
Liberia 89
Libya 165
Life expectancy *see* Mortality
Lifestyle change 1, 3
Low birth weight 58, 141, 176, **242**, 246
  developing world 130
  obesity relationship **139–140**, 142
Low fat food consumption 118

Mad cow disease (bovine spongiform
    encephalopathy; BSE) 43, 61
Maintenance diet 12
Malaria 241
Malaysia 44
Malnutrition (undernutrition) 23, 55, 241,
    **242**, 246
  affluent countries 36–37
  Brazilian children
    stunting/wasting 227, 228–229, 235
    underweight in older children/
      adolescents 229, 230, *230*
  China 206, 217
  developing world **38–39**
  early nutritional deprivation 19, 148
    impact on brain development 38
  India 37
  late-eighteenth century Europe 12, *13*
  micronutrient deficiencies 38–39
  sub-Saharan Africa 37
  traditional farming societies 30
  work capacity impact 12, 16
Manuring 115
  historical aspects 29
Market share 53, 54
Market-driven growth 56
Mass media 3, **126**, *127*
  globalization 4
  influence in urban versus rural
    populations 123
Maturity-onset-type diabetes of youth
    (MODY) 170
Mauritius 174
  cardiovascular disease preventive
    interventions 200
  Interhealth program 243
Meat consumption 32, 53, 58, 59, 118,
    119
  China 211, *212*
  current dietary shifts 120, 160
  dietary fat intake 116–117
  early agricultural societies 115
  hunting societies 114
Meat production 42, 43
  global levels 35
Mediterranean diet 43
Mega-cities (urban agglomerations) 100,
    **103–105**, *104*
Metabolically obese, normal-weight
    (MONW) women 173
Metformin 174

Mexico
  obesity 155–156, *156*
    school-age children 160
  population aging 94
  population growth 89
Micronutrient deficiencies 36, 38–39, 241
Middle East
  obesity 152, 155
    preschool children 158, 159
    school-age children 159
Migrant/transplanted populations 124,
    199–200
  diabetes type 2 165
Milk 42, 118
  Chinese consumption trends 217
  feed conversion efficiency 45
  global production 35
  production targets 56
Millet 28, 29, 30, 118, 123, 210
Morbidity
  body height relationship 18
  cardiovascular disease 191, *192*
  labor productivity impact 20
Mortality
  AIDS impact 75, 80, 82–83, *83*, 90, 91
  body height relationship 18, *18*, *19*
  body mass index (BMI) relationship 17,
    *17*, 18, *19*
  cardiovascular disease 191
  Chinese nutrition transition study 207,
    208, **216**, *217*
  developing world 195
    least-developed regions 80
  developmental malnutrition-related risk
    19
  labor productivity impact 20
  obesity-related risk 149
  projections for population growth
    prediction 75, **80**, *81*, **82**, 83, 90–91
  secular trends 9, *10*, 19–20, 71, 72, 73, 74
Mortality decline index 82
Multicropping 29
Multilevel governance 56

National Gross Domestic Product (GDP)
    *52*, 53
Naurua 169
  diabetes 165, 166
Neolithic Revolution 26
Nephropathy, diabetes type 2 166, 171, 182,
    183, 184
Neuropathy, diabetes type 2 166, 171, 182,
    183, 184
New Zealand
  fertility trends 76
  food trade disputes 65
Niger
  median age of population 95
  population growth prediction 89
Nigeria
  agricultural resources for population
    growth 40, 41
  fetal programming studies 132, 133
  population growth prediction 89
Nitrate contamination 62

Nitrogen fertilizers 31–32, *31*
Noncommunicable diseases (NCD) 191
  *see also* Nutrition-related
      noncommunicable diseases
North Africa
  obesity 152, 155, 156–157, *157*
  preschool children 158, 159
North Karelia Project 243
Norway 65
  behavioral dietary change 118
  meat consumption 43
Nutrition transition
  dynamics **111–127**
  globalization relevance **52–53**
  poverty 4–5
  rapidity of shift 2, 3
  stages 2, *2*, *3*, **112**, *113*, **114–118**
    China 206
  urbanization 196–197
  *see also* Dietary intake
Nutrition-related noncommunicable diseases
    (NR-NCD) 2, 61, 114, 130, 241
  fetal programming hypothesis 129
  prevention strategies in developing world
    242–243
Nutritional cardiomyopathy 194
Nutritional status
  body height relationship 17–18
  measurement (net nutrition) 11
  productivity impact **11–16**
  secular trend 16–17
Nuts 26, 27, 114

Oats 29, 30
Obesity 3, 22, 36, 37, 58, 61, 196
  assessment 147–149
  body fat distribution 170–171
  Brazil 231, *231*, *232*, 233, 235, 236,
    237–238
  cancer risk 149
  cardiovascular disease risk 140, 149
  childhood malnutrition association 5, 150
  China 207, 217, 218, 219
  consequences 149–150
  definition 148
  developing world 130, **147–162**, 175
    men **156–157**
    preschool children **157–159**, *158*
    school-age children 148, **159–160**
    social mapping 153–155, *153*, *154*
    trends 155–156
    women **150–156**, *151*, *152*, *153*
  diabetes type 2 association 140, 149,
    166, **168**, 170, 175, 179
  energy balance discrepancy 147–148
  energy density of diet 179–180
  Europe 177
  hypertension association 149
  impaired glucose tolerance 197
  intrauterine factors 175
  low birth weight relationship **139–140**,
    142
  mortality risk 149
  prevention at population level 184–185
  public health implications 171

stroke association 149
sweetened drinks consumption 180–181
thrifty genotype hypothesis 139, 140,
  141, 199
  diabetes type 2 **169–170**
urbanization association 170
USA 22
*see also* Overweight
Oceania
  fertility trends 80
  obesity 155, 156
  population aging 94
  population growth rate 85
  urbanization 99, 100, 101, 103
Oil crops 33
Oils consumption 125, *126*
Organic agricultural products 23
Organic recycling 31
Orr, John Boyd 56
Osteoporosis 118
Output per capita 14
Overfishing 35–36
Overweight
  Brazilian children 227, 228–229, 230,
    *230*, 235, 236
  definitions 148
    childhood 149
  diabetes type 2 association 166
  low birth weight relationship **139–140**
  *see also* Obesity

Packaging waste 58–59
Pakistan 53
  agricultural resources for population
    growth 40, 41
  obesity in children 157
  population aging 94
  population growth prediction 89
Peanuts 29
Peas 29
Pellagra 116
Peppers 30
Period of receding famine 2, *113*, **115–116**
Pesticides 31, 32, 62
  pollution 58
Philippines, Cebu Longitudinal Health and
    Nutrition Survey (CLHNS) 131,
    134–135, *135*, *136*
Phosphate fertilizers 31, 32
Physical activity *see* Exercise
Physical inactivity 1, 58, 116, 129, 161,
    242
  cardiovascular disease risk 196, 197, 201
  children 161
  diabetes risk 168, **171–173**
  leisure time 161
  television in promotion 4
Pima Indians 169, 174, 183, 198, 199
  diabetes type 2 165, 166, 183
  effects of diabetic pregnancy 175
Plowing 28
Poland 59
Pollution 55, 58
Polyunsaturated fatty acids (PUFA) 116, 181,
    182

Population age/sex distribution
    standardization 12
Population aging **91–96**, *92*, *93*, *95*
Population growth 71, *72*, **73–91**, *74*
  developing world 73, 75, *84*, **84–86**, *86*,
    *87*, *88*, **88**, **89**
  population momentum 75
  projections for future **75–76**, **78**, **80**,
    **83–86**, *84*, *86*, *87*, *88*, **88–90**
  negative growth rates 84, 85, 86, *88*,
    **88**, 89
Population momentum 75
Pork 118
  Chinese consumption 219
  feed conversion efficiency 45
  global production 35
  income-related consumption 125, *125*
Potatoes 28, 30, 124
Poultry 42, 119
  Chinese consumption 211, *212*, 217, 219
  feed conversion efficiency 45
  global production 35
Poverty 51, 57–58, **242**
  cardiovascular disease risk in developing
    world 196
  health inequalities 58
  nutrition transition **4–5**
  post-Industrial Revolution 116
  USA 36–37
Premature birth 58
Processed foods 4, 116, 160, 238
  nutrition labeling 162
  urban versus rural populations 123, 124
Productivity
  agricultural advances impact 14
  body size relationship 10, 16
    self-reinforcing cycle **16–20**
  definition 13–14
    output per capita 14
  demographic/economic impact in USA
    20–21
  effect of improved nutrition **11–16**
  modern farming 32–33, *33*
  mortality/morbidity reduction impact 20
  nutritional status-related increase **13–16**,
    *15*
    empirical estimate 15–16
    secular trends **9–23**
  *see also* Work capacity
Profits 53
Protein, global per capita food supply 36
Pune Maternal Nutrition Study 131,
    138–139, 141

Recycling waste 28, 46, 58–59
Retinol 5
Retinopathy, diabetes type 2 166, 171, 182,
    183, 184
Rheumatic heart disease 191, 194
Rice 29, 47, 118, 119, 123
  bioengineering advances 48
  Chinese traditional diet 206
  global mean harvest 33
  high-yielding varieties 32
  historical aspects 28

Rural population dynamics 98, 99–100
Russia
  demography 40
  fetal programming studies 139
  mortality trends 82
  population decline 89
Rye 29

Salmon aquaculture 46
*Salmonella* 61
Salt intake 196, 199
  reduction in Finland 244–245
Saturated fat intake 5, 116
  coronary heart disease 178
  diabetes 177, 178, 181
Saudi Arabia 53
Scandinavian diet 43
Seasonality of food supply 37, 114
Sedentary lifestyle *see* Physical inactivity
Seeds 26, 27, 114
Selenium 5
Self-reliance policies 56, 57, 65
Self-report dietary intake studies
    178–179
Sen, Amartya 57
Seven Countries Study 198
Shifting farming 28
Shopping by car 60
Siege of Leningrad 176
Singapore 165
Sino-MONICA 195
Skinfold measurement *see* Fat fold
    measurements
Soil structure 46, 58
Somalia 38
Sorghum 118, 210
South Africa 53
  Birth to Ten (BTT) study 131, 134,
    138
  cardiovascular disease precursor changes
    in children 133
  fetal programming studies 132, 134,
    137, 138, 139
South Asian migrant groups 199, 200
Soybeans 29, 37, 118
  animal feed 45
  global production 35
Spain
  diabetes 181
  population aging 95
State-led self-reliance policies 56, 57
STEPwise approach 245
Straw:grain ratio 32
Stroke 58, 191, 192
  developing world 198
    health transition model 194
    projections for 2020 192
  ethnic variability 167, 198
  obesity association 149
Sub-Saharan Africa 60
  animal protein consumption 42
  food supply 37, 42
  hypertension 197
  obesity 152, 155, 157, 158, 159
  population growth prediction 89

Sugar intake 37, 116, 117
  childhood obesity 180–181
  current dietary shifts 119–122, *120*, 122, *122*
  urban versus rural populations 123
Sugar production 33
  global levels 35
Surveillance systems 245–246
Sustainable consumption 51, **58–60**
  appropriate localism approach 57
Sweden
  diabetes type 2 182
    lifestyle interventions 169
  fetal programming studies 133, 134
Sweet potato 48
Sweetened drinks–obesity relationship 180–181
Sweets consumption 118

Taiwan 42, 44
Tanzania
  diabetes type 2 165
  obesity levels 153, *153*
Technophysio evolution 10
Television 4, **126**, *127*, 161, 242
  Brazil 237, 238
  China 213, 214–215, *214*, 219
Tobacco 58, 243
  cardiovascular disease risk 196, 197–198, 201
Tomatoes 30
Torres Straits Islanders 166
Total energy requirement 12
Trade power 54
Traditional farming 26, **27–30**
  intensification 29
  renewability 28
Transgenic pigs 48
Transgenic seed 47
Transnational food corporations 55
  Codex meetings participation 64
  turnover *52*, 53, *53*
Transport of food 60, 124
Tuberculosis 91
Tubers 28, 114
Turkey
  meat consumption 44
  obesity levels 153, *153*, 154

Uganda 95
UK
  diabetes in children/adolescents 165
  diet-related health inequalities 57
  ethnic variability in disease 167
  fruit imports 60
  life expectancy 9, *10*

malnutrition (undernutrition) 56
  late-eighteenth century 12, *13*
  mean cereal harvest 33
  migrant groups 200
  poverty 57–58
  secular trends
    body size 16
    energy available for work 14, 15, *15*
    food intake (calories per capita) 13, *13*, 15
Undernutrition *see* Malnutrition
United Kingdom Prospective Diabetes Study (UKPDS) 183
Urban agglomerations (mega-cities) 100, **103–105**, *104*
Urbanization 3, 31, 55, 58, **59**, *101*, 196
  Brazil 234, 237
  cardiovascular disease association 195–196
  demographic trends 72, *73*, *96*, **96–105**, *97*
  developing world 98–99
  size of settlements 100, 101, *101*, *102*, 103
  diet composition impact 119, 121, **122–124**, *123*
  hypertension association 170
  local food production 59
  low-income countries 122, 124
  obesity association 170
  patterns of migration 124
  stress response 141
  urban agglomerations 100, 103
Uruguay 76
USA
  agricultural mechanization 32
  agricultural output 20–21, 22
  animal protein consumption 42, 44
  behavioral dietary change 118
  cardiovascular disease precursor changes in children 133
  demography 40
  diabetes type 2 166, 177–178, 182, 183–184, 185
    children/adolescents 165
    lifestyle interventions 174–175
  fat intake 36
  fertility trends 76, 80
  fetal programming studies 132
  food packaging 58
  food production 34, 36–37
    dairy products 35
    mean cereal harvest 33
    soybeans 35
  life expectancy 9, *10*
  micronutrient deficiencies 36

obesity 22
  children 158, 159, 180
  social mapping *154*, 155
  trends 155
population aging 94
population growth rate 85, 89
poverty 36–37
productivity 10
  demographic/economic change 20–21
  trade disputes 64, 65
  urbanization 99, 100, 101, 103
    mega-cities 104

Value-adding 53, 54
Vegetable oils/fats 4, 160, 181, 182, 196
Vegetables 118, 119, 196, 245
  Chinese consumption **211**, 217
    traditional diet 206
  local urban/peri-urban production 59
  production targets 56
Vitamin A 48
  deficiency 38

Weight loss
  body fat distribution 171
  diabetes management 174
  physical activity 172
Wheat 29, 30, 47, 119, 123
  Chinese traditional diet 206
  global mean harvest 33
  high-yielding varieties 32
  historical aspects 28
  world market prices 65
WHO-MONICA 177
Work capacity
  energy available for work
    agricultural advances impact 14
    secular trends 14, *15*
  food supply relationship **13–14**, *15*
    empirical estimates **15–16**
    late-eighteenth century Europe 12
  output per capita 14
Work changes 3
World Food Summit 65
World Health Organization (WHO) 63
World Trade Organization (WTO) 60, 63, 65, 66

Xerophthalmia syndrome 38

Yemen
  median age of population 95
  population growth prediction 89

Zinc 5, 36

# Food Science and Technology
## International Series

Maynard A. Amerine, Rose Marie Pangborn, and Edward B. Roessler, *Principles of Sensory Evaluation of Food*. 1965.

Martin Glicksman, *Gum Technology in the Food Industry*. 1970.

Maynard A. Joslyn, *Methods in Food Analysis*, second edition. 1970.

C. R. Stumbo, *Thermobacteriology in Food Processing*, second edition. 1973.

Aaron M. Altschul (ed.), *New Protein Foods*: Volume 1, *Technology, Part A* – 1974. Volume 2, *Technology, Part B* – 1976. Volume 3, *Animal Protein Supplies, Part A* – 1978. Volume 4, *Animal Protein Supplies, Part B* – 1981. Volume 5, *Seed Storage Proteins* – 1985.

S. A. Goldblith, L. Rey, and W. W. Rothmayr, *Freeze Drying and Advanced Food Technology*. 1975.

R. B. Duckworth (ed.), *Water Relations of Food*. 1975.

John A. Troller and J. H. B. Christian, *Water Activity and Food*. 1978.

A. E. Bender, *Food Processing and Nutrition*. 1978.

D. R. Osborne and P. Voogt, *The Analysis of Nutrients in Foods*. 1978.

Marcel Loncin and R. L. Merson, *Food Engineering: Principles and Selected Applications*. 1979.

J. G. Vaughan (ed.), *Food Microscopy*. 1979.

J. R. A. Pollock (ed.), *Brewing Science*, Volume 1 – 1979. Volume 2 – 1980. Volume 3 – 1987.

J. Christopher Bauernfeind (ed.), *Carotenoids as Colorants and Vitamin A Precursors: Technological and Nutritional Applications*. 1981.

Pericles Markakis (ed.), *Anthocyanins as Food Colors*. 1982.

George F. Stewart and Maynard A. Amerine (eds.), *Introduction to Food Science and Technology*, second edition. 1982.

Malcolm C. Bourne, *Food Texture and Viscosity: Concept and Measurement*. 1982.

Hector A. Iglesias and Jorge Chirife, *Handbook of Food Isotherms: Water Sorption Parameters for Food and Food Components*. 1982.

Colin Dennis (ed.), *Post-Harvest Pathology of Fruits and Vegetables*. 1983.

P. J. Barnes (ed.), *Lipids in Cereal Technology*. 1983.

David Pimentel and Carl W. Hall (eds.), *Food and Energy Resources*. 1984.

Joe M. Regenstein and Carrie E. Regenstein, *Food Protein Chemistry: An Introduction for Food Scientists*. 1984.

Maximo C. Gacula, Jr., and Jagbir Singh, *Statistical Methods in Food and Consumer Research*. 1984.

Fergus M. Clydesdale and Kathyrn L. Wiemer (eds.), *Iron Fortification of Foods*. 1985.

Robert V. Decareau, *Microwaves in the Food Processing Industry*. 1985.

S. M. Herschdoerfer (ed.), *Quality Control in the Food Industry*, second edition. Volume 1 – 1985. Volume 2 – 1985. Volume 3 – 1986. Volume 4 – 1987.

F. E. Cunningham and N. A. Cox (eds.), *Microbiology of Poultry Meat Products*. 1987.

Walter M. Urbain, *Food Irradiation*. 1986.

Peter J. Bechtel, *Muscle as Food*. 1986.

H. W.-S. Chan, *Autoxidation of Unsaturated Lipids*. 1986.

Chester O. McCorkle, Jr., *Economics of Food Processing in the United States*. 1987.

Jethro Jagtiani, Harvey T. Chan, Jr., and William S. Sakai, *Tropical Fruit Processing*. 1987.

J. Solms, D. A. Booth, R. M. Dangborn, and O. Raunhardt, *Food Acceptance and Nutrition*. 1987.

R. Macrae, *HPLC in Food Analysis*, second edition. 1988.

A. M. Pearson and R. B. Young, *Muscle and Meat Biochemistry*. 1989.

Dean O. Cliver (ed.), *Foodborne Diseases*. 1990.

Marjorie P. Penfield and Ada Marie Campbell, *Experimental Food Science*, third edition. 1990.

Leroy C. Blankenship, *Colonization Control of Human Bacterial Enteropathogens in Poultry*. 1991.

Yeshajahu Pomeranz, *Functional Properties of Food Components*, second edition. 1991.

Reginald H. Walter, *The Chemistry and Technology of Pectin*. 1991.

Herbert Stone and Joel L. Sidel, *Sensory Evaluation Practices*, second edition. 1993.

Robert L. Shewfelt and Stanley E. Prussia, *Postharvest Handling: A Systems Approach*. 1993.

R. Paul Singh and Dennis R. Heldman, *Introduction to Food Engineering*, second edition. 1993.

Tilak Nagodawithana and Gerald Reed, *Enzymes in Food Processing*, third edition. 1993.

Dallas G. Hoover and Larry R. Steenson, *Bacteriocins*. 1993.

Takayaki Shibamoto and Leonard Bjeldanes, *Introduction to Food Toxicology*. 1993.

John A. Troller, *Sanitation in Food Processing*, second edition. 1993.

Ronald S. Jackson, *Wine Science: Principles and Applications*. 1994.

Harold D. Hafs and Robert G. Zimbelman, *Low-fat Meats*. 1994.

Lance G. Phillips, Dana M. Whitehead, and John Kinsella, *Structure–Function Properties of Food Proteins*. 1994.

Robert G. Jensen, *Handbook of Milk Composition*. 1995.

Yrjö H. Roos, *Phase Transitions in Foods*. 1995.

Reginald H. Walter, *Polysaccharide Dispersions*. 1997.

Gustavo V. Barbosa-Cánovas, M. Marcela Góngora-Nieto, Usha R. Pothakamury, and
Barry G. Swanson, *Preservation of Foods with Pulsed Electric Fields*. 1999.

Ronald S. Jackson, *Wine Science: Principles, Practice, Perception*, second edition. 2000.

R. Paul Singh and Dennis R. Heldman, *Introduction to Food Engineering*, third
edition. 2001.

Ronald S. Jackson, *Wine Tasting: A Professional Handbook*. 2002.

Malcolm C. Bourne, *Food Texture and Viscosity: Concept and Measurement*, second
edition. 2002.

Dean O. Cliver and Hans P. Riemann (eds.), *Foodborne Diseases*, second edition. 2002.

| Country | Map Abbreviation | Country | Map Abbreviation | Country | Map Abbreviation |
|---|---|---|---|---|---|
| Afghanistan | Afg. | Greece | Grc. | Pakistan | Pak. |
| Austria | Aut. | Guatemala | Gtm. | Panama | Pan. |
| Azerbaijan | Aze. | Guinea | Gin. | Poland | Pol. |
| Bangladesh | Bgd. | Guinea Bissau | Gnb. | Portugal | Prt. |
| Belarus | Blr. | Guyana | Guy. | Qatar | Qat. |
| Benin | Ben. | Haiti | Hti. | Republic of Moldova | Mda. |
| Bhutan | Btn. | Honduras | Hnd. | Romania | Rom. |
| Botswana | Bwa. | Ireland | Irl. | Rwanda | Rwa. |
| Bulgaria | Bgr. | Israel | Isr. | Senegal | Sen. |
| Burkina Faso | Bfa. | Italy | Ita. | Sierra Leone | Sle. |
| Burundi | Bdi. | Jordan | Jor. | Somalia | Som. |
| Cambodia | Khm. | Kenya | Ken. | South Korea | S. Kor. |
| Cameroon | Cmr. | Kuwait | Kwt. | Spain | Esp. |
| Central African Republic | C.A.R. | Kyrgyzstan | Kgz. | Suriname | Sur. |
| Congo | Cog. | Laos | Lao. | Swaziland | Swz. |
| Costa Rica | Cri. | Latvia | Lva. | Sweden | Swe. |
| Cote d'Ivoire | Civ. | Lebanon | Lbn. | Syria | Syr. |
| Democratic Republic of the Congo | Drg. | Liberia | Lbr. | Tajikistan | Tjk. |
| Denmark | Dnk. | Lithuania | Ltu. | Thailand | Tha. |
| Djibouti | Dji. | Madagascar | Mdg. | Tunisia | Tun. |
| Dominican Republic | Dom. | Malawi | Mwi. | Turkmenistan | Tkm. |
| East Timor | Etm. | Malaysia | Mys. | Uganda | Uga. |
| Equatorial Guinea | Gnq. | Mauritania | Mrt. | Ukraine | Ukr. |
| Eritrea | Eri. | Morocco | Mar. | United Arab Emirates | U.A.E. |
| Estonia | Est. | Mozambique | Moz. | United Kingdom | U.K. |
| Finland | Fin. | Myanmar | Mmr. | United Republic of Tanzania | Tza. |
| France | Fra. | Namibia | Nam. | Uzbekistan | Uzb. |
| French Guiana | Guf. | Nepal | Npl. | Vietnam | Vnm. |
| Gabon | Gab. | Netherlands | Nld. | Western Sahara | W. Sah. |
| Georgia | Geo. | Nicaragua | Nic. | Yemen | Yem. |
| Germany | Deu. | North Korea | N. Kor. | Yugoslavia | Yug. |
| Ghana | Gha. | Norway | Nor. | Zambia | Zmb. |
| | | Oman | Omn. | Zimbabwe | Zwe. |